AF566906

ERRATUM

On page 106, Table 6.1 and page 108, Table 6.5 the drug used in the LIPID trial should read Pravastatin and not Lovastatin.

PREVENTION OF ISCHEMIC STROKE

PREVENTION OF ISCHEMIC STROKE

Edited by

Cesare Fieschi MD
Professor of Neurology
Department of Neurological Sciences
Università degli Studi di Roma
'La Sapienza'
Rome 00185
ITALY

Marc Fisher MD
Chief of Neurology
Memorial Health Care and
Professor of Neurology
University of Massachusetts
Medical School
Worcester
MA 01605
USA

MARTIN DUNITZ

First published in the United Kingdom in 2000 by
Martin Dunitz Ltd
The Livery House
7-9 Pratt Street
London NW1 0AE

Tel:	+44-(0)20-7482-2202
Fax:	+44-(0)20-7267-0159
E-mail:	**info@mdunitz.globalnet.co.uk**
Website:	http://www.dunitz.co.uk

A CIP catalogue record for this book is available from the British Library

ISBN 1-85317-738-5

Distributed in the United States by:
Blackwell Science Inc.
Commerce Place, 350 Main Street
Malden MA 02148, USA
Tel: 1-800-215-1000

Distributed in Canada by:
Login Brothers Book Company
324 Salteaux Crescent
Winnipeg, Manitoba R3J 3T2
Canada
Tel: 1-204-224-4068

Distributed in Brazil by:
Ernesto Reichmann Distribuidora de Livros, Ltda
Rua Coronel Marques 335, Tatuape 03440-000
Sao Paulo,
Brazil

Composition by Wearset, Boldon, Tyne and Wear
Printed and bound in Great Britain by Biddles Ltd, Guildford and King's Lynn.

Contents

List of Contributors

Corrado Argentino MD PhD
Department of Neurological Sciences, Università degli Studi di Roma, 'La Sapienza', 00185 Rome, Italy.

Richard C Becker MD
Professor of Medicine, University of Massachusetts Medical School, Director, Cardiovascular Thrombosis Center, Director, Anticoagulation Services and Director, Coronary Care Unit, University of Massachusetts,Memorial Medical Center,Worcester, MA 01655, USA.

José Biller MD
Professor and Chairman, Department of Neurology, Indiana University School of Medicine, Indianapolis, IN 46202-5124, USA.

Julien Bogousslavsky MD
Professor and Chairman, Department of Neurology, University Hospital, University of Lausanne, Lausanne, Switzerland.

Marie-Germaine Bousser MD
Professor, Neurologie Hôpital Lariboisière, 75475 Paris,France.

Natan M Bornstein MD
Head of Stroke Unit, Department of Neurology, Sackler Faculty of Medicine, Tel-Aviv 64239, Israel.

Gudrun Boysen MD
Professor of Neurology, Department of Neurology, Bispebjerg Hospital, Copenhagen NV, Denmark.

Antonio Carolei MD
Professor of Neurology, Clinica Neurologica, Università degli Studi di l'Aquila, 67100 l'Aquila-Coppito, Italy.

Olli Carpén MD PhD
Senior Investigator of the Academy of Finland, Consultant in Pathology, Department of Pathology, Haartman Institute, University of Helsinki, Helsinki, Finland.

Geoffrey A Donnan MBBS MD FRACP
Professor of Neurology, Director of Research, National Stroke Research Institute, Boronia Centre, Austin and Repatriation Medical Centre, Banksia Street, Heidelberg West , Victoria, 3081, Australia.

Christopher F Dowd MD
Associate Professor of Radiology and Neurological Surgery, Departments of Radiology and Neurological Surgery, University of California at San Francisco, San Francisco, CA 94143, USA.

Timo Erkinjuntti MD PhD
Chief, Memory Research Unit, Department of Clinical Neurosciences, Helsinki University Central Hospital, Helsinki, Finland.

Anne Falcou MD
Stroke Unit, Department of Neurological Sciences, Università degli Studi di Roma, 'La Sapienza', 00185 Rome, Italy.

Cesare Fieschi MD
Professor of Neurology, Department of Neurological Sciences, Università degli Studi di Roma, 'La Sapienza', 00185 Rome, Italy.

Marc Fisher MD
Chief of Neurology, Memorial Health Care and Professor of Neurology, University of Massachusetts Medical School, Worcester, MA 01605, USA.

Bhuwan P Garg MD
Professor of Neurology, Director of Paediatric Neurology, Indiana University School of Medicine, Indianapolis, IN 46202-5200, USA.

Amanda K Gilligan BSc MBBS (Hons) FRACP
Neurologist, National Stroke Research Institute, Boronia Centre, Austin and Repatriation Medical Centre, Banksia Street, Heidelberg West, Victoria 3081, Australia.

Van V Halbach MD
Professor of Radiology and Neurological Surgery, Department of Radiology and Neurological Surgery, University of California at San Francisco, San Francisco, CA 94143, USA.

Michael G Hennerici MD
Professor and Chairman, Department of Neurology, University of Heidelberg, Universitatsklinikum Mannheim, Mannheim, Germany.

Randall T Higashida MD
Clinical Professor of Radiology and Neurological Surgery, Chief, Division of Interventional Neuroradiology, University of California at San Francisco, San Francisco, CA 94143, USA.

Richard Kay MD FRCP
Professor, Division of Neurology, Department of Medicine and Therapeutics, The Chinese University of Hong Kong, Prince of Wales Hospital, Shatin, Hong Kong, China.

Markku Kaste MD PhD
Professor and Chairman, Department of Clinical Neurosciences, Helsinki University Central Hospital, Helsinki, Finland.

Petri T Kovanen MD PhD
Professor and Director, Wihuri Research Institute, Helsinki, Finland.

Todd E Lempert MD
Assistant Clinical Professor, Department of Radiology, University of California at San Francisco, San Francisco, CA 94143, USA.

Riitta Lassila MD PhD
Division of Cardiology, Helsinki University Central Hospital, Assistant Scientific Director, Wihuri Research Institute, Helsinki, Finland.

Adel M Malek MD PhD
Clinical Instructor, Department of Radiology, University of California at San Francisco, San Francisco, CA 94143, USA.

Carmine Marini MD
Clinica Neurologica, Università degli Studi di l'Aquila, 67100 l'Aquila-Coppito, Italy.

Philip M Meyers MD
Clinical Instructor, Department of Radiology, University of California at San Francisco San Francisco, CA 94143, USA.

Michael F Oliver MD FRCP FESC FRSE
Professor Emeritus, Cardiac Medicine , National Heart and Lung Institute, Imperial College School of Medicine, Dovehouse Street, London, UK.

Giuseppe Di Pasquale MD FESC FACC
Director, Divison of Cardiology, Bentivoglio Hospital, Bologna, Italy.

Constantine C Phatouros MBBS FRACR
Clinical Instructor, Department of Radiology, University of California at San Francisco, San Francisco, CA 94143, USA.

Andrea Pozzati MD FESC
Divison of Cardiology, Bentivoglio Hospital, Bologna, Italy.

Massimiliano Prencipe MD PhD
Department of Neurological Sciences, Università degli Studi di Roma, 'La Sapienza', 00185 Rome, Italy.

Maurizia Rasura MD
Stroke Unit, Department of Neurological Sciences, Università degli Studi di Roma, 'La Sapienza', 00185 Rome, Italy.

David G Sherman MD
Professor and Chief, Division of Neurology, University of Texas Health Science Center, San Antonio, Texas 78284-7883, USA.

Ingmar Skoog MD PhD
Institute of Clinical Neuroscience, Department of Psychiatry, Sahlgrenska University Hospital, Göteborg, Sweden.

Frederick A Spencer MD
Assistant Professor of Medicine, University of Massachusetts Medical School, Director, Thrombophilia Center, Associate Director, Coronary Care Unit, University of Massachusetts Memorial Medical Center, Worcester, MA 01655, USA.

Amanda G Thrift BSc (Hons) PhD
Epidemiologist, National Stroke Research Institute, Boronia Centre, Austin and Repatriation Medical Centre, Banksia Street, Heidelberg West, Victoria 3081, Australia.

Danilo Toni MD PhD
Stroke Unit, Department of Neurological Sciences, Università degli Studi di Roma, 'La Sapienza', 00185 Rome, Italy.

Michel Torbey MD
University of Massachusetts Health Care, Department of Neurology, Worcester, MA 01655-0318, USA.

François J G Vingerhoets MD
Privat-Docent, Maître d'enseignement et de recherche, Department of Neurology, University Hospital, University of Lausanne, Lausanne, Switzerland.

Preface

The worldwide burden of stroke is enormous, affecting both the health care delivery system and financial expenditure. In many developed countries, stroke remains a leading cause of death and disability and a similar trend is now evident in developing countries. It is therefore critical for physicians, patients and government agencies involved with health care delivery to be cognisant of recent developments targeted at preventing stroke.

Advances in diagnostic methodologies have provided fast and accurate insights into the mechanisms of stroke. Rapid intervention is now proven to reduce the threat of functional dependence in a number of stroke patients. New therapeutic approaches are being tested, based on a growing understanding of the immediate pathophysiology, and we can envision a day in the not too distant future when multiple therapies will be available for acute stroke.

Nevertheless, prevention remains of paramount importance and the prospects for stroke prevention continue to advance. Long term antiplatelet or anticoagulant therapy in selected individuals at risk can safely reduce the incidence of stroke. Risk factor management, surgical and, potentially, other vascular interventional techniques may also be effective.

This volume provides both the specialist and primary care physician with an up-to-date review of the emerging opportunitites for management and prevention of stroke. We thank all the authors of the book for sharing their knowledge and hope that those who read it will be both educated and stimulated by these valuable contributions.

We would also like to thank Aleth Patrassi and Linda Dickman for their help and collaboration in the preparation of this title.

C Fieschi
M Fisher

1

The burden of stroke: a need for stroke prevention

Corrado Argentino and Massimiliano Prencipe

INTRODUCTION

Stroke is the most common disease causing disability, the most common neurological life-threatening disease and the third leading cause of death in industrialized countries, accounting for one in every 15 deaths.[1]

The burden of stroke and the need for prevention can be measured in public health terms by epidemiological data (incidence, prevalence, mortality) and economic impact.

EPIDEMIOLOGY OF STROKE

Incidence

Current estimates from the American Heart Association are that almost 500 000 new strokes occur in the United States each year.[1] In the world, age-adjusted incidence rates range between 100 and 300 per 100 000 per year, depending on the population demographics, country of origin and study methodology.[2]

In a community-based prospective cohort study carried out in Umbria, Italy[3] using a methodology similar to the Oxfordshire Community Stroke Project,[4] the crude average annual stroke incidence was 254 per 100 000, and the age-adjusted rates to the Italian and European populations were 181 and 155 per 100 000, respectively. In the Copenhagen City Heart study,[5] the stroke incidence rate was 214 per 100 000, which is very similar to the rate calculated in the registry carried out in Malmo, Sweden (225 per 100 000).[6] The Perth Community Study found an incidence of 258 per 100 000.[7] In Taiwan, 8562 stroke-free people, followed for 4 years, had a disease incidence of 330 per 100 000, which is higher than in the US and the UK but similar to Japan.[8]

The high incidence of stroke in various countries documents the burden of the disease on a worldwide scale, but the studies so far conducted contain numerous methodological biases. Epidemiological information should actually be based on population studies with sample projections at an interval of at least 10 years.[9] All cases of stroke should be recorded, i.e., both cases followed by admission to hospital and cases not referred, with particular attention being paid to relapsing patients. There is a need for an accurate register and a file of neuroimages to assure data quality. Unfortunately, the available data do not fulfil these criteria and have numerous methodological faults. Many studies are based on Caucasian samples, with little information available on eastern European countries and, above all, on Asian populations and on the whole African continent.[10]

Direct evidence of a decline in stroke incidence is difficult to collect;[11,12] rates did decline in Rochester, Minnesota, but are now increasing again,[13] although this was not observed in Soderhamn, Sweden.[14] Assuming that the incidence of stroke is decreasing,[15] the burden will remain substantial for the foreseeable future given the aging of the population. In fact, the burden of stroke will fall on the acute hospital services, rather than on rehabilitation facilities, because strokes are more likely to be fatal in elderly people than in younger subjects.[9]

Prevalence

In 1997 in the US, the American Heart Association estimated that there were 3 890 000 stroke survivors, many of whom required long-term care.[1] A typical estimate of prevalence is 500/100 000, although this clearly depends on the population age structure.[16] Stroke prevalence is not a particularly useful statistic; incidence, and even mortality, data provide more information on etiology, geographical and time trends, as well as the influence of various risk factors. For health-service planning purposes, the prevalence of disability in general is far more important than stroke-related disability alone, particularly when one comes to consider elderly populations that have so many additional causes of disability, such as arthritis, breathlessness, angina and deafness. In any event, prevalence is difficult to measure because a large sample of the population has to be identified as the denominator, a large proportion of that sample must be seen and questioned, and many past stroke episodes are forgotten by patients.

Mortality

Altogether, stroke accounts for almost 10% of all deaths in industrialized countries, the vast majority of deaths involving people over the age of 65.[2] The average age-adjusted stroke mortality in industrialized countries is 50–100 per 100 000 per year,[2] but death rates vary greatly around the world. There are wide differences from country to country, with the highest rates being reported in eastern Europe and Portugal, and the lowest rates reported in Switzerland, Canada and the US.[17] Stroke mortality has been decreasing since the early 1900s at a rate of 1% per year until 1968 and at a rate of 5% per year during the last few years.[17] Unfortunately, mortality data may not provide a complete description of the magnitude of stroke for many reasons: (1) not all patients die; (2) death certificates may not provide accurate determination of the cause of death; and (3) changes in the international coding of diseases (e.g., the assumption of sudden death has been modified: in the past, sudden death was often recorded as stroke, while more recently it has been attributed to an unknown coronaropathy).[18,19]

In addition, well-conducted epidemiological studies have supported the hypothesis that the drop in stroke mortality is associated with an improved survival,[20–22] which is, in turn, unfortunately associated with an increase in the number of disabled people.[23]

COST OF STROKE

Globally, stroke accounts for 2–4% of total healthcare costs, and for more than 4% of direct healthcare costs in industrialized countries.[24] In 1997, the economic cost of stroke in the US was $40.9 billion. The direct cost (hospital care, drugs, professional care) was $26.2 billion; the indirect cost, mostly represented by loss of output, was $14.7 billion.[1]

It is important to distinguish between the lifetime cost of the first stroke and acute and subacute care costs, as well as between the direct and indirect costs of the disease. The direct costs are related to the diagnosis, treatment and rehabilitation of stroke, while the indirect costs are related to the economic and social changes of patients, as well as to substantial modifications in the lives of caregivers. Furthermore, the estimates of stroke costs depend on the conditions of the patient's life before the disease, in terms of residual abilities and long-term survival probabilities.

The lifetime cost per person varies depending on the type of stroke and degree of neurological deficit. In the US, in 1996, it was estimated that the lifetime cost per person was $103 576, with a higher cost associated with subarachnoid hemorrhage due to a higher direct cost and earlier mean age of onset which, in turn, results in far greater indirect costs.[25]

The direct costs of stroke

The direct cost of stroke in the US is approximately $30 billion per year, with an average cost per case of $50 000. A consistent part is represented by in-patient hospital costs during the first year of disease, which range from 40% to 85% of the direct cost.[24–28]

In one analysis of the hospital expenses alone,[29] the burden of the individual elements was reported: nursing costs accounted for about 81%, while 19% covered the remaining costs (of which 19% was for physicians, 10% for specific drugs, 31% for general treatment and 40% for instrumental examinations).

Obviously, the direct cost of disease varies from country to country depending on the type of assistance and the length of stay in hospital, the rehabilitation unit and nursing home. The average length of stay in hospital is relatively short in the Netherlands (27 days),[30] if compared with Sweden (59 days) and Scotland (65 days).[31] Very little information is available on rehabilitation unit costs, and all is based on isolated experiences. As regards the nursing home, in the US 101 900 admissions were attributable to stroke in 1990, at a net present value of more than $29 296 per patient admission, with a mean length of stay of 432 days,[25] which is comparable to the Netherlands (470 days).

A major cost not reflected directly in current studies is nursing-home care, which is particularly significant for stroke patients with more severe disability.[32]

The indirect costs of stroke

Indirect costs account for a consistent part of the lifetime cost for all types of stroke[25] and are related not only to the patient's condition, but also to the lives of the family and caregiver.

The first indirect cost to consider is loss of productivity, which is very difficult to evaluate. Cornes and Roy (1991)[33] reported that only a minority of patients of working age return to work. Angeleri and co-workers (1993)[34] showed that 20.6% return to work, but not always to the same job, and often after readapting to new conditions. Moreover, language disturbances can be a hindrance at work.

Another indirect cost is related to residual social activity of stroke patients, resulting in various changes of quality of life. Depression, social support, functional status, social class, age and cardiovascular diseases can predict the quality of life after stroke.[35] King and co-workers[35] found that satisfaction of the next-of-kin is the most important item related to the quality of life in long-term stroke survivors, while health and functional satisfaction are less important.

Few studies have focused on the burden of stroke for family and caregivers. A well-conducted Australian study found that, 1 year after stroke, 43% of patients were moderately handicapped and lived at home. Globally, 55% of the caregivers of these patients showed evidence of emotional distress, particularly if patients were affected by dementia and/or abnormal behavior. The disorders of caregivers and relatives included anxiety (58%), depression (50%), fear (35%), frustration (32%), resentment (29%), impatience (25%) and guilt (10%).[36] In this regard, it should be kept in mind that family members play an important role in promoting behavioral changes in patients after stroke.

CONCLUSIONS

The burden of stroke, measured in terms of medical, social and economic impact, highlights the need for an urgent amelioration in primary and secondary prevention and treatment. Since stroke is very expensive, particularly severe strokes, treatments to prevent stroke and to reduce stroke disability are likely to be of excellent value.

REFERENCES

1. American Heart Association. *Heart and Stroke Facts Statistics: 1997 Statistical Supplement.* Dallas; American Heart Association: 1997.
2. Wolf PA, D'Agostino RB. Epidemiology of stroke. In: *Stroke: Pathophysiology, Diagnosis, and Management* (Barnett HJM, Mohr JP, Stein BM, Yatsu FM, eds.) 3rd edn, pp. 3–28. New York; Churchill Livingstone: 1998.
3. Ricci S, Celani MG, La Rosa F *et al.* SEPIVAC: a community based study of stroke incidence in Umbria, Italy. *J Neurol Neurosurg Psych* 1991; **54:**695–8.
4. Bamford J, Sandercock P, Dennis M, Burn J, Warlow C. A prospective study of acute cerebrovascular disease in the community: the Oxfordshire Community Stroke Project—1981–1986. 2. Incidence, case fatality rates and overall outcome at one year of cerebral infarction, primary intracerebral haemorrhage, and subarachnoid haemorrhage. *J Neurol Neurosurg Psych* 1990; **53:**16–22.
5. Lindenstrom E, Boysen G, Nyboe J, Appleyard M. Stroke incidence in Copenhagen, 1976–1988. *Stroke* 1992; **23:**28–32.
6. Jerntorp P, Berglund G. Stroke registry in Malmo, Sweden. *Stroke* 1992; **23:**357–61.
7. Anderson C, Jamrozik K, Stewart-Wynne E. Ascertaining the true incidence of stroke. 1: the Perth Community Stroke Study [abstract]. *J Stroke Cerebrovasc Dis* 1992; **2**(Suppl 1):100.
8. Hu H-H, Sheng W-Y, Chu F-L *et al.* Incidence of stroke in Taiwan. *Stroke* 1992; **23:**1237–41.
9. Malmgren R, Bamford J, Warlow C, Sandercock P, Slattery J. Projecting the number of patients with first-ever strokes and patients newly handicapped by stroke in England and Wales. *Br Med J* 1989; **298:**656–60.
10. Sudlow C, Warlow C. Comparing stroke incidence worldwide. What makes studies comparable? *Stroke* 1996; **27:**550–8.
11. Bonita R, Beaglehole R, North JDK. The long-term monitoring of cardiovascular disease: is it feasible? *Comm Hlth Studies* 1983; **7:**111.
12. Malmgren R, Warlow C, Bamford J, Sandercock P. Geographical and secular trends in stroke incidence. *Lancet* 1987; **ii:**1196.
13. Broderick JP, Phillips SJ, Whisnant JP *et al.* Incidence rates of stroke in the eighties: the end of the decline of stroke? *Stroke* 1989; **20:**577–82.
14. Terent A. Increasing incidence of stroke among Swedish women. *Stroke* 1988; **19:**423.
15. Bonita R. Epidemiology of stroke. *Lancet* 1992; **339:**342.
16. Wade DT, Langton Hewer R, Skilbeck CE, David RM. *Stroke, a Critical Approach to Diagnosis, Treatment and Management.* London; Chapman and Hall: 1985.
17. National Institutes of Health. *Morbidity and Mortality: 1996 Chartbook on Cardiovascular, Lung, and Blood Disease.* Bethesda, Maryland; NIH: 1996.
18. Phillips LH, Whisnant JP, Reagan TJ. Sudden death from stroke. *Stroke* 1977; **8:**392–5.
19. Thomas AC, Knapman PA, Krikler DM, Davies MJ. Community study of the causes of "natural" sudden death. *Br Med J* 1988; **297:**1453–6.
20. Howard G, Craven TE, Sanders L, Evans GW. Relationship of hospitalized stroke rate and in-hospital mortality to the decline in US stroke mortality. *Neuroepidemiology* 1991; **10:**251–9.
21. Modan B, Wagener DK. Some epidemiologic aspects of stroke: mortality/morbidity trends, age, sex, race, socioeconomic status. *Stroke* 1992; **23:**1230–6.
22. Harmsen P, Tsipogianni A, Wilhelmsen L. Stroke incidence rates were unchanged, while fatality rates declined, during 1971–1987 in Goteborg, Sweden. *Stroke* 1992; **23:**1410–5.
23. Bonita R, Beaglehole R. Stroke mortality. In: *Stroke, Populations, Cohorts and Clinical Trials* (Whisnant JP, ed.), pp. 39–79. Oxford; Heinemann: 1993.
24. Drummond MF, Ward GH. The financial burden of stroke and the economic evaluation of treatment alternatives. In: *Stroke: Epidemiological, Therapeutic and Socioeconomic Aspects* (Rose FC, ed.). London; Royal Society of Medicine Services Ltd: 1987.
25. Taylor TN, Davis PH, Torner JC, Holmes J, Meyer JW, Jacobson MF. Lifetime cost of stroke in the United States. *Stroke* 1996; **27:**1459–66.
26. Persson U, Silvberg R, Lindgren B *et al.* Direct cost of stroke for a Swedish population. *Int J Tech Assess Hlth Care* 1990; **6:**125–37.
27. Adelman SN. National survey of stroke: economic impact. *Stroke* 1981; **12**(Suppl I):69–87.
28. Smurawska LT, Alexandrov AV, Bladin CF, Norris JW. Cost of acute stroke care in Toronto, Canada. *Stroke* 1994; **25:**1628–31.
29. Dennis M, Wellwood I, McGregor K, Dent J, Forbes J. What are the major components of the cost of caring for stroke patients in hospital in the UK? *Cerebrovasc Dis* 1995; **5:**243.
30. Arraway W, Whisnant J, Drury I. The continuing

decline in the incidence of stroke. *Mayo Clin Proc* 1983; **58:**520–3.
31. Isard PA, Forbes JF. The cost of stroke to the National Health Service in Scotland. *Cerebrovasc Dis* 1992; **2:**47–50.
32. Leibson CL, Ransom J, Brown RD, O'Fallon WM, Hass SL, Whisnant JP. Stroke-attributable nursing home use: a population-based study. *Neurology* 1998; **51:**163–168.
33. Cornes P, Roy CW. Vocational Rehabilitation Index assessment of rehabilitation medicine service patients. *Int Disabil Studies* 1991; **13:**5–8.
34. Angeleri F, Angeleri VA, Foschi N, Giaquinto S, Nolfe G. The influence of depression, social activity, and family stress on functional outcome after stroke. *Stroke* 1993; **24:**1478–83.
35. King RB. Quality of life after stroke. *Stroke* 1996; **27:**1467–72.
36. Anderson CS, Linto JRN, Stewart-Wynne EGGS. A population-based assessment of the impact and burden of caregiving for long-term stroke survivors. *Stroke* 1995; **26:**843–9.

2

Major risk factors and protective factors: how to improve primary prevention of cerebrovascular disease

Amanda G Thrift, Amanda K Gilligan and Geoffrey A Donnan

CONTENTS • Risk factors and protective factors • Primary prevention of ischemic stroke: how can it be improved?

RISK FACTORS AND PROTECTIVE FACTORS

The etiology of acute ischemic stroke can be delineated into the broad categories of cardioembolic, large vessel disease (artery to artery emboli, hemodynamic mechanisms), and small vessel disease. Consequently, the major factors predisposing to ischemic stroke directly relate to risk factors for atherosclerosis, lipohyalinosis, thrombosis and embolic phenomena. Conversely, protective factors are those that may have an influence on either preventing, arresting, or reversing these conditions.

These risk and protective factors may be modifiable or non-modifiable (Table 2.1). Non-modifiable risk factors are those that cannot be altered by intervention. Advancing age, male

Table 2.1 Current status of risk factors for ischemic stroke

Non-modifiable risk factors	*Modifiable risk factors*	
	Established	*Possible*
Age	Hypertension	Physical inactivity
Gender	Diabetes	Obesity
Heart disease	Smoking	Dietary factors
Family history	Atrial fibrillation	Oral contraceptive use
Ethnicity	Hypercholesterolemia	Lack of hormone replacement therapy
Socioeconomic status	Alcohol consumption	Infection
	Prothrombotic factors	Stress
	Prior transient ischemic attack	
	Prior stroke	

gender, ethnic background, socioeconomic status, family history and genetic conditions are all examples of which, given our current state of medical knowledge, are fixed in terms of risk profile. Modifiable risk factors are those for which either treatment is available or in which alterations in behavior can reduce the proportion of the population exposed (i.e., reduce the risk factor prevalence). A reduction in the population exposure then influences the disease in question (in this instance, ischemic stroke).

Established, modifiable risk factors for ischemic stroke currently include hypertension, cigarette smoking, carotid and aortic arch atherosclerosis, atrial fibrillation, hypercholesterolemia, diabetes, transient ischemic attack (TIA), previous stroke, prothrombotic conditions (see Chapter 4) and hyperhomocysteinemia. There are a number of other less well-established risk factors and protective factors that are also modifiable. Such 'possible' factors include alcohol consumption, regular exercise, obesity, oral contraception, hormone replacement and illicit drug use (Table 2.1). In this chapter we will review the current status of risk factors for each category and then attempt to put this information in the context of suggested methods to reduce the impact of stroke by improvements in primary prevention.

Non-modifiable risk factors

Advancing age

The incidence of ischemic stroke increases dramatically with age, approximately doubling for each decade of life.[1] The risk profile for older people differs from the younger stroke population as will be discussed in Chapters 5 and 6.

Male gender

Within each age group, the incidence of ischemic stroke (expressed as the number of first-ever events per 100 000 population per year) is greater among men than women.[1] In the older age categories, the overall number of ischemic stroke events, however, is greater in women simply because of the larger number of women surviving to these ages.

Ethnicity

Several investigators have observed differences in stroke incidence and subtypes in people of different races. It is well accepted that Asian populations have a lower rate of ischemic stroke (approximately 70% of all strokes)[2,3] compared with European, Australian or American populations (80–85%).[1,4–10] There is evidence that blacks are at more than twice the risk of stroke than whites of the same age.[11–13] There is also evidence that ischemic stroke incidence is greater in an Hispanic population.[13]

Socioeconomic status

Increased stroke incidence occurs among people of lower socioeconomic status.[14–16] This group has been shown to have a high prevalence of risk factors (expressed as the number of people with the disease per 100 000 population per year) for stroke, including hypertension (especially uncontrolled hypertension), smoking and obesity.[15] They are also more likely to consume low fiber, high fat, high salt diets with low levels of antioxidants, as well as undertaking less physical activity.[15] Social isolation in men has also been found to increase the risk of stroke about two-fold (adjusted odds ratio (OR) 2.02, 95% confidence interval (CI) 1.00–4.08).[17]

Family history

Parental history of stroke has a small but significant impact on stroke risk,[18,19] as does a parental history of ischemic heart disease.[18] In a cohort of British men aged 40–59 years, the risk of stroke in those with a parent dying from stroke or heart trouble was 1.4 (95% CI 1.1–2.0) and 1.3 (95% CI 1.0–1.7), respectively, when compared to those without this family history.[18] In a Russian case–control study the presence of any family history of stroke increased the risk of stroke by 2.7 (95% CI 1.42–5.09).[19] Other recent studies have provided less impressive figures.[20,21]

The increased risk of stroke among family members has also been shown to occur among siblings of stroke patients. Living brothers and sisters of stroke patients were more likely to have had a stroke than siblings of the patients' spouses.[22]

Genetic factors

Evidence for a genetic contribution to stroke prevalence is provided by the results of a twin study. Concordance rates of twins self-reporting a stroke were 17.7% for monozygotic twins and 3.6% for dizygotic twins, resulting in a five-fold increase in risk among monozygotic twins.[23] Although genetic factors appear to be associated with stroke, many of these genetic factors are likely to be influenced by lifestyle factors. Specific genetic risk factors for stroke are currently being explored.

Clinical syndromes with Mendelian inheritance, such as cerebral autosomal dominant arteriopathy with subcortical infarcts and leukoencephalopathy (CADASIL) have now been described.[24] Further research with other genetic markers has expanded as the human genome project has accelerated towards the year 2000.

Potential genetic factors for increased risk of ischemic stroke include thrombotic and procoagulant gene mutations (platelet adhesion factors, Factor V Leiden, prothrombin, fibrinogen, plasminogen activator inhibitor 1), lipid metabolism molecules (apolipoproteins, lipoprotein receptors and lipolytic enzymes) and homocysteine metabolism (C677T methylene tetrahydrofolate reductase (MTHFR) mutation). Detailed discussions of procoagulant factors can be found in Chapter 4.

Angiotensin I converting enzyme (ACE) is a potential genetic marker for stroke. It is intimately related to the renin–angiotensin system which provides control of renal arteriolar perfusion pressure and systemic blood pressure. ACE influences angiotensin activity, which has been shown to promote arterial intimal hyperplasia and potentially the progression of atherosclerosis. In a recent meta-analysis it has been shown that the D allele for the ACE gene, acting recessively, may be a moderate and independent risk factor for ischemic stroke.[25]

Modifiable risk factors and protective factors

Hypertension

Hypertension is probably the most clearly established modifiable risk factor for ischemic stroke. In a recent meta-analysis of 45 prospective cohorts in which the influence of the level of diastolic blood pressure on the risk of stroke was investigated, the authors showed that for each 10 mmHg increase in diastolic blood pressure there was an increase in stroke risk of 1.84 (95% CI 1.80–1.90; Table 2.2).[26] No separate association was reported for ischemic stroke (stroke was used as a generic term to include all types) and the majority of these studies used mortality as an endpoint. Consequently, this result may not be representative of ischemic strokes *per se*. In a meta-analysis of a number of Chinese studies, the risk of ischemic stroke associated with hypertension was 5.25 (95% CI 3.95–6.98).[27]

This issue has also been addressed in a number of recent epidemiological studies, in which ischemic stroke has been investigated separately. In these studies hypertension has been reported to increase the risk of ischemic stroke between 2.4- and 8-fold (Table 2.3).[19,28–32] Moreover, when different levels of baseline blood pressure have been assessed the risk of ischemic stroke has been found to be greater at higher levels of systolic blood pressure.[29,32–34] Interestingly, the association between past history of hypertension and ischemic stroke appears to be greater in younger individuals than older patients.[35] This finding is supported by the results of other studies limited to younger people where the point estimate of ischemic stroke risk associated with hypertension was found to be about six- to seven-fold.[36–37] Lacunar stroke has been reported to have a greater association with hypertension than ischemic stroke in general, with an adjusted odds ratio of 8.9 (95% CI 4.2–18.8) being recorded in one study.[38]

Evidence for a benefit of antihypertensive therapy has been provided by a number of studies and, in meta-analyses of these, therapy was reported to reduce the risk of stroke by between 29% and 51% (Table 2.4).[39–41] Low- and high-dose diuretics and beta-blockers were all found to be of benefit in reducing the number of strokes, as was therapy among patients older than 59 years of age.[40,41] One could speculate that the relatively lower impact of hypertension

Table 2.2 Meta-analyses of risk factors for stroke

Reference	Factor	Number of studies	Events	Risk ratio (and 95% CI)
Prospective Studies Collaboration[26]	Diastolic blood pressure	45 cohorts†	13 397	1.84 (1.80–1.90) for each 10 mmHg increase
He *et al.*[27]	Hypertension	12 Chinese studies	2379	5.43 (4.62–6.39) stroke
		6 Chinese studies	NR	5.25 (3.95–6.98) ischemic stroke
Shinton and Beevers[64]*	Smoking	22	NR	1.92 (1.71–2.16)
Qizilbash *et al.*[68]	Hypercholesterolemia	10	778	1.31 (1.11–1.54)
Prospective Studies Collaboration[26]	Hypercholesterolemia	45 cohorts†	13 397	0.98 (0.94–1.01) for each 1 mmol/l increase
WHO Collaborative Study[119]	Oral contraceptive pill	22 centers	2242	1.53 (0.71–3.31) < 50 µg
				5.30 (2.56–11.0) ≥ 50 µg

* Analysis is restricted to patients with ischemic stroke; † 33 studies—majority are mortality studies; NR, not reported.

Table 2.3 Prevalence rates, relative risks and potential relative impact of targeting/treating selected risk factors for ischemic stroke

Risk factor*	Prevalence	Relative risk (range)†	Relative impact
Hypertension[146]	18% men 14% women	2.4–8.0	High
Atrial fibrillation[148]		2.0–5.8	Low
aged ≥ 40 years	2.3%		
aged ≥ 65 years	4.7%		
men aged ≥ 75 years	10%		
women aged ≥ 75 years	5.6%		
Smoking[146]	24% men 21% women	1.4–5.7	High
Hypercholesterolemia[146]‡	16% men 14% women	1.3	Low
Diabetes[147]	4%	1.5–4.0	Low
Heavy alcohol consumption[147]§	2.4%	2.2–2.4	Low

* Prevalence data obtained from the references indicated.
† The range of relative risk point estimates were obtained from the following sources: hypertension,[19,28–32] diabetes,[19,28–32] smoking,[19,28–30,32,54,58–61,85] hypercholesterolemia,[68] atrial fibrillation,[19,31,53–55,149] and heavy alcohol consumption.[28,84] With the exception of atrial fibrillation, studies are only included if a wide age bracket is included. The prevalence of atrial fibrillation is reported for people aged 40 years or more.
‡ Hypercholesterolemia is defined as a plasma cholesterol level of ≥6.5 mmol/l.
§ Heavy alcohol consumption is defined as drinking on average five or more standard drinks per day.

on the risk of ischemic stroke in some communities[11,28,32,42] when compared to others,[19,29,30,36,37] might be partly due to improved control of hypertension. However, there is no direct evidence for this, and it is just as likely that the differences in relative risk are attributable to differences in subject age, or prevalence of other risk factors.

Atherosclerosis

Atherosclerosis, the disease of aging arteries, is accelerated in multiple medical conditions, which are, in themselves, risk factors for ischemic stroke. Hypertension, diabetes, hypercholesterolemia and diabetes are the major factors implicated. Importantly, smoking is also associated with atherosclerotic stenosis of the carotid artery.[43] More recently, such factors as homocysteine levels have also been identified as risk factors.[44–47]

Although there appears to be a difference in the distribution of atherosclerosis between individuals, there is also significant overlap. For example, ischemic heart disease and peripheral vascular disease are common in patients with ischemic stroke.[48]

In the 1990s aortic arch atheroma has emerged as an important risk factor for ischemic stroke in people without carotid disease or cardioembolic source of stroke. In a study conducted by Amarenco *et al.* between 1991 and 1993, the odds ratio for ischemic stroke among patients with aortic arch atherosclerotic plaques ≥4 mm was 9.1 (95% CI 3.3–25.2) after adjustment for atherosclerotic risk factors.[49] In the 31% of ischemic stroke

Table 2.4 Meta-analyses of treatment effects to reduce the prevalence of stroke risk factors

Reference	Risk factor	Treatment	Number of studies	Events	Risk ratio (95% CI)	Relative risk reduction with treatment
Collins *et al.*[39]	Hypertension	Antihypertensive medication	16	773	0.6 (0.5–0.7)	40%
Psaty *et al.*[40]	Hypertension	High dose diuretics	9	320	0.49 (0.39–0.62)	29–51%
		Low dose diuretics	4	538	0.66 (0.55–0.78)	
		Beta-blockers	4	482	0.71 (0.59–0.86)	
Insua *et al.*[41]	Hypertension	Antihypertensive medication in patients over 59 years of age	9	243	0.64 (0.49–0.82)*	34–35%
				629	0.65 (0.55–0.76)†	
Barnett *et al.*[57]	Atrial fibrillation	Warfarin and non-valvular AF	6	190	0.36 (0.26–0.49)	64%
Barnett *et al.*[57]	Atrial fibrillation	Aspirin and non-valvular AF	3	228	0.78 (0.61–1.01)	22%
Bucher *et al.*[72]	Hypercholesterolemia	HMGCoA reductase inhibitors	8	NR	0.76 (0.62–0.92)	24%ǂ
		Cholestyramine or colestipol	3		1.07 (0.57–2.00)	
		Clofibrate or Gemfibrozil	5		1.12 (0.84–1.48)	
		Diet	10		0.98 (0.82–1.18)	
Blauw *et al.*[77]	Hypercholesterolemia	HMGoA reductase inhibitors	13	442	0.69 (0.57–0.83)	31%

* Stroke mortality; † stroke morbidity; NR, not reported; ǂ with HMGCoA reductase inhibitors.

patients without any known predisposing cause, 28.2% had aortic plaques ≥4 mm, compared with 8.1% among patients having atrial fibrillation or significant carotid stenosis (OR 4.7, 95% CI 2.2–10.1). In more recent studies the odds ratio for complex or thick aortic arch atheroma (≥5 mm thickness) associated with ischemic stroke has been reported to be 2.6 (95% CI 1.1–5.9) and 7.1 (95% CI 2.7–18.4) in the United States and Australia, respectively.[50,51] There are, as yet, no randomized, controlled trials of therapy for aortic arch atherosclerosis.

Patients with a history of ischemic heart disease have been reported to be about twice as likely to suffer an ischemic stroke than patients without coronary artery disease.[11,48] Whether this might be attributable to an overlap of atherosclerotic disease in both vascular territories, a more direct mechanistic association (embolism from the heart), or both, is unclear. Similarly, atherosclerosis affecting the carotid arteries and ascending aortic arch are independent risk factors for stroke, either because of intracranial atherosclerotic association or because of the presence of atheroma in these regions as sources of embolism and/or hemodynamic compromise.[50,51]

Atherosclerotic disease may be influenced by surgical or medical therapy. For symptomatic carotid stenoses (with 70% or more stenosis), carotid endarterectomy has been shown to be of benefit when performed by surgeons with major complication rates of 2–3% or less.[52] The evidence for the beneficial effect of surgery for asymptomatic and less severe symptomatic stenosis is less definitive and is discussed in detail in Chapters 14 and 15.

Atrial fibrillation

Atrial fibrillation, either valvular or nonvalvular, is associated with a major increase in the risk of embolic events. The relative risk point estimate of ischemic stroke has been reported to vary between 2.0 and 5.8 (Table 2.3).[19,31,53–55] Age may increase the risk of ischemic stroke independent of other risk factors in a population with atrial fibrillation.[56] Treatment with anticoagulants and antiplatelet agents has been shown to be effective in reducing the risk of stroke (Table 2.4). A meta-analysis of anticoagulant treatment in atrial fibrillation, and involving a total of 190 strokes, provided evidence for a 64% reduction in ischemic stroke with treatment.[57] The effect of treatment with aspirin was not so marked: a 22% reduction in ischemic events was reported, although the 95% confidence interval crossed unity.[57]

Cigarette smoking

There have been many studies that have shown an increase in the risk of ischemic stroke associated with smoking.[19,28,32,33,36,37,42,58–63] In a meta-analysis of 22 studies, the risk of ischemic stroke associated with smoking was found to be 1.92 (95% CI 1.71–2.16; Table 2.2).[64] The evidence for this association is strengthened by the demonstration of a positive dose–response relationship.[28,32,42] Ex-smokers tend to be at lower risk of ischemic stroke than current smokers, and in many studies past smoking does not reach statistical significance as an independent risk factor for ischemic stroke.[19,36,37,42,65] After 12 years of follow-up in the Honolulu Heart Program, an increased risk of ischemic stroke was observed among those who continued to smoke at the 6th year follow-up, and a reduced risk was observed among those who had ceased smoking at the 6th year of follow-up.[66] This provides some further support that smokers can reduce their risk of ischemic stroke after ceasing smoking.

Cigarette smoking may be a more important risk factor for lacunar stroke than for other forms of ischemic stroke.[38,61] The odds ratio of lacunar stroke associated with cigarette smoking was observed to be 6.6 (2.9–14.8) in a case–control study.[38]

A possible mechanism for the increased risk of ischemic stroke associated with smoking is that of accelerated carotid artery atherosclerosis. This notion is supported by an ultrasonic Doppler study in which carotid artery plaque thickness was positively associated with pack-years of smoking, and in another study where smoking was independently associated with severe carotid stenosis.[43,67]

Hypercholesterolemia

Hyperlipidemia and, in particular, hypercholesterolemia has recently been highlighted as a risk factor for stroke because of the beneficial effects of statin drugs in reducing stroke risk among subjects with prior cardiovascular disease. Paradoxically, elevated serum cholesterol has always been considered to be a weak or non-existent risk factor for stroke. The Prospective Studies Collaboration group analyzed 45 cohort studies and found no increase in stroke risk with increased serum cholesterol.[26] However, the potential biases of using fatal stroke only as an endpoint in most studies should be recognized.[26] In a prior meta-analysis, in which equivalent cut-off points for hypercholesterolemia were used (of roughly 5.7 mmol/l), the risk of stroke increased 1.3-fold for subjects with total cholesterol levels above about 5.7 mmol/l.[68] Similar levels of association have been provided in more recent studies,[33,42,69] unless serum cholesterol level has been used as a continuous variable, when these positive associations have not been demonstrated.[11,62,70] However, the role of cholesterol in increasing the risk of ischemic stroke is biologically plausible, with a report of a significant positive correlation between plasma total cholesterol-HDL cholesterol ratio and carotid bifurcation atherosclerosis.[71]

Given these weak and variable associations between cholesterol level and ischemic stroke, what have been the effects of lipid lowering? A meta-analysis of 10 randomized trials on the effect of cholesterol-lowering with dietary intervention did not provide evidence for an overall benefit on the risk of stroke (Table 2.4).[72] Meta-analysis of the trials using cholestyramine, colestipol, clofibrate and gemfibrozil also showed no improvement in stroke risk.[72] When meta-analysis of the 3-hydroxy-3-methylglutaryl coenzyme A (HMGCoA) reductase inhibitors (the 'statins') was considered, an overall reduction of 24% (relative risk 0.76, 95% CI 0.62–0.92) was observed among patients treated with these agents.[72] In one more recent trial using pravastatin, the stroke risk was reduced by 19% ($P = 0.048$).[73] These drugs do not appear to be as effective in primary prevention as in secondary prevention which might be explained by the larger number of the latter trials undertaken (and consequent larger patients numbers), thus increasing the power to observe a difference.[74] The disparity between the dramatic effects of the statins in reducing stroke risk compared to the more modest effects of other methods of lowering cholesterol levels may be due, in part, to the greater efficiency of the former, but also may be due to other pharmacological effects of the statins such as plaque stabilization, amelioration of endothelial dysfunction, and improvement on platelet coagulation abnormalities.[75]

None of the meta-analyses have provided separate data for stroke subtype.[72,74,76,77] This may have resulted in an underestimate of the overall effect of cholesterol-lowering because there is some evidence that lower serum cholesterol may increase the risk of cerebral hemorrhage.[78] The risk reduction for ischemic stroke alone may, consequently, be even larger than these estimates.

Diabetes

Diabetes, diagnosed according to a fasting serum glucose ≥7.8 mmol/l or a random sample 11.1 mmol/l, is associated with a two-fold increase in incidence of hypertension and cardiac disease.[79] Diabetics are also at increased risk of asymptomatic carotid artery disease and hyperlipidemia.[79] Because these other factors are also independent risk factors for ischemic stroke it is more difficult to determine the level of association between diabetes and ischemic stroke *per se*.

Diabetes has been reported to increase the risk of ischemic stroke between 1.5- and 4-fold (Table 2.3).[19,28–32] In the largest published population-based case–control study, in which stroke subtype is CT-verified in 86% of patients, the increased risk of ischemic stroke among diabetics compared to non-diabetics was 2.3 (95% CI 1.3–4.0), adjusting for multiple known risk factors.[28] Larger cohort studies involving 9565 and 5017 participants provided similar results (odds ratio of 2.12 and 2.47, respectively).[11,34]

Benefit from strict control of blood glucose has been shown to reduce the common diabetic complications such as nephropathy, neuropathy and retinopathy in Type 1 and Type 2 diabetes.[80,81] As yet, longitudinal studies have not provided evidence for a decreased risk of stroke among diabetics with strict glycemic control.[80,81]

Alcohol consumption

The issue of alcohol consumption and risk of ischemic stroke is still unclear.[11,28,30,33,82,83] Heavy alcohol consumption has been associated with an increased risk of ischemic stroke in some studies,[36,42,83,84] but not in others.[28,85,86] There is also some evidence that small amounts of alcohol, and specifically wine, may provide some degree of protection from stroke.[84,87,88] Although some investigators have postulated a J-shaped relationship between alcohol consumption and ischemic stroke,[84,89] it has also been suggested that this relationship is a possible artefact of inclusion of past drinkers (a group at risk of ischemic stroke) together with abstainers in the reference category.[90] Binge drinking has been positively associated with ischemic stroke in a Finnish study and has been associated with stroke mortality among men in a Swedish study (relative risk 1.6, 95% CI 1.1–2.5).[82,91]

Transient ischemic attack and prior stroke

Transient ischemic attacks (TIAs) are transient focal neurological symptoms due to focal cerebral ischemia and last less than 24 h. There is a 12% risk of stroke within 12 months of a TIA and the highest risk is in the first month (8%).[92] These patients need urgent assessment, diagnosis and preventative treatment and their needs are similar to those of the patient who has suffered only a mild stroke. In cohort and case–control studies, the point estimate of ischemic stroke risk varies from 2.7 to 3.9.[19,93] Patients with prior stroke are also at an increased risk.[28,29] Recurrent stroke will be discussed in more detail in Chapter 10.

Hyperhomocysteinemia

Homocysteine is a highly reactive sulphur containing amino acid and hyperhomocysteinemia has been associated with premature atherosclerosis.[45,47] Hypertension and smoking have also been associated with an increased serum homocysteine level, but hyperhomocysteinemia has been shown to be an independent risk factor for peripheral vascular, cerebrovascular and coronary artery disease. There is clear evidence that homocysteine increases with low folate levels, increasing age and is higher in males.[44,45,72] Recent studies have provided evidence that folate supplementation will decrease serum homocysteine levels and reduce the risk of progressive atherosclerosis,[44,94–96] but this therapeutic approach has not, as yet, been extended to stroke prevention.

Possible risk factors and protective factors

Dietary factors

A number of dietary factors have been implicated as protective or risk factors for stroke. These factors include dietary fats,[14,97] fish consumption,[14] consumption of fresh fruit and vegetables,[16,98,99] various micronutrients (such as vitamin C, carotene and calcium[14]), salt intake,[28,29] and coffee consumption.[100] None of these studies have provided conclusive evidence for either a positive or negative association with ischemic stroke. However, the positive association between coffee consumption (three or more cups per day) and ischemic stroke among hypertensive middle-aged men (OR 2.1, 95% CI 1.2–3.7) might be worthy of further investigation.[100] Issues related to dietary folate have already been discussed.

Physical activity

Physical exercise improves cardiovascular fitness, aids weight reduction and lowers resting blood pressure.[101–103] The specific effect of physical activity on stroke risk is less clear, in part because the amount and pattern of physical activity over time is difficult to quantify. Early studies provided inconclusive evidence for an association between physical activity and stroke.[104–106] In the Tilburg hospital-based case–control study the risk of stroke associated with heavy physical activity was 0.4 (95% CI 0.2–0.9).[107] In a more recent study by Sacco *et al.*[108] conducted in patients aged 39 years and over, the odds ratio associated with light, moderate or heavy physical activity in the 2-week period prior to the ischemic event (or interview for controls) was 0.37 (0.25–0.55). Similarly, in a British study of ischemic stroke, increasing levels of physical activity afforded reduced risks of ischemic stroke.[109] This protective effect was also evident in a case–control study of lacunar stroke among people exercising at least three times per week (OR 0.3, 95% CI 0.1–0.7).[38] In contrast, there have been other reports of no benefit from physical activity on the risk of ischemic stroke.[29,36] The reason for conflicting findings may relate to the difficulty in obtaining an accurate and consistent measurement of exposure.

Obesity

There are several studies that have demonstrated an association between obesity (as measured by body mass index, BMI, measured in kg/m^2) and stroke,[19,37,62,107,110–112] and the association may be greater in women.[37,110,111] Other investigators, however, have reported no such association.[70,113] There is, as yet, no evidence that weight reduction reduces stroke risk.

Oral contraceptive pill and hormone replacement therapy

Following the wide availability of the oral contraceptive pill in the 1960s, an association between oral contraceptive use and cerebral ischemia became evident.[114,115] Later investigators did not replicate these findings.[37,63,116–118] In a more recent international multicenter study, oral contraceptives were again associated with ischemic stroke in Europe, developing countries and Latin America (Table 2.2).[119] When separate analyses were conducted for users of low-dose estrogen (<50 μg) and high-dose estrogen, there was an increased risk of ischemic stroke among the high-dose users but not among the low-dose users.[119] It is possible that the decline in dose of hormone in the oral contraceptive pill over time may account for the decline in risk of ischemic stroke with use of the pill. Furthermore, a potentiation of risk of ischemic stroke has been observed among women taking the oral contraceptive pill who are also hypertensive[119] and among women taking the oral contraceptive pill who also smoke.[119,120]

There is conflicting evidence regarding the possibility that hormone replacement therapy is negatively associated with ischemic stroke risk.[121–123] There has been one report that hormone replacement therapy provides protection from ischemic stroke in smokers, although there is the possibility of bias given that there were a small number of observations in this category (11 ischemic strokes).[124] As reported in a recent review, although hormone replacement therapy appears to provide protection from cardiovascular disease, the beneficial effect of hormone replacement therapy in preventing strokes is unconvincing, and there remains some concern that hormone replacement may increase the risk of cancer.[125]

Hemostatic factors

Factors that enhance thrombosis and reduce fibrinolysis may account for the paradox of a high risk of stroke in populations with low risk of coronary heart disease.[126] Prothrombotic states account for only a small percentage of ischemic stroke with no other causes found. It is estimated that it occurs in about 4% of young stroke patients, the more common factors relating to protein C, antithrombin III, activated protein C deficiency or lupus anticoagulant.[127] Other conditions such as polycythemia rubra vera sickle cell disease and essential thrombocythemia are rare.

Temperature and seasonal variation

Ambient temperature has been shown to correlate negatively with ischemic stroke incidence,[128] with more ischemic strokes occurring during winter.[129] It is unknown whether these meteorological changes are real risk factors for stroke, or whether there are some other variables that are influenced by seasonal variations (e.g. increases in blood pressure, platelets, red blood cells and blood viscosity during winter, and seasonal variation in fibrinogen and high density lipoprotein cholesterol in elderly people).[128] In the Framingham study more atherothrombotic brain infarctions were found to occur at home and were concentrated between 8:01 a.m. and noon.[130]

Cocaine

Cocaine is an emerging risk factor for ischemic stroke, with the number of reported events rising dramatically during the 1980s as it became cheaper, purer and easier to obtain.[131] Whether crack cocaine, an alkaloidal form of cocaine that can be smoked,[132] is also associated with ischemic stroke is less clear. There is some disagreement for such an association, with one report of a positive temporal association between crack cocaine use and ischemic stroke in a series of 18 patients,[133] while in a case–control study involving 39 ischemic stroke and 99 controls there was no observed temporal association (OR 1.2, 95% CI 0.4–3.8).[134]

Infection

There are possible associations between infection as an acute precipitant of stroke. In a case–control study of 166 patients with cerebrovascular ischemia (TIA and ischemic stroke) and 166 controls, infection within the preceding week was observed to be associated with an increased risk of ischemic stroke (OR 3.5, 95% CI 1.6–7.7).[135] On the death-certificate diagnosis of the condition, bronchopneumonia was found to be more common in people dying from cerebral infarction than in controls (OR 1.49; 1.15–1.93),[112] but it is likely that this is a secondary phenomenon. In a case–control study involving 68 cases of cerebral infarction and 68 controls, the risk associated with HIV infection was 3.2 (95% CI 1.1–8.9).[136]

PRIMARY PREVENTION OF ISCHEMIC STROKE: HOW CAN IT BE IMPROVED?

The main aim of primary prevention is to reduce the incidence of stroke in a given population. There are two main approaches that can be adopted to achieve this aim. The high-risk approach relates to the identification of persons at high risk and either introducing treatment strategies or minimizing risky behaviors. The mass, or population, approach involves either mass screening for identification of individuals at risk or media and education campaigns to alter risky behaviors on a population basis. This latter approach may result in an overall small reduction in the exposure variable on an individual basis, but may have a significant impact on the whole population.

The effectiveness of primary prevention strategies are influenced by three important aspects of each risk factor. These are whether the risk factor is modifiable; whether there is a strong association between the factor and the disease; and whether the risk factor is common within the population.

Which risk factors can be modified?

Modifiable risk factors are those that can be altered either by changes in behavior or via treatment. Such risk factors might include hypertension, coronary artery disease, smoking, hypercholesterolemia, obesity, atrial fibrillation, transient ischemic attacks, and physical inactivity. Ceasing smoking, introducing exercise, or reducing alcohol or fat intake would be ways in which changes in behavior might modify these factors. Modification could also be achieved by treatment with medication, such as antihypertensive agents to reduce blood pressure levels or use of antilipidemic drugs to reduce cholesterol levels.

The benefits of antiplatelet therapy for treating transient ischemic attacks has been demonstrated;[137–139] these treatments include antiplatelet agents such as aspirin, dipyridamole, ticlopidine or clopidogrel. Combinations of some antiplatelet agents may increase overall antithrombotic action.[140]

Hypertension is modifiable via a multitude of available medications[39–41] as well as regular exercise to control diastolic and systolic levels,[101–103] and reducing salt intake.[141] Many believe that the falling age-related mortality from stroke is a direct consequence of better blood pressure control,[142–143] although others suggest that other factors may contribute.[144,145]

There have been a number of meta-analyses of antihypertensive agents, HMGCoA reductase inhibitors, and warfarin in non-valvular atrial fibrillation, all of which have shown a benefit in reducing the risk of stroke

(Table 2.4).[39,57,77] The role of aspirin in non-valvular atrial fibrillation is less well established.[57]

Strength of association

The strength of the association is indicated by the relative risk or odds ratio of the exposure variable. The higher the relative risk, the stronger is the association. The relative risks for a number of factors are given in Table 2.3. Because the relative risks vary between studies, the range of point estimates reported have been provided. For example, the point estimates for the association between hypertension and ischemic stroke range from 2.4 to 8.0.[19,28–32] A relative risk of 8.0 would be considered a very strong association, while that for hypercholesterolemia (1.3) would not. Hypertension has the strongest association with ischemic stroke of all factors listed (Table 2.4).

Prevalence of risk factors

The prevalence of a risk factor is the proportion within the population in whom the factor is present. The more common the risk factor within the population, the greater is its prevalence. Estimates for the prevalence of a number of risk factors are provided in Table 2.3.[146–148] Because prevalence rates of many of these factors differ between populations, these data should not be considered to be definitive, but will be used for illustrative purposes only. As shown in Table 2.4, the prevalences of smoking (21% for women and 24% for men) and hypertension (14% for women and 18% for men) are relatively high when compared to prevalence rates of diabetes (4%), atrial fibrillation (2.3%) and heavy alcohol consumption (2.4%). Although the estimated prevalence of atrial fibrillation is quite low for the population as a whole, it increases with age, increasing to 10% in men aged 75 plus.[149]

Attributable risk

The attributable risk is the proportion of a disease (in this instance, ischemic stroke) that is associated with exposure to a particular risk factor. It is mathematically derived from both the relative risk and the prevalence of the risk factor under investigation. The formula for calculation of the attributable risk for a given population is:

$$\text{Population attributable risk} = \frac{P(RF) \times (RR - 1)}{[P(RF) \times (RR - 1)] + 1}$$

where P(RF) is the prevalence of the risk factor in the population and RR is its relative risk. Figure 2.1 shows the relationship for a series of prevalence rates of people exposed at various relative risks. As shown in the graph, a high attributable risk is achieved when both the relative risk and the prevalence rate of the exposure variable are relatively high: if only one of these variables is high, the attributable risk is unlikely to be high. This can be illustrated using the prevalence rates and estimated relative risks provided in Table 2.4. Supposing that the relative risk of smoking is 3.0 and the prevalence of smoking is 24%, the proportion of ischemic stroke that is attributable to smoking is

$$\text{Population attributable risk for smoking} = \frac{0.24 \times (3 - 1)}{[0.24) \times (3 - 1)] + 1} = 0.32$$

Thus, 32% of ischemic stroke would be considered to be attributable to smoking. If, however, an exposure variable has a high relative risk and a low prevalence rate, the attributable risk will not be so marked. For example, supposing that the relative risk of ischemic stroke with atrial fibrillation is 3.6, and the prevalence of atrial fibrillation in the population is 2.3%, the proportion of ischemic stroke attributable to atrial fibrillation is 5.64%. Consequently, treatment of all people with atrial fibrillation is unlikely to have an appreciable impact on the incidence of ischemic stroke. However, if one considers males aged over 75 years (i.e., a stroke-prone age group),

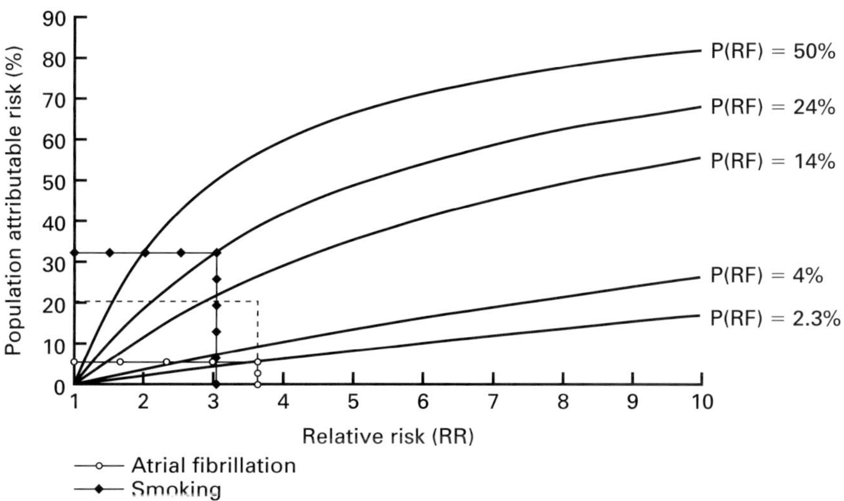

Figure 2.1 Relationship between population attributable risk, relative risk (RR) and prevalence of risk factor (P(RF)). (Adapted from Whisnant.[153]) For smoking, the relative risk used is 3.0, the smoking prevalence is 24%, and the consequent proportion of ischemic stroke that is attributable to smoking is 32% (—♦—). For atrial fibrillation the relative risk used is 3.6, the prevalence is 2.3%, and the consequent attributable risk is 5.64% (—○—). When the same relative risk is used for atrial fibrillation, but a prevalence value of 10% is utilized instead (i.e., for men aged 75 years and over), the population attributable risk for this age group of men is 21% (------).

where the prevalence of atrial fibrillation has been reported to be 10%, the population attributable risk (using a relative risk of 3.6) would be 21% in males of this age. Consequently, treatment of this group of men is likely to result in a considerable reduction in stroke incidence.

Multiplicity of risk factors

The individual at high risk of ischemic stroke often has multiple risk factors. In a recent review, the importance of multiple risk factors was discussed.[150] First, the interactive effect of the presence of risk factor combinations was considered. Important interactions have been shown to occur between transient ischemic attacks and age, hypertension and age, and cigarette smoking and age; all risk factors have shown a declining risk of stroke with increasing age. An interaction was also observed between atrial fibrillation, hypertension and age; hypertension potentiated the risk of stroke among those with intermittent atrial fibrillation, and this declined with age.[150] A potentiation of stroke risk has also been observed among smokers with hypertension.[151] Second, the presence of more than one independent risk factor collectively was shown to increase the population attributable risk. As an example, the presence of hypertension with any two of the other risk factors (smoking, transient ischemic attack, or ischemic heart disease) was associated with a population attributable risk of about 40%.

What are the best strategies to improve prevention?

As discussed, the two main primary prevention strategies are the population and high-risk approaches. It would obviously be foolish to take either approach in isolation because both strategies can provide benefit. Consequently, to improve primary prevention we need to combine high-risk and population approaches. The high-risk approach may involve screening patients for particular risk factors opportunistically, and then providing treatment for those individuals at high risk. An example of this might be the screening of all patients presenting to general practice for hypertension. Because the population-attributable risk for hypertension is relatively high, treating hypertensives identified in this way is likely to be effective in reducing ischemic stroke incidence. Interestingly, in a study of mainstream practice for risk-factor control, investigators have reported that only about 60% of ischemic stroke patients with hypertension were being treated for their elevated blood pressure.[152] This illustrates the potential for improvement in this area.

To complement this strategy, the population approach should also be used. Here one tries to bring about a small reduction in a particular risk factor in each individual in the whole population. Two examples of how this might be achieved are: by educating people on the benefits of exercise; or by reducing their salt intake (either by educating people on which high-salt foods to avoid, or by introducing taxes for high-salt processed foods).

In order to have the greatest impact on reducing the incidence of ischemic stroke, targeted risk factors must have a strong association with ischemic stroke, be relatively common in the population, and be modifiable. Table 2.3 summarizes the relative impact of a number of risk factors for ischemic stroke. When the attributable risk of ischemic stroke that is associated with exposure to a risk factor is at least 20%, the relative impact of treatment of that factor is considered to be high. A low relative impact is listed for all factors where the attributable risk is less than 10%. It must be noted that, although diabetes is listed in the table, there is still no evidence that its treatment reduces the incidence of ischemic stroke.

In conclusion, a combined strategy, utilizing the high-risk and population approaches, to improve primary prevention of ischemic stroke is advocated. To reduce the stroke burden in a population, one might aim to reduce those factors that contribute most to stroke, i.e., by reducing the mean blood pressure levels and by reducing the consumption of cigarettes. In addition to this approach, those at high risk of stroke, either with excessive levels of a particular risk factor, with multiple risk factors or with certain conditions such as prior transient ischemic attacks, should be treated to reduce their individual risk. Treatments that have been shown to reduce risk in these patients include antihypertensive medications, HMGCoA reductase inhibitors, and anticoagulants. Further improvement might also be achieved with the identification and modification of, as yet, unknown risk factors.

REFERENCES

1. Anderson CS, Jamrozik KD, Burvill PW, Chakera TMH, Johnson GA, Stewart-Wynne EG. Determining the incidence of different subtypes of stroke: results from the Perth Community Stroke Study, 1989–1990. *Med J Aust* 1993; **158:**85–9.
2. Tanaka H, Ueda Y, Hayashi M *et al.* Risk factors for cerebral hemorrhage and cerebral infarction in a Japanese rural community. *Stroke* 1982; **13:**62–73.
3. Udea K, Hasuo Y, Kiyohara Y *et al.* Intracerebral hemorrhage in a Japanese community, Hisayama: incidence, changing pattern during long-term follow-up, and related factors. *Stroke* 1988; **19:**48–52.
4. Ricci S, Celani MG, La Rosa F *et al.* SEPIVAC: a community-based study of stroke incidence in Umbria, Italy. *J Neurol Neurosurg Psychiatr* 1991; **54:**695–8.
5. D'Alessandro G, Di Giovanni M, Roveyaz L *et al.* Incidence and prognosis of stroke in the Valle d'Aosta Italy. *Stroke* 1992; **23:**1712–5.
6. Bamford J, Sandercock P, Dennis M, Burn J, Warlow C. A prospective study of acute cerebrovascular disease in the community: the Oxfordshire Community Stroke Project, 1981–6. 2. Incidence, case fatality rates and overall outcome at one year of cerebral infarction, primary intracerebral and subarachnoid haemorrhage. *J Neurol Neurosurg Psychiatr* 1990; **53:**16–22.

7. Brown RD, Whisnant JP, Sicks JD, O'Fallon WM, Wiebers DO. Stroke incidence, prevalence, and survival. Secular trends in Rochester, Minnesota, through 1989. *Stroke* 1996; **27:**373–80.
8. Wolf PA, D'Agostino RB, O'Neal A *et al.* Secular trends in stroke incidence and mortality. The Framingham Study. *Stroke* 1992; **23:** 1551–5.
9. Tuomilehto J, Sarti C, Narva EV *et al.* The FINMONICA Stroke Register. Community-based stroke registration and analysis of stroke incidence in Finland, 1983–1985. *Am J Epidemiol* 1992; **135:**1259–70.
10. Giroud M, Milan C, Beuriat P *et al.* Incidence and survival rates during a two-year period of intracerebral and subarachnoid haemorrhages, cortical infarcts, lacunes and transient ischaemic attacks. The stroke registry of Dijon: 1985–1989. *Int J Epidemiol* 1991; **20:** 892–9.
11. Giles WH, Kitter SJ, Hebel JR, Losonczy KG, Sherwin RW. Determinants of black–white differences in the risk of cerebral infarction. *Arch Intern Med* 1995; **155:**1319–24.
12. Kittner SJ, White LR, Losonczy KG, Wolf PA, Hebel JR. Black–white differences in stroke incidence in a national sample: the contribution of hypertension and diabetes mellitus. *J Am Med Assoc* 1990; **264:**1267–70.
13. Sacco RL, Boden-Albala B, Gan R *et al.* Stroke incidence among white, black and Hispanic residents of an urban community. The Northern Manhattan Stroke Study. *Am J Epidemiol* 1998; **147:**259–68.
14. Ross RK, Jian-Min Y, Henderson BE, Park J, Gao Y-T, Yu MC. Prospective evaluation of dietary and other predictors of fatal stroke in Shanghai, China. *Circulation* 1997; **96:**50–5.
15. James WPT, Nelson M, Ralph A, Leather S. Socioeconomic determinants of health: the contribution of nutrition in inequalities in health. *Br Med J* 1997; **314:**1545–9.
16. Artalejo FR, Guallar-Castillón P, Banegas JRB, Manzano BdA, Calero JdR. Consumption of fruit and wine and the decline in cerebrovascular disease mortality in Spain (1975–1993). *Stroke* 1998; **29:**1556–61.
17. Kawachi I, Colditz GA, Ascherio A *et al.* A prospective study of social networks in relation to total mortality and cardiovascular disease in men in the USA. *J Epid Comm Hlth* 1996; **50:**245–51.
18. Wannamethee GS, Shaper GA, Ebrahim S. History of parental death from stroke or heart trouble and the risk of stroke in middle-aged men. *Stroke* 1996; **29:**1492–8.
19. Feigin VL, Wiebers DO, Nikitin YP, O'Fallon WM, Whisnant JP. Risk factors for ischemic stroke in a Russian community: a population-based case–control study. *Stroke* 1998; **29:** 34–9.
20. Jousilahti P, Rastenyte D, Tuomilehto J, Sarti C, Vartiainen E. Parental history of cardiovascular disease and risk of stroke. A prospective follow-up of 14,371 middle-aged men and women in Finland. *Stroke* 1997; **28:**1361–6.
21. Barrett-Connor E, Khaw KT. Diabetes mellitus: an independent risk factor for stroke? *Am J Epidemiol* 1998; **128:**116–23.
22. Diaz JF, Hachinski VC, Pederson LL, Donald A. Aggregation of multiple risk factors for stroke in siblings of patients with brain infarction and transient ischemic attacks. *Stroke* 1986; **17:**1239–42.
23. Brass LM, Issacsohm JL, Merikangas KR, Robinette DC. A study of twins and stroke. *Stroke* 1991; **23:**221–8.
24. Mohr JP. CADASIL and white matter syndromes. *Ann Neurol* 1998; **44:**715–6.
25. Sharma P. Meta-analysis of the ACE gene in ischaemic stroke. *J Neurol Neurosurg Psychiatr* 1997; **64:**227–30.
26. Prospective Studies Collaboration. Cholesterol, diastolic blood pressure, and stroke: 13,000 strokes in 450,000 people in 45 prospective cohorts. *Lancet* 1995; **346:** 1647–53.
27. He J, Klag MJ, Wu Z, Whelton PK. Stroke in the People's Republic of China. 2. Meta-analysis of hypertension and risk of stroke. *Stroke* 1995; **26:**2228–32.
28. Jamrozik K, Broadhurst RJ, Anderson CS, Stewart-Wynne EG. The role of lifestyle factors in the etiology of stroke. A population-based case–control study in Perth, Western Australia. *Stroke* 1994; **25:**51–9.
29. Ellekjaer EF, Wyller TB, Sverre JM, Holmen J. Lifestyle factors and risk of cerebral infarction. *Stroke* 1992; **23:**829–34.
30. Kim JS, Yoon SS, Yo HJ, Kim CY, Choi-Kwon S, Lee BC. Type A behavior and stroke: high tenseness dimension may be a risk factor for cerebral infarction. *Eur Neurol* 1998; **39:** 168–73.
31. Woo J, Lau E, Lam CWK *et al.* Hypertension, lipoprotein (a), and apolipoprotein A-1 as risk factors for stroke in the Chinese. *Stroke* 1991; **22:**203–8.
32. Berger K, Schulte H, Stögbauer F, Assman G.

Incidence and risk factors for stroke in an occupational cohort. The PROCAM Study. *Stroke* 1998; **29:**1562–6.
33. Benfante R, Yano K, Hwang L-J, Curb D, Kagan A, Ross W. Elevated serum cholesterol is a risk factor for both coronary heart disease and thromboembolic stroke in Hawaiian Japanese men. *Stroke* 1994; **25:**814–20.
34. Manolio TA, Kronmal RA, Burke GL, O'Leary DH, Price TR. Short-term predictors of incident stroke in older adults. *Stroke* 1996; **27:**1479–86.
35. Petrovich H, Curb D, Bloom-Marcus R. Isolated systolic hypertension and risk of stroke in Japanese-American men. *Stroke* 1995; **26:** 25–9.
36. You RX, McNeil JJ, O'Malley HM, Davis SM, Thrift AG, Donnan GA. Risk factors for stroke due to cerebral infarction in young adults. *Stroke* 1997; **28:**1913–8.
37. Petitti DB, Sidney S, Bernstein A, Wolf S, Quesenberry C, Ziel HK. Stroke in users of low-dose oral contraceptives. *N Engl J Med* 1996; **335:**8–15.
38. You R, McNeil JJ, O'Malley HM, Davis SM, Donnan GA. Risk factors for lacunar infarction syndromes. *Neurology* 1995; **45:**1483–7.
39. Collins R, Peto R, MacMahon S *et al.* Blood pressure, stroke, and coronary heart disease. Part 2: short-term reductions in blood pressure: overview of randomised drug trials in their epidemiologic context. *Lancet* 1990; **335:**827–38.
40. Psaty BM, Smith NL, Siscovick DS *et al.* Health outcomes associated with antihypertensive therapies used as first-line agents. A systematic review and meta-analysis. *J Am Med Assoc* 1997; **277:**739–45.
41. Insua JT, Sacks HS, Lau T-S *et al.* Drug treatment of hypertension in the elderly: a meta-analysis. *Arch Intern Med* 1994; **121:**355–62.
42. Lee T-K, Huang Z-S, Ng S-K *et al.* Impact of alcohol consumption and cigarette smoking on stroke among the elderly in Taiwan. *Stroke* 1995; **26:**790–4.
43. Dempsey RJ, Moore RW. Amount of smoking independently predicts carotid artery atherosclerosis severity. *Stroke* 1992; **23:** 693–6.
44. Rimm EB, Willett WC, Hu FB *et al.* Folate and vitamin B_6 from diet and supplements in relation to risk of coronary heart disease among women. *J Am Med Assoc* 1998; **279:** 359–64.
45. Welch GN, Loscalzo J. Homocysteine and atherosclerosis. *N Engl J Med* 1998; **338:** 1042–50.
46. Perry IJ, Refsum H, Morris RW, Ebrahim SB, Ueland PM, Shaper AG. Prospective study of serum total homocysteine concentration and risk of stroke in middle-aged men. *Lancet* 1995; **346:**1395–8.
47. Graham IM, Daly LE, Refsum HM *et al.* Plasma homocysteine as a risk factor for vascular disease: The European Concerted Action Project. *J Am Med Assoc* 1997; **277:**1775–81.
48. Wolf PA, Kannel WB, McGee DL, Meeks SL, Barucha NE, McNamara PM. Duration of atrial fibrillation and imminence of stroke: the Framingham Study. *Stroke* 1983; **14:** 664–7.
49. Amarenco P, Cohen A, Tzourio C *et al.* Atherosclerotic disease of the aortic arch and the risk of ischemic stroke. *N Engl J Med* 1994; **331:**1474–9.
50. Di Tullio MR, Sacco RL, Gersony D *et al.* Aortic atheromas and acute ischaemic stroke: a transoesophageal echocardiographic study in an ethnically mixed population. *Neurology* 1996; **46:**1560–6.
51. Jones EF, Kalman JM, Calafiore P, Tonkin AM, Donnan GA. Proximal aortic atheroma. An independent risk factor for cerebral ischemia. *Stroke* 1995; **26:**218–24.
52. Goldstein LB, Hasselblad V, Matchar DB, McCrory DC. Comparison and meta-analysis of randomized trials of endarterectomy for symptomatic carotid artery stenosis. *Neurology* 1995; **45:**1965–70.
53. Wolf PA, Dawber TR, Thomas E, Kannel WB. Epidemiologic assessment of chronic atrial fibrillation and risk of stroke: the Framingham Study. *Neurology* 1978; **28:** 973–7.
54. Abu-Zeid HAH, Choi NW, Maini KK, Hsu PH, Nelson NA. Relative role of risk factors associated with cerebral infarction and cerebral hemorrhage. A matched pair case–control study. *Stroke* 1977; **8:**106–12.
55. Yuan Z, Bowlin S, Einstadter D, Cebul R, Conners AR, Rimm AA. Atrial fibrillation as a risk factor for stroke: a retrospective cohort study of hospitalized medicare beneficiaries. *Am J Pub Hlth* 1998; **88:**395–400.
56. Feinberg WM. Anticoagulation for the prevention of stroke. *Neurology* 1998; **51** (Suppl 3):20–22.
57. Barnett HJM, Eliasziw M, Meldrum HE. Drugs and surgery in the prevention of ischemic stroke. *N Engl J Med* 1995; **332:** 238–48.
58. Colditz GA, Bonita R, Stampfer MJ *et al.* Cigarette smoking and risk of stroke in middle-aged women. *N Engl J Med* 1988; **318:**937–41.
59. Gill JS, Shipley MJ, Tsementzis SA *et al.*

Cigarette smoking: a risk factor for hemorrhagic and nonhemorrhagic stroke. *Arch Intern Med* 1989; **149:**2053–7.
60. Wolf PA, D'Agostino RP, Kannel WB, Bonita R, Belanger AJ. Cigarette smoking as a risk factor for stroke: the Framingham Study. *J Am Med Assoc* 1988; **259:**1025–9.
61. Donnan GA, McNeil JJ, Adena MA, Doyle AE, O'Malley HM, Neill GC. Smoking as a risk factor for cerebral ischaemia. *Lancet* 1989; **ii:**643–7.
62. Yano K, Popper JS, Kagan A, Chyou P-H, Grove JS. Epidemiology of stroke among Japanese men in Hawaii during 24 years of follow-up. The Honolulu Heart Program. *Health Rep* 1994; **6:**28–38.
63. Lidegaard O. Oral contraception and risk of thromboembolic attack: results of a case–control study. *Br Med J* 1993; **306:**956–63.
64. Shinton R, Beevers G. Meta-analysis of relation between cigarette smoking and stroke. *Br Med J* 1989; **298:**789–94.
65. Love BB, Jones MP, Adams HP, Bruno A. Cigarette smoking: a risk factor for cerebral infarction in young adults. *Arch Neurol* 1990; **47:**693–8.
66. Abbott RB, Yin Y, Reed DM, Yano K. Risk of stroke in male cigarette smokers. *N Engl J Med* 1986; **315:**717–20.
67. Mast H, Thompson JLP, Lin I-F *et al.* Cigarette smoking as a determinant of high-grade carotid stenosis in Hispanic, black, and white patients with stroke or transient ischaemic attack. *Stroke* 1998; **29:**908–12.
68. Qizilbash N, Duffy SW, Warlow C, Mann J. Lipids are risk factors for ischaemic stroke: overview and review. *Cerebrovasc Dis* 1991; **2:**127–36.
69. Vasuvat A, Towanabut S. Blood lipids, the risk factor of cerebral infarction. *J Med Assoc Thai* 1993; **76:**109–16.
70. Nakayama T, Date C, Yokoyama T, Yoshiike N, Yamaguchi M, Tanaka H. A 15.5-year follow-up study of stroke in a Japanese provincial city. *Stroke* 1997; **28:**45–52.
71. Ford SC, Crouse JR, Howard G, Toole JF, Ball MR, Frye J. The role of plasma lipids on carotid bifurcation atherosclerosis. *Ann Neurol* 1985; **17:**301–3.
72. Bucher HC, Griffiths LE, Guyatt GH. Effect of HMGCoA reductase inhibitors on stroke: a meta-analysis of randomized, controlled trials. *Ann Intern Med* 1998; **128:**89–95.
73. The long-term Intervention with Pravastatin in Ischaemic Disease (LIPID) Study Group. Prevention of cardiovascular events and death with pravastatin in patients with coronary heart disease and a broad range of initial cholesterol levels. *N Engl J Med* 1998; **339:** 1349–57.
74. Hebert PR, Gaziano JM, Chan KS, Hennekens CH. Cholesterol lowering with statin drugs, risk of stroke, and total mortality. *J Am Med Assoc* 1997; **278:**313–21.
75. Delanty N, Vaughan CJ. Vascular effects of statins in stroke. *Stroke* 1997; **28:**2315–20.
76. Atkins D, Psaty BM, Koepsell TD, Longstreth WT, Larson EB. Cholesterol reduction and the risk for stroke in men: a meta-analysis of randomized, controlled trials. *Ann Intern Med* 1993; **119:**136–45.
77. Blauw GJ, Lagaay AM, Smelt AHM, Westendorp RGJ. Stroke, statins, and cholesterol: a meta-analysis of randomized, placebo-controlled, double-blind trials with HMG-CoA reductase inhibitors. *Stroke* 1997; **28:**946–50.
78. Eastern Stroke and Coronary Heart Disease Collaborative Research Group. Blood pressure, cholesterol, and stroke in eastern Asia. *Lancet* 1998; **352:**1801–7.
79. Biller J, Love BB. Diabetes and stroke. *Med Clin North Am* 1993; **77:**95–111.
80. DCCT Research Group. The effect of intensive treatment of diabetes on the development and progression of long-term complications of insulin-dependent diabetes mellitus. *N Engl J Med* 1993; **329:**977–86.
81. UK Prospective Diabetes Study (UKPDS) Group. Intensive blood-glucose control with sulphonylureas or insulin compared with conventional treatment and risk of complications in patients with type 2 diabetes (UKPDS 33). *Lancet* 1998; **352:**837–53.
82. Hansagi H, Romelsjö A, Gerhardsson de Verdier M, Andréasson S, Leifman A. Alcohol consumption and stroke mortality: 20 year follow-up of 15,077 men and women. *Stroke* 1995; **26:**1768–73.
83. Kiyohara Y, Kato I, Iwamoto H, Nakayama K, Fujishima M. The impact of alcohol and hypertension on stroke incidence in a general Japanese population. The Hisayama Study. *Stroke* 1995; **26:**368–72.
84. Gill JS, Shipley MJ, Tsementzis SA *et al.* Alcohol consumption: a risk factor for hemorrhagic and non-hemorrhagic stroke. *Am J Med* 1991; **90:**489–97.

85. Gorelick PB, Rodin MB, Langenberg P, Hier DB, Costigan J. Weekly alcohol consumption, cigarette smoking, and the risk of ischemic stroke: results of a case control study at three urban medical centres in Chicago, Illinois. *Neurology* 1989; **39**:339–43.
86. Shinton R, Sagar G, Beevers G. The relation of alcohol consumption to cardiovascular risk factors and stroke. The West Birmingham Stroke Project. *J Neurol Neurosurg Psychiatr* 1993; **56**:458–62.
87. Knuiman MW, Vu HTV. Risk factors for stroke mortality in men and women: the Busselton Study. *J Cardiovasc Risk* 1996; **3**: 447–52.
88. Truelsen T, Grønbæk M, Schnohr P, Boysen G. Intake of beer, wine, and spirits and risk of stroke. *Stroke* 1998; **29**:2467–72.
89. Herman B, Schmitz PI, Leyten AC *et al.* Multivariate logistic analysis of risk factors for stroke in Tilburg. The Netherlands. *Am J Epidemiol* 1983; **118**:514–25.
90. Shaper AG, Wannamethee SG, Walker M. Alcohol and mortality in British men: explaining the U-shaped curve. *Lancet* 1988; **ii**: 1267–73.
91. Hillbom M, Kaste M. Ethanol intoxication: a risk factor for ischemic brain infarction. *Stroke* 1983; **14**:694–9.
92. Sacco RL. Identifying patient population at high risk for stroke. *Neurology* 1998; **51** (Suppl 3):27–30.
93. Davis PH, Dambrosia JM, Schoenberg BS *et al.* Risk factors for ischemic stroke: a prospective study in Rochester, Minnesota. *Ann Neurol* 1987; **22**:319–27.
94. Giles HW, Kittner JS, Anda FR, Croft BJ, Casper LM. Serum folate and risk for ischemic stroke: First National Health and Nutrition Examination Survey Epidemiologic Follow-up Study. *Stroke* 1995; **26**:1166–70.
95. Selhub J, Jacques PF, Wilson PW, Rush D, Rosenberg IH. Vitamin status and intake as primary determinants of homocysteinemia in an elderly population. *J Am Med Assoc* 1993; **270**:2693–8.
96. Malinow MR, Duell PB, Hess DL *et al.* Reduction of plasma homocyst(e)ine levels by breakfast cereal fortified with folic acid in patients with coronary heart disease. *N Engl J Med* 1998; **338**:1009–15.
97. Gillman WM, Cupples A, Millen EB, Ellison RC, Wolf AP. Inverse association of dietary fat with development of ischemic stroke in men. *J Am Med Assoc* 1997; **278**:2145–50.
98. Gillman MW, Cupples A, Gagnon D *et al.* Protective effect of fruits and vegetables on development of stroke in men. *J Am Med Assoc* 1995; **273**:1113–7.
99. Key TJA, Thorogood M, Appleby PN, Burr ML. Dietary habits and mortality in 11 000 vegetarians and health conscious people: results of a 17 year follow up. *Br Med J* 1996; **313**:775–9.
100. Hakim AA, Ross GW, Curb JD *et al.* Coffee consumption in hypertensive men in older middle-age and the risk of stroke: the Honolulu Heart Program. *J Clin Epidemiol* 1998; **51**:487–94.
101. Duncan JJ, Farr JE, Upton J, Hagan RD, Oglesby ME, Blair SN. The effects of aerobic exercise on plasma catecholamines and blood pressure in patients with mild essential hypertension. *J Am Med Assoc* 1985; **254**:2609–13.
102. Jennings G, Nelson L, Nestel P *et al.* The effects of changes in physical activity on major cardiovascular risk factors, haemodynamics, sympathetic function, and glucose utilization in man: a controlled study of four levels of activity. *Circulation* 1986; **73**:30–40.
103. Seals DR, Hagberg JM. The effect of exercise training on human hypertension: a review. *Med Sci Sports Exerc* 1984; **16**:207–15.
104. Salonen JT, Puska P, Tuomilehto J. Physical activity and risk of myocardial infarction, cerebral stroke and death: a longitudinal study in Eastern Finland. *Am J Epidemiol* 1982; **115**:526–37.
105. Kannel WB, Sorlie P. Some health benefits of physical activity. The Framingham Study. Arch Intern Med 1979; **139**:857–61.
106. Paffenbarger RS, Wing AL. Characteristics in youth predisposing to fatal stroke in later years. *Lancet* 1967; **i**:753–4.
107. Herman B, Leyten ACM, van Luijk JH, Frenken CWGM, Op de Coul AAW, Schulte BPM. An evaluation of risk factors for stroke in a Dutch community. *Stroke* 1982; **13**: 334–8.
108. Sacco RL, Gan R, Boden-Albala B *et al.* Leisure-time physical activity and ischemic stroke risk. The Northern Manhattan Stroke Study. *Stroke* 1998; **29**:380–7.
109. Wannamethee G, Shaper AG. Physical activity and stroke in British middle aged men. *Br Med J* 1992; **304**:597–601.
110. Rexrode KM, Hennekens CH, Willett WC *et al.* A prospective study of body mass index, weight change, and risk of stroke in women. *J Am Med Assoc* 1997; **19**:1539–45.
111. Folsom AR, Prineas RJ, Kaye SA, Munger RG.

Incidence of hypertension and stroke in relation to body fat distribution and other risk factors in older women. *Stroke* 1990; **21:** 701–6.

112. Ogunniyi A, Chandra V, Shoenberg BS. Conditions associated at death with specific types of completed stroke in patients with and without hypertension: a case–control study. *Neuorepidemiology* 1989; **8:**24–31.
113. Walker SP, Rimm EB, Kawachi I, Stampfer MJ, Willett WC. Body size and fat distribution as predictors of stroke among US men. *Am J Epidemiol* 1996; **144:**1143–50.
114. Sartwell PE, Masi AT, Arthes FG, Greene GR, Smith HE. Thromboembolism and oral contraceptives: an epidemiological case–control study. *Am J Epidemiol* 1969; **90:**365–80.
115. Vessey P, Doll R. Investigation of relation between use of oral contraceptives and thromboembolic disease. A further report. *Br Med J* 1969; **2:**651–7.
116. Vessey MP, Villard-Mackintosh L, McPherson K, Yeates D. Mortality among oral contraceptive users: 20 year follow up of women in a cohort study [comment]. *Br Med J* 1989; **299:**1487–91.
117. Colditz GA. Oral contraceptive use and mortality during 12 years of follow-up: the nurses' health study. *Ann Intern Med* 1994; **120:**821–6.
118. Schairer C, Adami H-O, Hoover R, Persson I. Cause-specific mortality in women receiving hormone replacement therapy. *Epidemiology* 1997; **8:**59–65.
119. WHO Collaborative Study of Cardiovascular Disease and Steroid Hormone Contraception. Ischaemic stroke and combined oral contraceptives: results of an international, multicentre, case–control study. *Lancet* 1996; **348:** 498–505.
120. Royal College of General Practitioners' Oral Contraception Study. Further analyses of mortality in oral contraceptive users. *Lancet* 1981; **i:**541–6.
121. Paganini-Hill A, Ross RK, Henderson BE. Postmenopausal oestrogen treatment and stroke: a protective study. *Br Med J* 1988; **297:**519–22.
122. Boysen G, Nyboe J, Appleyard M *et al.* Stroke incidence and risk factors for stroke in Copenhagen, Denmark. *Stroke* 1988; **19:**1345–53.
123. Petitti D, Sidney S, Quesenberry CP, Bernstein A. Ischemic stroke and use of estrogen and estrogen/progestogen as hormone replacement therapy. *Stroke* 1998; **29:**23–8.
124. Lindentrøm E, Boysen G, Nyobe J. Lifestyle factors and risk of cerebrovascular disease in women. The Copenhagen City Heart Study. *Stroke* 1993; **24:**1468–72.
125. Lip GYH, Beevers G, Zarifis J. Hormone replacement therapy and cardiovascular risk: the cardiovascular physicians viewpoint. *J Intern Med* 1995; **238:**389–99.
126. Gliksman M, Wilson A. Are hemostatic factors responsible for the paradoxical risk factors for coronary heart disease and stroke? *Stroke* 1992; **23:**607–10.
127. Barinagarrementeria F, Cantu-Brito C, De La Pena A, Izaguirre R. Prothrombotic states in young people with idiopathic stroke. A prospective study. *Stroke* 1994; **25:**287–90.
128. Azevedo E, Riberio JA, Martins R, Barros H. Cold: a risk factor for stroke. *J Neurol* 1995; **242:**217–21.
129. Giroud M, Beuriat P, Vion P, D'Athis PH, Dusserre L, Dumas R. Stroke in a French prospective population study. *Neuroepidemiology* 1989; **8:**97–104.
130. Kelly-Hayes M, Wolf PA, Kase CS, Brand FN, McGuirk JM, D'Agostino RB. Temporal patterns of stroke onset. *Stroke* 1995; **26:** 1343–7.
131. Cregler LL. Cocaine: the newest risk factor for cardiovascular disease. *Clin Cardiol* 1991; **14:**449–56.
132. Cregler LL, Mark H. Medical complications of cocaine abuse. *N Engl J Med* 1986; **315:** 1495–500.
133. Levine SR, Brust JCM, Futrell N *et al.* Cerebrovascular complications of the use of the 'crack' form of alkaloidal cocaine. *N Engl J Med* 1990; **323:**699–704.
134. Qureshi AI, Akbar MS, Czander E, Safdar K, Janseen RS, Frankel MR. Crack cocaine use and stroke in young patients. *Neurology* 1997; **48:**341–5.
135. Grau AJ, Buggle F, Becher H *et al.* Recent bacterial and viral infection is a risk factor for cerebrovascular ischemia: clinical and biochemical studies. *Neurology* 1998; **50:** 196–203.
136. Qureshi A, Janssen RS, Karon JM *et al.* Human Immunodeficiency Virus infection and stroke in young patients. *Arch Neurol* 1997; **54:**1150–3.
137. Antiplatelet Trialists' Collaboration. Secondary prevention of vascular disease by prolonged antiplatelet treatment. *Br Med J [Clin Res]* 1988; **296:**320–31.
138. Medical Research Council Working Party. Medical Research Clinical trial of treatment of hypertension in older adults: principal results. *Br Med J* 1992; **304:**405–12.

139. Medical Research Council Working Party. Stroke and coronary heart disease in mild hypertension: risk factors and the value of treatment. *Br Med J* 1988; **296:**1565–70.
140. Diener H, Cunha L, Forbes C, Sivenius J, Smets P, Lowenthal A. European Stroke Prevention Study 2. Dipyridamole and acetylsalicylic acid in the secondary prevention of stroke. *J Neurol Sci* 1996; **143:**1–13.
141. Law MR, Frost CD, Wald NJ. Analysis of data from trials of salt reduction. *Br Med J* 1991; **302:**819–24.
142. Garraway WM, Whisnant JP. The changing pattern of hypertension and the declining incidence of stroke. *J Am Med Assoc* 1987; **258:**214–7.
143. Whisnant JP. The decline of stroke. *Stroke* 1984; **15:**160–8.
144. Klag MJ, Whelton PK, Seidler AJ. Decline in US stroke mortality. Demographic trends and antihypertensive treatment. *Stroke* 1989; **20:**14–21.
145. Bonita R, Beaglehole R. Increased treatment of hypertension does not explain the decline in stroke mortality in the United States, 1970–1980. *Hypertension* 1989; **13**(Suppl I):69–73.
146. Risk Factor Prevalence Study Management Committee. *Risk Factor Prevalence Study: Survey Number 3, 1989.* Canberra: National Heart Foundation of Australia and Australian Institute of Health; 1990.
147. Australian Institute of Health and Welfare. *Australia's Health 1994: the Fourth Biennial Health Report of the Australian Institute of Health and Welfare.* Canberra: Australian Government Publishing Service, 1994.
148. Feinberg WM, Blackshear JL, Laupacis A, Kronmal R, Hart RG. Prevalence, age distribution, and gender of patients with atrial fibrillation. Analysis and implications. *Arch Intern Med* 1995; **155:**469–73.
149. Sudlow M, Thomson R, Thwaites B, Rodgers H, Kenny RA. Prevalence of atrial fibrillation and eligibility for anticoagulants in the community. *Lancet* 1998; **352:**1167–71.
150. Whisnant JP. Modelling of risk factors for ischaemic stroke: the Willis lecture. Stroke 1997; **28:**1839–43.
151. Bonita R, Scragg R, Stewart A, Jackson R, Beaglehole R. Cigarette smoking and risk of premature stroke in men and women. *Br Med J* 1986; **293:**6–8.
152. Kalra L, Perez I, Melbourn A. Stroke risk management. *Stroke* 1998; **29:**53–7.
153. Whisnant JP. *Stroke: Populations, Cohorts, and Clinical Trials.* Oxford: Butterworth-Heinemann; 1993.

3

Heart disease and stroke

Giuseppe Di Pasquale and Andrea Pozzati

CONTENTS • **Introduction** • **Cardioembolic stroke** • **Coexisting ischemic heart disease**

INTRODUCTION

The need for a multidisciplinary evaluation of patients with stroke has been firmly established in recent years. In this framework the role of the cardiologist is of utmost relevance because of the multiple interactions between cardiovascular and cerebrovascular disease.[1–4]

There are two major reasons for the cardiologist to look after patients with transient ischemic attack (TIA) or stroke. First of all, TIA or ischemic stroke may be cardioembolic in nearly one-quarter of cases. Second, more than one-half of cerebrovascular patients may have coexisting coronary artery disease (CAD) and the risk of coronary events in the long-term follow-up exceeds the risk of cerebrovascular recurrences. Thus the search for cardiac sources of embolism and for coexisting CAD should be performed in many patients with cerebral ischemia.

CARDIOEMBOLIC STROKE

Nearly 20% of all ischemic strokes, and probably more, are cardioembolic; non-valvular atrial fibrillation (NVAF) accounts for about 50% of cardioembolic strokes[5,6] and it has been established that oral anticoagulant therapy (OAT) in these patients can reduce the embolic risk by two-thirds.

The widespread use of transesophageal echocardiography (TEE) allows the detection of potential cardiac sources of embolism in many cases of cryptogenic stroke which accounts for up to 40% of the cases in some series of young adults.[7–19] In patients with ischemic stroke studied within the first six hours potential embolic sources were found in more than 80% of cases.[10]

However, the diagnosis of cardioembolic stroke is often difficult and frequently remains uncertain. Diagnosis of cardioembolic stroke should be done by exclusion, i.e., only when there is no coexistent carotid artery disease. Carotid artery disease and potential embolic cardiac diseases frequently coexist and it is often difficult to determine whether the cardiac or cerebrovascular source is responsible for the cerebral ischemic event. In many series potential cardioembolic lesions were found in about 30% of patients with ischemic stroke, but carotid artery disease coexisted in nearly 10% of cases. Moreover the etiology remained unknown in about 30% of cases and up to 40% in younger patients with normal cardiac clinical findings.[11–17] Many authors have considered most of these cases to be of possible cardioembolic etiology.

Neurological symptoms of stroke and neuroimaging findings may be suggestive but are not entirely specific for the diagnosis of cardioembolic stroke. Also lacunar strokes, commonly attributed to small vessel disease, have recently been associated with cardioembolic disease (in some cases).

Cardiac sources of embolism

The cardiac lesions more frequently detected in patients with TIA or stroke include:

1. lesions at high embolic risk, i.e., ventricular thrombi (detectable in acute myocardial infarction and dilatative cardiomyopathies), left atrial appendage thrombi (detectable in patients with atrial fibrillation (AF), sick sinus syndrome and atrial flutter), endocarditic vegetations (both infective and degenerative or marantic), rheumatic mitral valve disease, thrombosis of prosthetic heart valves, cardiac tumors; and
2. lesions at low or uncertain embolic risk, i.e., mitral valve prolapse, mitral annular calcification, aortic valve calcification or calcified aortic valve stenosis (Table 3.1).

Beside physical examination, echocardiography is the technique of choice for the confirmation of cardiac sources of embolism suspected at clinical examination and for the detection of occult cardiac lesions in patients with a normal clinical examination.

Table 3.1 Risk stratification of cardiac sources of embolism

High embolic risk
Atrial fibrillation
Rheumatic mitral stenosis
Prosthetic cardiac valves
Recent myocardial infarction
Dilated cardiomyopathy
Cardiac tumors
Infective endocarditis
Low or uncertain embolic risk
Atrial flutter
Mitral valve prolapse
Mitral annular calcification
Valvular strands
Patent foramen ovale
Atrial septal aneurysm
Chiari's network
Aortic valve calcification
Calcified aortic stenosis
Hypertrophic cardiomyopathy
Remote myocardial infarction
Ventricular aneurysm
Aortic plaques

Transthoracic echocardiography

Transthoracic echocardiography (TTE) was first introduced into clinical practice in the 1970s and then regularly used in the cardiological investigation of patients with ischemic stroke.[18]

Echocardiographic studies showed that transesophageal echocardiography (TEE) was effective in detecting potential cardiac sources of embolism in many patients with a history and clinical evidence of heart disease.[19,20] Conversely, in patients with normal cardiac findings a negative echocardiographic result was found in nearly 95% of cases. In these patients the yield of TTE was only 1.5% (range 0–6%). An exception is represented by patients younger than 45 years. For these patients, who have a low prevalence of cerebrovascular disease, a hidden cardioembolic lesion is detectable in about 35% of cases by TTE.[15,17,21–24]

In conclusion, TTE is an adequate tool for searching for potential cardioembolic lesions in patients with known cardiac disease, whereas it has a very low sensitivity in patients without overt cardiac disease.

Transesophageal echocardiography

An important improvement for detecting possible sources of cardioembolic stroke has been achieved with the routine use of TEE.[7,8,10] TEE provides a detailed visualization of the morphology and function of cardiac structures, that

Table 3.2 Cardiac sources of systemic embolism: diagnostic yield of TEE vs. TTE

Cardiac lesions	*TEE*	*TTE*
Mass lesions		
LA thrombus	+++	−
LAA thrombus	+++	−
LA myxoma	+++	++
Mitral valve vegetations	++	+
Aortic valve vegetations	+	+
LV thrombus	−	++
Other conditions		
LA SEC	+++	−
Atrial septal defect	+++	+
Patent foramen ovale	+++	−
Atrial septal aneurysm	+++	+
Mitral valve prolapse	++	++
Aortic plaques	+++	−

− insufficient; + sufficient; ++ good; +++ excellent.
TEE, transesophageal echocardiography; TTE, transthoracic echocardiography; LA, left atrial; LAA, left atrial appendage; LV, left ventricular; SEC, spontaneous echo contrast.

cannot be obtained by the transthoracic approach. The superiority of the transesophageal approach is related to the proximity of the probe to the heart chambers with the absence of intervening structures. TEE gives an unimpaired view of the right and left atrial chambers, the interatrial septum and the atrioventricular valves, and allows for exploration of the left atrial appendage. This structure is inaccessible with the transthoracic approach and is frequently occupied by thrombi. The search for potential cardiac sources of embolic stroke actually represents one of the major indications for transesophageal echocardiography in most institutions.[20]

Several studies compared TEE and TTE in the detection of potential cardiac sources of embolism. The cardiac lesions more frequently detected in patients with ischemic stroke and the diagnostic yield of the two echocardiographic techniques are summarized in Table 3.2.[26–28]

Other cardiac imaging techniques

Cardiac ultrafast CT, magnetic resonance imaging (MRI), and ^{111}Indium-labeled platelet scintigraphy are supplementary techniques that can be used when echocardiographic studies are non-diagnostic. ^{111}Indium-labeled platelet scintigraphy is an imaging technique for detecting the ongoing platelet deposition on the surfaces of thrombi. Therefore thrombus activity can be evaluated, particularly in unstable conditions such as prosthetic cardiac valve thrombosis and acute myocardial infarction. The high cost and long duration of the study are the main limitations of this technique.

ECG Holter monitoring

Holter monitoring in patients with TIA or stroke discloses potentially embologenic arrhythmias in less than 4% of cases. These data suggest that Holter monitoring should be reserved only for those patients with suspected paroxysmal AF or sick sinus syndrome. Although the mechanism of stroke in patients with sick sinus syndrome is not yet clear, episodes of transient AF or severe bradycardia, in the presence of critical atherosclerotic carotid lesions, can be involved.

Patients with overt cardiac disease

In patients with overt cardiac disease the sensitivity of TTE was 76%, but increased to 85% with the TEE. TEE provides additional information about cardiac disease and can disclose left atrial or appendage thrombi, spontaneous echocontrast and left atrial appendage dysfunction, which are significant predictors of high thromboembolic risk.

Atrial fibrillation

Among the possible cardiac sources of embolism, non-valvular atrial fibrillation (NVAF) is the most frequent, accounting for the 45% of cardioembolic strokes.[5]

NVAF carries a high risk of systemic embolism, in particular stroke. However, the risk of stroke is not uniform, widely ranging between 0.4%[29] and 12% per year[30] with an average of 4.5% per year observed in the pooled analysis of five randomized controlled trials.[31–36]

The efficacy of OAT for the prevention of stroke has definitely been assessed by large randomized clinical trials. Overall, warfarin decreased the frequency of all strokes by 68% and the risk of bleeding was quite low (1.3% in warfarin-treated patients).[31] However, the bleeding risk is probably higher in patients treated in general clinical practice. Patients included in these trials were carefully selected, representing only 7–39% of screened patients. Moreover the safety of long-term OAT at conventional levels has not been completely defined among patients older than 75 years. A risk stratification is therefore warranted for identifying patients at high and low risk of stroke in order to plan optimal antithrombotic treatment.

A number of clinical and two-dimensional echocardiographic risk factors have been identified and prospectively validated.[28,31,37] Current practice recommendations for OAT or antiplatelet treatment are based on thromboembolic risk factors, including recent congestive heart failure or left ventricular dysfunction, previous thromboembolism, systolic blood pressure greater than 160 mmHg, or advanced age (>75 years for females).[39] In the presence of any of these risk factors patients with NVAF have a high risk of stroke if untreated with adjusted-dose warfarin.[40] Patients without any of these risk factors have low to moderate rates of stroke when treated with aspirin.[41] The low risk category includes patients who have no thromboembolic risk factors or history of hypertension. According to these criteria approximately 60% of patients with NVAF should be treated with OAT and maybe more if also considering patients with a history of hypertension.

TEE allows the detection of other markers of thromboembolism in patients with NVAF that are not detectable by the transthoracic approach. These markers include left atrial and left atrial appendage thrombi, spontaneous echo contrast, and left atrial appendage dysfunction.[42,43] The prevalence of these findings is significantly higher in AF patients who have suffered stroke or systemic embolism. The predictive role of these new markers has been validated in prospective studies.[44,45] Finally, the safety of cardioversion of AF without prolonged anticoagulation, with the use of TEE to exclude atrial thrombi, has been established in several studies.[46,47]

Atrial flutter

Only in recent years has it been established that in patients with atrial flutter the risk of stroke is not negligible. Similar to AF, evidence exists in atrial flutter of left atrial and left atrial appendage dysfunction either with persistent atrial flutter or after electrical cardioversion or radio-frequency ablation.[48–52] Moreover, the prevalence of left atrial thrombi and spontaneous echo contrast of 10% and 30%, respectively, has been documented in patients with atrial flutter by TEE.[53–56]

The prevalence of systemic thromboembolism and stroke is about 7% with an estimated risk of 1.8% per year which is less than that observed in patients with AF.[57–60]

Effective OAT is associated with a significant reduction of the embolic risk.[59,60] In the absence of controlled clinical trials the indications for OAT may be the same as those established in the guidelines for AF.

Acute myocardial infarction

Since the 1980s several studies focused on the risk of stroke and systemic thromboembolism in patients with recent myocardial infarction (MI). Embolic risk is high in patients with anterior infarction and in those with left ventricular thrombosis.[61–65] The risk of ischemic stroke is presumed to be 1–3% for all MI patients and 2–6% for anterior MI.[66]

Echocardiographic studies have reported a high incidence of left ventricular thrombi following MI. In a meta-analysis of several echocardiographic studies including 2018 patients with recent MI, the prevalence of left ventricular thrombi was 27%.[67] This finding is almost exclusively patients with anterior MI (39%), whereas for inferior MI the prevalence of thrombus is very low (0–5%). About 90% of mural thrombi occur when the ventricular apex is involved. In most cases thrombosis occurs within 48 h after the acute MI, although it may be found even after 1–2 weeks.[68]

The risk of stroke is undoubtedly high when left ventricular thrombus is detected. Indeed, the rate of embolic events was 18% in 921 patients with thrombus, compared with 2% in patients without. Furthermore, a meta-analysis from 11 echocardiographic studies performed in patients with acute MI showed a five-fold increase of embolic risk in the presence of left ventricular thrombosis.[69] The morphological characteristics of thrombi have clinical importance because thrombi with mobility and protrusion into the left ventricular cavity have higher embolic potential. The prevalence of embolic events is 55% for a mobile thrombus vs. 10% for a stratified thrombus, and 47% for a protruding thrombus vs. 7% for stratified thrombi.[65–67] Most embolic events, including stroke, occur within 3 weeks from acute MI. It has been shown that OAT is able to reduce the prevalence of intracardiac thrombus (odds ratio 0.32), as well as decreasing the risk for systemic embolism. In the previously mentioned pooled review of echocardiographic studies, patients with left ventricular thrombosis who were on OAT exhibited a relative risk of 0.3 to suffer an embolic event.[67] This means that OAT decreases the embolic risk by 70% in patients with MI and echocardiographic documentation of thrombus.

Despite the lack of definite guidelines, the use of OAT is recommended following MI in patients at high risk for embolic events. Patients with large anterior MI or with apex involvement should receive heparin treatment, independently from the use of thrombolytics. In those with mural thrombus or at high risk for embolism (heart failure, previous embolic event, AF) warfarin is given in order to reach a value of international normalized ratio (INR) between 2 and 3. OAT has to be continued for at least 3 months, because the embolic risk declines thereafter; anticoagulation has to be continued in patients with chronic AF or other documented risk factors.

Recent studies, however, have demonstrated that the risk of stroke may also persist after the first few months following MI. An observational study performed on 2231 patients with postinfarct left ventricular dysfunction enrolled in the SAVE study, demonstrated that the annual incidence of stroke in the 5 years following acute MI is rather high, equal to 1.5% per year.[70] Independent risk factors for stroke resulted in a lower ejection fraction (18% increase of the risk of stroke for each 5% reduction of the ejection fraction), older age and absence of treatment with aspirin or anticoagulation. A retrospective analysis has shown an 81% reduction of the risk of stroke by OAT and a 56% reduction with aspirin. The results of these studies, even if preliminary, to evaluate the efficacy of OAT, demonstrate the efficacy of OAT in stroke prevention after MI is enhanced in the presence of significant left ventricular dysfunction.

Long-term trials with antiplatelet agents or OAT following MI show a significant reduction in the occurrence of stroke. Because of the low embolic risk after 3 weeks from MI, it is conceivable that antithrombotic therapy prevents athero-thrombotic stroke due to carotid artery disease, rather than from cardioembolic sources. In particular, treatment with aspirin is able to reduce non-fatal stroke by 25% at 27 months.[71]

It is interesting to note that clinical investigations with OAT vs. placebo show a higher reduction of stroke (from 40% in Sixty Plus[72] and 42% in ASPECT,[74] to 55% in WARIS[73]), in spite of a reasonably low hemorrhagic risk. However, the intensity of anticoagulation in these studies was higher (INR 2.7–4.8) than that recommended in clinical practice. A subsequent analysis from ASPECT investigators has shown that the optimal intensity of OAT has an INR value between 3 and 4, because the mildly increased risk of bleeding complications is offset by a marked reduction of ischemic events during a 3-year period.[75]

Comparison between aspirin and OAT following MI has been tested by two trials, but no conclusive results are available.[76,77] Comparison between aspirin and OAT has recently been investigated in clinical trials. The first available study is CARS,[78] which has compared aspirin alone with aspirin plus warfarin at two fixed regimens (1 or 3 mg/day) in patients following MI. Mortality was similar among the three groups, whereas ischemic stroke was higher in patients treated with warfarin, when compared to those receiving aspirin alone (1.5% and 1.1% vs. 0.5%). Thus, warfarin at a fixed dosage is not better than aspirin.

Finally, long-term OAT is not indicated in patients with left ventricular postinfarction aneurysm. The prevalence of intracardiac thrombus is quite high (48–66% in surgical series, 49% at autopsy), but the risk of systemic embolism is low (0.35 per 100 patients/year), presumably because the thrombus is contained within the non-contractile aneurysmal cavity.[79] OAT is recommended only in patients with thrombus presenting any previously described high risk morphological findings.

Prosthetic cardiac valves

Patients with prosthetic cardiac valves are at high risk of systemic embolism and stroke is the most common clinical presentation.[80] In patients with a mechanical valve the incidence of major embolic events is about 4% per year in the absence of antithrombotic treatment, whereas it is 2% during antiplatelet therapy and 1% with anticoagulants.[81]

The embolic risk is different according to the prosthetic model and the position. The risk is two-fold higher for a mechanical mitral prosthesis when compared to the aortic position. Also, embolic risk is higher for the caged-ball type (e.g. Starr–Edwards) than for the single tilting disk (Bjork Shiley) or the bileaflet model (e.g. St. Jude Medical). Patients at highest embolic risk are those with multiple prosthetic valves, AF, advanced age (>70 years), and poor left ventricular function.

In patients with a bioprosthetic valve the embolic risk is moderately high during the first 3-month period following surgery. Thereafter, endothelization of the bioprosthetic ring has a protective role and the risk of thromboembolism approximates that of patients with mechanical prosthetic valves who are receiving anticoagulants.[82,83]

Patients with mechanical prosthetic valves require long-term OAT, which has to be initiated as soon as possible following surgery (within 6–12 h).[84] The prevalence of major bleeding during OAT is 1.4% per year.[81] In selected patients with aortic valve replacement without additional embolic risk factors, low-intensity OAT (INR 2.0–3.0) is adequate for the prevention of thromboembolic events, while reducing the incidence of thromboembolic complications. The overall incidence of adverse events, either thromboembolic or hemorrhagic, is minimal when the INR value is between 2.5 and 4.9 according to a European study[85] and between 2.5 and 3.6 according to a meta-analysis from 12 North American studies.[84]

The use of antiplatelet therapy with OAT has been proposed in order to reduce the risk of thromboembolism further. Dipyridamole has been associated with conflicting results.[86,87] The combination of high dose aspirin (500–1000 mg/day) with low intensity OAT (INR 1.8–2.3) has decreased embolic events, but increased the incidence of gastroenteric bleeding.[88,89] Otherwise the combination of low dose aspirin (100 mg/day) with warfarin (INR 3.0–4.5) has been beneficial in patients with prosthetic valves at high embolic risk (coexisting AF or previous embolism).[90] Indeed such a regimen significantly decreased systemic embolism and death, but increased minor (but not major) hemorrhagic complications. Finally, the combination of low-dose aspirin (100 mg/day) plus lower-intensity OAT (INR 2.3–3.5) showed similar antithrombotic protection and fewer bleeds in comparison with high intensity OAT (INR 3.5–4.5) alone.[91] In conclusion, the association of aspirin with OAT is advisable in patients who have suffered an embolic event during adequate OAT, in those with additional embolic risk factors (AF, previous thromboembolism, left atrial thrombosis, poor left ventricular function), or in patients with a strong indication for aspirin treatment (i.e., coexisting coronary artery disease, previous TIA or stroke).

In patients with bioprosthetic valves, low intensity anticoagulation (INR 2.0–3.0) is indicated during the first 3 months following surgery; thereafter aspirin is sufficient prophylaxis.[92,93] Long-term OAT treatment is warranted only in patients at high risk for embolism.

Rheumatic mitral stenosis

Rheumatic mitral valve stenosis has the highest embolic risk in comparison with any other cardiac disorder. The embolic risk is even higher when AF is present, as well as in the elderly and in those with low cardiac output. The embolic risk is not related to the severity of stenosis, valvular calcification or New York Heart Association (NYHA) class.[94]

Despite the lack of randomized trials, OAT is undoubtedly useful to reduce systemic embolism and stroke. Definite indications for OAT (INR 2.0–3.0) are a previous thromboembolic event and AF, either paroxysmal or chronic. OAT is recommended in patients with sinus rhythm and moderate left atrial enlargement (>5 cm) who are at high risk for AF. Also, OAT is recommended in elderly patients and in those with severe stenosis.

In patients suffering from embolism despite OAT, two options are available: either increase the intensity of anticoagulation (INR up to 3.5), or combine OAT with low dose aspirin or dipyridamole.

Aortic valve calcification and calcified aortic stenosis

Aortic valve calcification and calcified aortic stenosis are reported in about 1% of patients with TIA or stroke undergoing echocardiography. Case reports provide evidence of brain infarction, retinal ischemia or peripheral vascular occlusion due to calcific emboli from aortic valves.[95,96] Embolism can complicate cardiac catheterization and valvuloplasty.[97] Primary oxalosis with calcium infiltration in the aortic valve and left ventricle has been reported as a cause of cardioembolic stroke.[98] However, in a prospective controlled study of 815 patients with aortic valve calcification or calcified aortic valve stenosis, stroke was not significantly associated with aortic valve disease, but hypertension and any carotid stenosis were.[99]

Cardiomyopathies

In patients with dilated cardiomyopathy the prevalence of ventricular thrombi is substantial, ranging from 11 to 60% among non-anticoagulated patients.[100–103]

Stroke and systemic thromboembolism are reported in 8.4–18% of the patients. The embolic risk is significantly higher in the presence of AF and advanced congestive heart failure.[65,104,105] There are no prospective studies of the risk/benefit ratio of OAT in patients with dilatative cardiomyopathy. However, non-randomized observational studies show efficacy of anticoagulant treatment for the prevention of embolism in these patients. The annual incidence of thromboembolism in four non-randomized studies was 0 in patients undergoing anticoagulation and 1.6–4.5% in non-treated patients.[106–108]

In the absence of definite guidelines based on prospective randomized trials, OAT should be indicated in patients with dilated cardiomyopathy at higher embolic risk such as those with AF, advanced congestive heart failure and left ventricular thrombosis.[109]

In patients with hypertrophic cardiomyopathy systemic embolism and stroke represent recognized complications in the natural history of heart disease.[110–112] Hypertrophic cardiomyopathy per se is not an embologenic heart disease. The embolic risk is almost invariably related to the occurrence of one of three events: AF; infective endocarditis; and evolution towards a dilatative form with systolic dysfunction and congestive heart failure. The embolic risk is particularly high in the presence of paroxysmal or chronic AF, with a definite indication for OAT (INR 2.0–3.0).

Heart failure

In patients with heart failure the incidence of thromboembolism is 0.9–5.5% per year (average 1.9 per year), but no randomized studies are available to support the use of OAT in these patients.[113,114] AF and previous thromboembolism seem to be the major risk factors, whereas the effect of left ventricular dysfunction has not been independently evaluated; nonetheless several studies suggest that stroke and thromboembolism are more likely among those patients with lower ejection fraction and lower peak exercise oxygen consumption.[101,106,115]

In the absence of definite guidelines, OAT is warranted in patients with AF or previous thromboembolism and advisable in patients with postinfarction or idiopathic cardiomyopathy showing severe left ventricular dilatation (>7 cm) and markedly depressed left ventricular function (ejection fraction <30%).

Infective endocarditis

Ischemic stroke complicates the course of infective endocarditis in about 20% of patients.[116–119] The majority of strokes occur within the initial 48 h after diagnosis during uncontrolled infection; stroke occurs later in about 5% of patients.[116–118] The stroke rate is higher with endocarditis due to *Staphylococcus aureus*. The risk of stroke is reduced by control of the infection with specific antimicrobial therapy.

No evidence of benefit exists for OAT in patients with infective endocarditis of a native valve.[120] Moreover, several authors have reported a high incidence of cerebral bleeding during OAT. Thus OAT is not indicated for the prevention of stroke and systemic embolism in patients with infective endocarditis. The only exception is the case of patients with endocarditis of mechanical prosthetic valves already under OAT therapy.

Antiplatelet therapy has not been studied in patients with endocarditis.

Patients without overt cardiac disease

In patients with cryptogenic stroke and a normal clinical examination, echocardiography may allow the detection of silent embologenic cardiac lesions. Before the introduction of TEE, a series of studies showed a correlation between cerebral ischemia and hidden cardiac lesions such as mitral valve prolapse, atrial septal aneurysm and left atrial myxoma. However, only after the introduction of TEE, has the detection of silent potential cardiac sources of embolism been dramatically improved. Several studies showed that TEE may detect potentially cardioembolic lesions in about 30–60% of patients with a negative TTE result.

Atrial septal aneurysm

Atrial septal aneurysm (ASA), a localized bulging of the interatrial septum, is detected by TEE in about 1% (range 0.2–4%) of patients undergoing TEE and in about 10% (range 1–21%) of patients with TIA or stroke.[121–126] The prevalence in patients with cryptogenic stroke is even higher (range 16–28%). Nearly one-half of the ASAs detected by TEE are not visualized by routine TTE.[126]

Cerebral ischemia in patients with ASA could be secondary to embolism from thrombi in the aneurysmal sac or to paradoxical embolism through a patent foramen ovale (PFO) which coexists in 60–75% of cases. Other potential mechanisms of embolism in patients with ASA include coexistent myxomatous mitral valvulopathy and Chiari's network, which is a congenital residual of the sinus venosus. A Chiari's network has been discovered incidentally in up to 4% of autopsy studies and in 2% of patients undergoing TEE, but it is more common in patients with cryptogenic strokes.[127]

TEE studies have shown a strong association between interatrial septum thickness >5 mm and cerebrovascular events.[128] A thickened interatrial septum was found in 75% of patients with a history of ischemic stroke and only in 24% of those without a history of cerebral ischemia. ASA has been particularly associated with small lacunar infarcts.[129]

The risk of stroke in a patient with ASA is unknown. Similarly, when ASA is detected in a patient with stroke, the risk of cerebrovascular recurrences is unclear. Some data show that aspirin can prevent thromboembolism in these patients, but no long-term comparison between warfarin and aspirin for preventing stroke is available. It is likely that the size of ASA and the coexistence of PFO or mitral valve abnormalities influence the risk of stroke and possible recurrences.

Patent foramen ovale

PFO has been found in autopsy studies in 10–18% of cases in the general population and in 30–35% of patients with a history of cerebral ischemia. In 1998 two studies with contrast TTE detected PFO in 40–50% of young adults with cryptogenic cerebral ischemia and in about 10% of controls.[130,131] The initial observations have been confirmed by a large number of case–control studies which consistently showed an increased prevalence of PFO among young adults with TIA or ischemic stroke (about 40%, range 32–48%) and particularly cryptogenic stroke (about 50%, range 49–61%).[131–138]

The mechanism for stroke in patients with PFO is paradoxical embolism, defined as embolic material originating in the venous circulation or right cardiac chambers, migrating into the systemic circulation through vascular shunts that bypass the pulmonary capillary bed. In patients with PFO there is not a sustained right-to-left interatrial shunt, but paradoxical embolism could be induced by transient shunting particularly during elevation of right atrial pressure (provoked by cough or Valsalva's maneuver).[135,137]

Because of the high prevalence of PFO in the general population, caution is required for the diagnosis of paradoxical embolism. In many patients with stroke, the PFO will probably not be etiologically related to the cerebral ischemia. Also in patients with cryptogenic stroke, in more than one-third of cases the PFO is only incidentally associated.

The pathogenetic role of PFO is more likely when the following conditions are present: (1) no evidence of other sources of embolism; (2) coexistence of deep venous thrombosis or pulmonary embolism; (3) large PFO or larger amounts of interatrial shunting or both; and (4) association of PFO with ASA (25%) or with mitral valve prolapse (MVP), both potential cardioembolic sources.

Current therapeutic options for secondary prevention include antiplatelet therapy, chronic OAT, and invasive procedures such as surgical closure or transcatheter closure of the defect.[139]

The risk of stroke recurrence is relatively low (1% per year, range 0–4%) in treated patients with aspirin or short-term anticoagulation followed by aspirin, if concurrent venous thrombosis is absent.[140–144] However, the risk of recurrent stroke is unknown for patients with complicated PFO (PFO associated with ASA or MVP) or with coexisting venous thrombosis vs. patients with isolated PFO, as all PFO are combined in the few existing clinical studies. Preliminary studies suggest that the recurrence of cerebral ischemia in patients with PFO may be significantly lowered by mechanical closure (surgical or transcatheter technique) rather than with antithrombotic treatment.[145–149] However, other studies found that the closure of PFO does not prevent recurrence of ischemic events.[150] The recurrence appears to occur more frequently in older cryptogenic stroke patients who may harbor other undefined causes for their stroke rather than paradoxical embolism. Further studies are needed to stratify recurrent risk and to select appropriate treatment.[139]

In the absence of definite indications derivable by prospective studies (e.g. PFO in cryptogenic stroke study (PICSS)) the following recommendations have been proposed for the secondary prevention of stroke:

1. aspirin in patients with isolated PFO;
2. long-term anticoagulation in patients with complicated PFO or coexisting venous thrombosis; and
3. surgical closure of PFO including transcatheter techniques in selected patients (e.g. stroke recurrence during OAT).

Mitral valve prolapse

Since the early 1970s, MVP was postulated to be a possible source of cerebral emboli. Many reports, mainly concerning stroke in young adults, have suggested a high prevalence of MVP in stroke.[151,152] Nevertheless, if restrictive echocardiographic criteria are adopted, MVP is less frequently identified, its prevalence rate approximating that in a healthy population (4–6%).[13] Indeed, the prevalence of cerebral ischemia in patients with MVP is low, approximately 0.5% per year.[153]

Thickening of the mitral leaflets with myxomatous changes, and mitral insufficiency may increase the risk of systemic emboli,[153,154] although these data have not been confirmed.[155] The risk is further increased in patients with atrial fibrillation or endocarditis. Scarce data are available concerning the occurrence of thrombi on the leaflets.

Detection of MVP should not preclude a further search for other causes of emboli. MVP can be associated with an ASA, PFO, or rarely, with idiopathic lesions of cerebral arteries caused by systemic connective tissue disorders.[17] The associations of MVP with abnormalities of platelet activity and clotting disorders have been previously documented.[156–158]

Primary prevention of embolism with antiplatelet agents should not be recommended. Aspirin can be given to patients with MVP after transient ischemic attacks. OAT has been advocated if antiplatelet therapy fails and in patients with AF.

Mitral annular calcification

Mitral annular calcification, which is detectable by TTE, has been reported in association with ischemic stroke,[159–162] and in one epidemiological study[162] it was an independent risk factor. The presumed mechanism for stroke is the detachment of small calcific emboli from the degenerated mitral annulus. However, a causal relationship between mitral annular calcification and stroke is difficult to demonstrate because mitral annular calcification is often associated with advanced age, congestive heart failure and particularly with AF.[33,163]

Valvular strands

Mobile filamentous strands of the cardiac valves have been associated with stroke and systemic embolization.[164–166] The association with cerebral ischemia has been reported for strands on both the mitral and aortic valves.

In a recent case–control study the association was greatest in the younger patients.[167] However, their clinical significance is not yet certain.

Cardiac tumors

Atrial myxomas represent more than 50% of primary cardiac tumors; 75% of the myxomas occur in the left atrium.[168] Systemic embolism and stroke occur in 40% of cases. Emboli are of two types: platelet–fibrin and tumor fragments.[169] Most atrial myxomas can be detected by TTE, but only TEE and MRI allow a precise definition of the mass and its connections with the cardiac structures. Atrial myxomas are found in about one in 200 young adults with stroke or TIA, and in perhaps one of 750 older patients with cerebral ischemia.

Aortic plaques

The possible role of aortic atherosclerotic plaques as possible sources of embolism has been convincingly established in patients undergoing coronary artery bypass surgery.

Autopsy studies have demonstrated a high prevalence of ulcerated plaques in the ascending aorta and aortic arch in patients who died from ischemic stroke.

TEE has shown the presence of aortic atherosclerotic plaques in nearly 41–44% of patients with ischemic stroke.[170–173] Aortic plaques can be detected occasionally by TTE, but only TEE can systematically detect aortic plaques, providing a detailed definition of the intimal surface of the thoracic aorta. Aortic plaques are detected mainly in older patients and frequently associated with coexisting carotid lesions.

Stratification of the embolic risk of aortic plaques has been attempted in several studies. Amarenco *et al.* investigated the prevalence and the characteristics of high-risk aortic plaques.[172] They observed that the embolic risk was significantly higher if the atheroma protruded or had a thickness of more than 4 mm. The same authors demonstrated an increased recurrence of embolic events (nearly four-fold) in patients with ischemic stroke and aortic plaques.[174]

Aortic plaque was detected in 57% of patients with AF, and complex plaque was detected in 25%.[175] However, since the predominant location of complex plaque was in the descending aorta, the role of aortic plaque as a source of embolism in AF is uncertain.

Possible treatments in patients with stroke and aortic plaques include aspirin, OAT and surgical removal. Previous reports claimed that OAT is harmful and can precipitate systemic embolism.[176–178] Recent observations suggest that OAT could be beneficial, particularly in patients with mobile thrombotic components of the plaque, which has been noted to disappear during therapy.[180] Finally, in a prognostic non-randomized study a better outcome with fewer embolic events in the follow-up has been demonstrated among patients treated with OAT vs. antiplatelets.[181] Only prospective randomized studies of comparison between aspirin and warfarin in patients with stroke and aortic plaques may indicate the optimal treatment for the prevention of recurrences.

Protocol for the detection of cardiac sources of embolism

Cardiac evaluation integrated with echocardiography allows the detection of cardiac sources of embolism in many patients with cerebral ischemia. The following algorithm for the search of cardiac sources of embolism in patients with stroke is proposed.

1. The cardiac evaluation should be reserved for patients potentially eligible for OAT or cardiac surgery.
2. In patients aged less than 45 years and with unexplained stroke TEE is always warranted.
3. In patients aged over 45 years without a history of cardiac disease and with unexplained stroke TEE is warranted, whereas in those with a history of cardiac disease TTE is often sufficient, possibly followed by TEE in selected patients.
4. In patients with AF, echocardiography may be redundant because the indication for OAT after stroke is usually clear. TTE is occasionally needed to clarify underlying structural cardiac disease. TEE is appropriate in selected cases, mainly when a causal relationship between AF and stroke is debatable.

COEXISTING ISCHEMIC HEART DISEASE

The prognosis of patients with cerebral ischemia is critically influenced by the coexistence of ischemic heart disease (IHD). Myocardial infarction and sudden death are the leading long-term causes of death in patients with cerebrovascular disease.[182] One-third of patients with TIA or stroke have a history of previous myocardial infarction or angina pectoris.[183] A similar prevalence of symptomatic IHD may be found in patients with asymptomatic carotid disease.

Patients with carotid lesions have a significant risk of coronary events during follow-up. After a TIA the cerebrovascular mortality is nearly 2% per year, while the coronary mortality is nearly 5% per year. Hence, after a TIA, the risk of myocardial infarction or coronary death

Table 3.3 Relative risk of coronary events vs. cerebrovascular events in patients with cerebrovascular disease

Category	*Ratio of coronary vs. cerebrovascular events*
Carotid intima–media thickness[190–194]	1 : 1
Asymptomatic carotid stenosis[187]	3 : 1
TIA[184,185,195]	2.5 : 1
Stroke[186]	2 : 1
Patients submitted to CEA[189,208]	2.5 : 1

TIA, transient ischemic attack; CEA, carotid endarterectomy.

is 2.5-fold the occurrence of stroke or cerebrovascular death.[184,185] In patients with threatened stroke the cardiovascular mortality is two-fold the cerebrovascular mortality.[186] Even in patients with asymptomatic carotid bruits, which are detectable in nearly 5% of the population older than 45 years, the prevalence rate of coronary death is three-fold the cerebrovascular mortality. Moreover, the risk of coronary events in the follow-up correlates with the degree of carotid stenosis.[187]

TIA is therefore an independent risk factor for MI and the presence of a multifocal vascular disease should be considered per se as an unfavorable prognostic factor. In the Coronary Artery Surgery Study, at any time during follow-up, patients with IHD associated with peripheral or carotid artery disease had a 25% greater likelihood of death compared with patients with IHD alone.[188]

Even in patients undergoing carotid endarterectomy, myocardial infarction is the leading cause of early and late morbidity and mortality. The annual mortality rate by IHD after carotid revascularization is nearly 5% per year, the occurrence of fatal stroke being 2%.[189]

Finally, an association has been found between carotid artery intima–media thickness, as measured non-invasively by ultrasonography, and the incidence of cardiovascular events. Five studies have explored this possible association, demonstrating that an increase in the thickness of the intima and media of the carotid artery (both common and internal carotid artery) is a strong predictor not only of stroke but also of myocardial infarction.[190–194] In a recent study performed on participants in the Cardiovascular Health Study, the association between cardiovascular events during a 6.2 year follow-up remained significant even after statistical adjustment for other risk factors, showing an increased risk for each quintile of combined intima–media thickness from the second quintile (relative risk 1.54) to the third (relative risk 1.84), fourth (relative risk 2.01), and fifth (relative risk 3.15).[194] The results of separate analysis of myocardial infarction and stroke paralleled those for the combined endpoint.

All these data show that cardiac events often occur in patients with symptomatic or asymptomatic carotid disease (Table 3.3). TIA may be considered a possible harbinger of future myocardial infarction or coronary death.[195] Nevertheless, a cardiological screening for the detection of a coexisting IHD is not usually performed in most patients with cerebral ischemia.

Since IHD is often asymptomatic, a cardiological evaluation limited to cerebrovascular patients with angina or myocardial infarction fails to identify many cases with coexisting IHD. A routine cardiological evaluation of cerebrovascular patients could allow the identification of a high-risk subgroup which could be submitted to a more aggressive approach.

Table 3.4 Methods for the detection of asymptomatic IHD in patients with cerebrovascular disease

Non-invasive testing
Standard ECG
Exercise ECG testing
Radionuclide studies
exercise myocardial scintigraphy
dipyridamole myocardial scintigraphy
Stress echocardiography
dipyridamole echocardiography
dobutamine echocardiography
Invasive testing
Coronary angiography

Coronary angiography

Coronary angiography is the gold standard for the identification and the staging of coronary lesions. Hertzer *et al.*,[196] at the Cleveland Clinic, routinely submitted to coronary angiography 506 consecutive patients with symptomatic carotid lesions undergoing carotid endarterectomy. Coronary lesions were disclosed in 93% of cases, severe (≥70%) in 65%. In a subgroup of 200 patients without a clinical history of IHD, coronary lesions were detected in 86% of patients, severe in 40%. This study assessed a very high prevalence of asymptomatic, significant IHD in cerebrovascular patients.

However, coronary angiography is an invasive, expensive procedure, which is not available in every institution. A routine screening of vascular patients with coronary angiography has an unfavorable cost–effectiveness ratio.

Cardiological non-invasive testing

Routine cardiological evaluation of patients with cerebral ischemia or candidates for carotid revascularization should start with a non-invasive investigation. The cardiological evaluation should include clinical evaluation, exercise ECG testing, myocardial scintigraphy, and stress echocardiography (Table 3.4).

In patients unable to exercise, a variety of techniques have been proposed as alternatives to exercise.[197,198] In our experience, Tl-201 myocardial scintigraphy or echocardiography after dipyridamole infusion could be a valid alternative to exercise testing. Dipyridamole is a pyrimidine derivative which produces a powerful vasodilating effect on artery vessels by enhancing endogenous plasma adenosine levels. In the presence of a stenotic coronary artery, it can lead to a maldistribution of coronary flow producing a coronary perfusion steal from a stenotic to a preferentially dilated bed. Dipyridamole infusion has been shown to be safe in a recent investigation involving 400 cerebrovascular patients from seven institutions.[199] Only one TIA occurred after dipyridamole infusion in a patient with a history of severe hypertension and normal carotid Doppler study.

Dipyridamole scintigraphy has been widely used for predicting coronary events in patients undergoing vascular surgery, including carotid endarterectomy. Since Boucher *et al.*[200] in 1985 suggested dipyridamole scintigraphy as the test of choice for detecting IHD in patients undergoing vascular surgery, many studies confirmed the prognostic capacity of this test to predict perioperative coronary events; nevertheless, recent more rigorous studies challenged the predictive role of this test.[201,202]

Dipyridamole echocardiography is less expensive and more frequently available in cardiological institutions. A large Italian multicenter study of candidates for vascular surgery recently confirmed that dipyridamole–echocardiography can adequately stratify the coronary risk of these patients.[203] Finally, recent studies have proposed dobutamine–echocardiography as an alternative to dipyridamole echocardiography.[204,205]

Several studies are available on the non-invasive evaluation of cerebrovascular patients, looking at the prevalence of silent IHD.[206–210] Rokey *et al.*[206] using Tl-201 myocardial scintigraphy and radioisotope ventriculography, studied 50 cerebrovascular patients and detected IHD in 29 (58%) cases; 14 of these were out of 34 (41%) patients without cardiac symptoms. Di Pasquale *et al.*[207] studied 140 patients with recent TIA or minor stroke by exercise ECG testing followed, if abnormal, by Tl-201 myocardial scintigraphy; silent IHD was disclosed in 33 cases (24%). Using the same protocol Urbinati *et al.*[208] studied 106 consecutive candidates for carotid endarterectomy; silent IHD was detected in 27 cases (25%). Love *et al.*[209] studied 60 patients with recent TIA, minor stroke, or asymptomatic carotid disease, by Tl-201 myocardial scintigraphy disclosing IHD in 27 cases (45%); 16 of the 27 (59%) were patients without known IHD. Di Pasquale *et al.*[210] studied, using dipyridamole Tl-201 myocardial scintigraphy, 38 patients without IHD after a completed stroke. All patients were unable to exercise; silent IHD was disclosed in 21 cases (55%). The detection of large perfusion defects (mean 2.2/8 segments) suggests a multi-vessel IHD in most of the cases. The prevalence of silent IHD in these patients is higher than in patients able to exercise suggesting that patients with completed stroke have a more severe widespread vascular disease.

Other studies evaluated the prognostic importance of IHD in the long-term follow-up of cerebrovascular patients. Rihal *et al.*[211] from the Mayo Clinic, retrospectively stratified 177 patients submitted to carotid endarterectomy by the presence of a clinical history of IHD or a positive preoperative exercise ECG testing. IHD was identified in 84 cases (47%). The perioperative morbidity was not significantly different between the two groups. After a mean follow-up period of 8 years, the cumulative incidence of coronary events was 67% in patients with IHD, and 25% in those without IHD.

Urbinati *et al.*[212] studied 172 patients undergoing carotid endarterectomy, suggesting an easy, feasible and low-cost algorithm for stratifying the short- and long-term risk of coronary events. The patients were classified into four groups: patients without IHD (no history of IHD and normal exercise testing); patients with silent IHD (no history of IHD, abnormal exercise testing and myocardial scintigraphy); patients unable to exercise; and patients with known IHD (previous myocardial infarction or angina pectoris). During the perioperative period, events occurred only in patients with known IHD and in those unable to exercise. During a follow-up period of 7 years patients with no IHD had a very good prognosis, while those with silent IHD and those who were unable to exercise had a worse prognosis, similar to the prognosis of patients with known IHD. These data outline the poor long-term prognosis of patients with silent IHD and of those unable to exercise, who should be monitored and treated more aggressively.

Landesberg *et al.*[213] performed preoperative thallium scanning, by treadmill exercise or dipyridamole infusion, in 226 consecutive patients undergoing carotid endarterectomy. Seventy-seven (34%) patients with significant reversible defects on thallium scanning were referred for coronary angiography, and 42 (19%) had subsequent coronary revascularization (preoperative percutaneous coronary angioplasty or coronary artery bypass in 24, combined carotid endarterectomy plus bypass graft in 10, and post-carotid endarterectomy coronary bypass in eight patients). Six patients had preoperative non-fatal MI and eight had stroke. During the follow-up (40 ± 23 months) 47 patients (18%) died, 31 (66%) from cardiac disease and four (8%) from stroke. Preoperative moderate to severe thallium defect without coronary revascularization, independently predicted long-term cardiac mortality. Patients with preoperative coronary revascularization had a long-term survival rate similar to that of patients with normal or mild defects on myocardial scintigraphy and significantly better than that of patients with moderate to severe fixed and/or reversible defects who did not undergo coronary revascularization. This study confirms that preoperative myocardial scintigraphy predicts long-term survival, and that selective coronary revascularization based on the thallium results improves the survival rate of patients undergoing carotid endarterectomy.

Management

Patients with TIA or stroke and coexisting, even asymptomatic IHD should be treated with antiplatelet and anti-ischemic therapy. The angiographic detection of a coexisting severe single or multivessel IHD may determine decision-making problems especially in patients who are candidates for carotid endarterectomy. When indications for both carotid and coronary revascularization are established, the choice of staged or combined operations is determined by assessment of the relative severity of carotid and cardiac risk factors. A combined procedure is preferentially adopted in some institutions as in our Cardiovascular Surgery Department.[214] Staged operations are preferred at the Cleveland Clinic because the incidence of neurological complications with this approach (1.5%) compares favorably with carotid endarterectomy in all other elective patients.[215] However, simultaneous operations should be considered for patients with unstable angina and for those with left main IHD, or multivessel lesions without adequate collateral circulation, or in the presence of poor left ventricular function.

Finally, it should be pointed out that most neurological complications of coronary artery bypass graft operations are due to cerebral embolization during manipulation of the ascending aorta from unsuspected atherosclerotic aortic disease.[216] The importance of aortic plaques as a potential mechanism of stroke has been definitely assessed.[170–174] Recently it has been suggested that intraoperative use of TEE could be useful in planning alternative procedures, such as avoiding the aortic cross-clamp, or modifying the placement of aortic cannula.[217]

Protocol for the detection of coexisting IHD

The early and late prognosis of patients with symptomatic or asymptomatic cerebral ischemia is critically influenced by the presence of IHD. Available data show that more than one-half of cerebrovascular patients have a coexisting IHD, often asymptomatic. Therefore, a cerebrovascular event can be considered as a ‘warning’ signal for a future coronary event.

All patients with carotid artery disease should be submitted for cardiac evaluation in order to identify patients at higher risk of coronary events. A non-invasive evaluation including exercise ECG testing followed, if abnormal, by myocardial scintigraphy is a reliable protocol for identifying and staging IHD in these patients; as an alternative to exercise, dipyridamole myocardial scintigraphy or echocardiography are warranted. Patients at high risk include those with strongly positive exercise testing or large perfusion defects at myocardial scintigraphy or multiple transient asynergic segments at dipyridamole echocardiography. In addition, patients unable to exercise should always be considered at high risk of coronary events. Finally, patients at high risk should be submitted to coronary angiography in order to identify the severity of the IHD and to plan the best monitoring and management. The high prevalence of asymptomatic three-vessel or left main IHD in cerebrovascular patients suggests the need of a randomized study comparing coronary artery bypass surgery with optimal medical treatment.[218]

REFERENCES

1. Furlan AJ. *The Heart and Stroke.* Heidelberg; Springer-Verlag: 1987.
2. Kulbertus HE, Franck G. *Neurocardiology.* Mount Kisco, NY; Futura: 1988.
3. Di Pasquale G, Pinelli G. *Heart–Brain Interactions.* Heidelberg; Springer-Verlag: 1992.
4. Wilterdink JL, Furie KL, Easton JD. Cardiac evaluation of stroke patients. *Neurology* 1998; **51**(Suppl):23–6.
5. Cerebral Embolism Task Force. Cardiogenic brain embolism. The second report of the

Cerebral Embolism Task Force. *Arch Neurol* 1989; **46:**727–43.
6. Hart RG. Cardiogenic embolism to the brain. *Lancet* 1992; **339:**589–94.
7. Daniel WG, Angerman C, Engherding R *et al.* Transesophageal echocardiography in patients with cerebral ischemic events and arterial embolism. A European multicenter study. *Circulation* 1989; **80:**473.
8. De Rook FA, Comess KA, Albers GW, Popp RL. Transesophageal echocardiography in the evaluation of stroke. *Ann Intern Med* 1992; **117:**922–32.
9. O'Brien PJ, Thiemann DR, McNamara RL *et al.* Usefulness of transesophageal echocardiography in predicting mortality and morbidity in stroke patients without clinically known cardiac sources of embolus. *Am J Cardiol* 1998; **81:**1144–51.
10. Fieschi C, Argentino C, Lenzi GL, *et al.* Clinical and instrumental evaluation of patients with ischemic stroke within the first six hours. *J Neurol Sci* 1989; **91:**311–21.
11. Sacco RL, Ellenberg JH, Tatemichi TK, Price TR, Wolf PA. Infarcts of undetermined cause: the NINCDS Stroke Data Bank. *Ann Neurol* 1989; **25:**382–90.
12. Hart RG, Miller TV. Cerebral infarction in young adults: a practical approach. *Stroke* 1983; **14:**110–4.
13. Adams HP, Butler MJ, Biller J, Toffol GJ. Non hemorrhagic cerebral infarction in young adults. *Arch Neurol* 1986; **43:**793–6.
14. Biller J, Johnson MR, Adams HP *et al.* Echocardiographic evaluation of young adults with non hemorrhagic cerebral infarction. *Stroke* 1986; **17:**608–12.
15. Bogousslavsky J, Regli F. Ischemic stroke in adults younger than 30 years of age. Cause and prognosis. *Arch Neurol* 1987; **44:**479–82.
16. Alvarez J, Matias-Guju J, Sumalla J *et al.* Ischemic stroke in young adults. I. Analysis of the etiological subgroups. *Acta Neurol Scand* 1989; **80:**28–34.
17. Urbinati S, Di Pasquale G, Andreoli A *et al.* Role and indication of two-dimensional echocardiography in young adults with cerebral ischemia: a prospective study in 125 patients. *Cerebrovasc Dis* 1992; **2:**14–21.
18. Labovitz AJ. The increasing role of transthoracic echocardiography in unexplained cerebral ischemia. *Echocardiography* 1993; **10:**363–5.
19. Greenland P, Knopman DS, Mikell FL, Asinger RV, Anderson DC, Good DC. Echocardiography in diagnostic assessment of stroke. *Ann Intern Med* 1981; **95:**51–3.
20. Lovett JL, Sandok BA, Giuliani ER, Nasser FN. Two-dimensional echocardiography in patients with focal cerebral ischemia. *Ann Intern Med* 1981; **95:**1–4.
21. Bogousslavsky J, Van Melle G, Regli F. The Lausanne stroke registry: analysis of 1000 consecutive patients with first stroke. *Stroke* 1988; **19:**1089–92.
22. Millikan C, Futrell N. The fallacy of the lacune hypothesis. *Stroke* 1990; **21:**1251–7.
23. Lodder J, Bamford JM, Sadnercock PA, Jones LN, Warlow CP. Are hypertension or cardiac embolism likely causes of lacunar infarction? *Stroke* 1990; **21:**375–81.
24. Bevan H, Sharma K, Bradley W. Stroke in young adults. *Stroke* 1990; **21:**382–6.
25. Khanderia BK, Oh J. Transesophageal echocardiography: state of the art and future directions. *Am J Cardiol* 1992; **69:**61–75.
26. Lee RJ, Bartzokis T, Yeoh TK, Grogin HR *et al.* Enhanced detection of intracardiac sources of cerebral emboli by transesophageal echocardiography. *Stroke* 1991; **22:**734–9.
27. Pop G, Sutherland GR, Koudstaal PJ, Sit TW, De Jong G, Roelandt JR. Transesophageal echocardiography in the detection of intracardiac embolic sources in patients with transient ischemic attacks. *Stroke* 1990; **21:**560–5.
28. Hofmann T, Kasper W, Meinerzt T, Geibel A, Just H. Echocardiographic evaluation of patients with clinically suspected arterial emboli. *Lancet* 1990; **336:**1421–4.
29. Kopecky SL, Gersh BJ, McGoon MD *et al.* The natural history of lone atrial fibrillation: a population-based study over three decades. *N Engl J Med* 1987; **317:**669–74.
30. European Atrial Fibrillation Trial (EAFT) Study Group. Secondary prevention in nonrheumatic atrial fibrillation after transient ischaemic attack or minor stroke. *Lancet* 1993; **342:**1255–62.
31. Atrial Fibrillation Investigators. Risk factors for stroke and efficacy of antithrombotic therapy in atrial fibrillation: analysis of pooled data from five randomized controlled trials. *Arch Intern Med* 1994; **154:**1449–57.
32. Petersen P, Boysen G, Godtfredsen J, Andersen ED, Andersen B. Placebo-controlled, randomised trial of warfarin and aspirin for prevention of thromboembolic complications in

chronic atrial fibrillation. The Copenhagen AFASAK Study. *Lancet* 1989; **1:**175–9.

33. The Boston Area Anticoagulation Trial for Atrial Fibrillation Investigators. The effect of low-dose warfarin on the risk of stroke in patients with nonrheumatic atrial fibrillation. *N Engl J Med* 1990; **325:**1505–11.
34. Connolly SJ, Laupacis A, Gent M, Roberts RS, Cairns JA, Joyner C, for the CAFA Study Coinvestigators. Canadian Atrial Fibrillation Anticoagulation (CAFA) Study. *J Am Coll Cardiol* 1991; **18:**349–55.
35. The Stroke Prevention in Atrial Fibrillation Investigators. The Stroke Prevention in Atrial Fibrillation trial: final results. *Circulation* 1991; **84:**527–39.
36. Ezekowitz MD, Bridgers SL, James KE *et al.*, for the Veterans Affairs Stroke Prevention in Nonrheumatic Atrial Fibrillation Investigators. Warfarin in the prevention of stroke associated with nonrheumatic atrial fibrillation. *N Engl J Med* 1992; **327:**1406–12.
37. The Stroke Prevention in Atrial Fibrillation Investigators. Predictors of thromboembolism in atrial fibrillation: I. Clinical features of patients at risk. *Ann Intern Med* 1992; **116:**1–5.
38. The Stroke Prevention in Atrial Fibrillation Investigators. Predictors of thromboembolism in atrial fibrillation: II. Echocardiographic features of patients at risk. *Ann Intern Med* 1992; **116:**6–12.
39. Laupacis A, Albers G, Dalen J, Dunn M, Jacobson A, Singer DE. Antithrombotic therapy in atrial fibrillation. *Chest* 1998; **114**(Suppl): 579–89.
40. Stroke Prevention in Atrial Fibrillation Investigators. Adjusted-dose warfarin versus low-intensity, fixed-dose warfarin plus aspirin for high risk patients with atrial fibrillation: Stroke Prevention in Atrial Fibrillation III randomised clinical trial. *Lancet* 1996; **348:**633–8.
41. The SPAF III Writing Committee for the Stroke Prevention in Atrial Fibrillation Investigators. Patients with nonvalvular atrial fibrillation at low risk of stroke during treatment with aspirin. *J Am Med Assoc* 1998; **279:**1273–7.
42. Di Pasquale G, Urbinati S, Pinelli G. New echocardiographic markers of embolic risk in atrial fibrillation. *Cerebrovasc Dis* 1995; **5:**315–22.
43. Manning WJ, Douglas PS. Transesophageal echocardiography and atrial fibrillation: added value or expensive toy? *Ann Intern Med* 1998; **128:**685–7.
44. Zabalgoitia M, Halperin JL, Pearce LA, Blackshear JL, Asinger RW, Hart RG. Transesophageal echocardiographic correlates of clinical risk of thromboembolism in nonvalvular atrial fibrillation. *J Am Coll Cardiol* 1998; **31:**1622–6.
45. The Investigators of FASTER (Fibrillazione Atriale Studio Transesofageo Emiliano-Romagnolo, Italy) Study. Transesophageal echocardiographic correlates of prior thromboembolism in non-valvular atrial fibrillation: a multicentre study. *Eur Heart J* 1996; **17**(Suppl):442.
46. Klein AL, Grimm RA, Black IW *et al.*, for the ACUTE Investigators. Cardioversion guided by transesophageal echocardiography: the ACUTE pilot study: a randomized, controlled trial. *Ann Intern Med* 1997; **126:**200–9.
47. Manning WJ, Silverman DI, Keighley CS, Oettgen P, Douglas PS. Transesophageal echocardiographically facilitated early cardioversion from atrial fibrillation using short-term anticoagulation: final results of a prospective 4.5-year study. *J Am Coll Cardiol* 1995; **25:**1354–61.
48. Santiago D, Warshofsky M, Li Mandri G *et al.* Left atrial appendage function and thrombus formation in atrial fibrillation-flutter: a transesophageal echocardiographic study. *J Am Coll Cardiol* 1994; **24:**159–64.
49. Omran H, Jung W, Rabahieh R *et al.* Left atrial appendage function in patients with atrial flutter. *Heart* 1997; **78:**250–4.
50. Grimm RA, Stewart WJ, Arheart K, Thomas JD, Klein AL. Left atrial appendage ''stunning'' after electrical cardioversion of atrial flutter: an attenuated response compared with atrial fibrillation as the mechanism for lower susceptibility to thromboembolic events. *J Am Coll Cardiol* 1997; **29:**582–9.
51. Jordaens L, Missault L, Germonpré E *et al.* Delayed restoration of atrial function after conversion of atrial flutter by pacing or electrical cardioversion. *Am J Cardiol* 1993; **71:**63–7.
52. Sparks PB, Jayaprakash S, Vohra JK *et al.* Left atrial ''stunning'' following radiofrequency catheter ablation of chronic atrial flutter. *J Am Coll Cardiol* 1998; **32:**468–75.
53. Sgalambro A, Corrado G, Gentile F *et al.* Thromboembolic risk in atrial flutter: preliminary results of the Italian multicenter FLASIEC study. *Circulation* 1998; **98**(Suppl):I–703.
54. Irani WN, Willett DL, Grayburn PA, Brickner E,

Afridi I. Prevalence of atrial thrombi and spontaneous echo contrast in atrial flutter: a prospective study using transesophageal echocardiography. *Circulation* 1995; **92**(Suppl I): 537–8.

55. Black IW, Hopkins AP, Lee LCL, Walsh WF. Evaluation of transesophageal echocardiography before cardioversion of atrial fibrillation and flutter in nonanticoagulated patients. *Am Heart J* 1993; **126:**375–81.
56. Bikkina M, Alpert MA, Mulekar M, Shakoor A, Massey CV, Covin FA. Prevalence of intraatrial thrombus in patients with atrial flutter. *Am J Cardiol* 1995; **76:**186–9.
57. Mehta B, Baruch L. Thromboembolism following cardioversion of "common" atrial flutter. Risk factors and limitations of transesophageal echocardiography. *Chest* 1996; **110:**1001–3.
58. Wood KA, Eisenberg SJ, Kalman JM *et al.* Risk of thromboembolism in chronic atrial flutter. *Am J Cardiol* 1997; **79:**1043–7.
59. Lanzarotti CJ, Olshansky B. Thromboembolism in chronic atrial flutter: is the risk underestimated? *J Am Coll Cardiol* 1997; **30:**1506–11.
60. Seidl K, Hauer B, Schwick N, Zellner D, Zahn R, Senges J. Risk of thromboembolic events in patients with atrial flutter. *Am J Cardiol* 1998; **82:**580–3.
61. Keating EC, Gross SA, Schlamowitz RA *et al.* Mural thrombi in myocardial infarctions: prospective evaluation of two-dimensional echocardiography. *Am J Med* 1983; **74:**989–95.
62. Weinreich DJ, Burke JF, Pauletto FJ. Left ventricular mural thrombi complicating acute myocardial infarction: long-term follow-up with serial echocardiography. *Ann Intern Med* 1984; **100:**789–94.
63. Ezekowitz MD, Kellerman DJ, Smith EO *et al.* Detection of active left ventricular thrombosis during acute myocardial infarction using Indium-III platelet scintigraphy. *Chest* 1984; **86:**35–9.
64. Johannessen KA, Nordrehaug JE, von der Lippe G. Left ventricular thrombosis and cerebrovascular accident in acute myocardial infarction. *Br Heart J* 1984; **51:**553–6.
65. Stratton JR. Chronic left ventricular thrombi. *G Ital Cardiol* 1994; **24:**269–79.
66. Cairns JA, Theroux P, Lewis HD Jr, Ezekowitz M, Meade TW, Sutton GC. Antithrombotic agents in coronary artery disease. *Chest* 1998; **114**(Suppl):611–33.
67. Van Dantzig JM, Delemarre BJ, Bot H, Visser CA. Left ventricular thrombus in acute myocardial infarction [review article]. *Eur Heart J* 1996; **17:**1640–5.
68. Spirito P, Bellotti P, Chiarella F, Domenicucci S, Sementa A, Vecchio C. Prognostic significance and natural history of left ventricular thrombi in patients with acute anterior myocardial infarction: a two-dimensional echocardiographic study. *Circulation* 1985; **72:**774–80.
69. Vaitkus PT, Barnathau ES. Embolic potential, prevention and management of mural thrombus complicating anterior myocardial infarction: a meta-analysis. *J Am Coll Cardiol* 1993; **22:**1004–9.
70. Loh E, Sutton MSJ, Wun C-C. Ventricular dysfunction and the risk of stroke after myocardial infarction. *N Engl J Med* 1997; **336:**251–7.
71. Antiplatelet Trialists' Collaboration. Collaborative overview of randomised trials of antiplatelet therapy: 1. Prevention of death, myocardial infarction, and stroke by prolonged antiplatelet therapy in various categories of patients. *Br Med J* 1994; **308:**81–106.
72. Report of the Sixty Plus Reinfarction Study Research Group. A double-blind trial to assess long-term anticoagulant therapy in elderly patients after myocardial infarction. *Lancet* 1980; **ii:**989–94.
73. Smith P, Arnesen H, Holme I. The effect of warfarin on mortality and reinfarction after myocardial infarction. *N Engl J Med* 1990; **323:**147–52.
74. ASPECT Research Group. Effect of long-term oral anticoagulant treatment on mortality and cardiovascular morbidity after myocardial infarction. *Lancet* 1994; **343:**499-503.
75. Azar AJ, Cannegieter SC, Deckers JW *et al.* Optimal intensity of oral anticoagulant therapy after myocardial infarction. *J Am Coll Cardiol* 1986; **27:**1349–55.
76. Breddin D, Loew D, Lechner K *et al.* The German–Austrian Aspirin trial: a comparison of acetylsalicylic acid, placebo and phenprocoumon in secondary prevention of myocardial infarction. *Circulation* 1980; **62**(Suppl 5):63–72.
77. The EPSIM Research Group. A controlled comparison of aspirin and oral anticoagulants in prevention of death after myocardial infarction. *N Engl J Med* 1982; **307:**701–8.
78. Coumadin Aspirin Reinfarction Study (CARS). Randomized double-blind trial of fixed low-dose warfarin with aspirin after myocardial infarction. *Lancet* 1997; **350:**389–96.

79. Lapeyre AC III, Steele PM, Kazmier FV, Chesebro JH, Vliestra RE, Fuster V. Systemic embolization in chronic left ventricular aneurysm: incidence and the role of anticoagulation. *J Am Coll Cardiol* 1985; **6:**534–8.
80. Vongpatanasin W, Hillis LD, Lange R. Prosthetic heart valves [review article]. *N Engl J Med* 1996; **335:**407–16.
81. Cannegieter SC, Rosendaal FR, Briët E. Thromboembolic and bleeding complications in patients with mechanical heart valve prostheses. *Circulation* 1994; **89:**635–41.
82. Bloomfield P, Wheatley DJ, Prescott RJ *et al.* Twelve-year comparison of a Bjork–Shiley mechanical heart valve with porcine bioprostheses. *N Engl J Med* 1991; **324:**573–9.
83. Hammermeister KE, Sethi GK, Henderson WG, Oprian C, Kim T, Rahintoola S, for the Veterans Affairs Coooperative Study on Valvular Heart Disease. A comparison of outcomes in men 11 years after heart valve replacement with a mechanical valve or bioprosthesis. *N Engl J Med* 1993; **328:**1289–96.
84. Stein PD, Alpert JS, Copeland J, Dalen JE, Godman S, Turpie AGG. Antithrombotic therapy in patients with mechanical and biological prosthetic heart valves. *Chest* 1998; **114:**602–10.
85. Cannegieter SC, Rosendaal FR, Wintzen AR, Van der Meer FJM, Vandenbroucke JP, Briët E. Optimal oral anticoagulant therapy in patients with mechanical heart valves. *N Engl J Med* 1995; **333:**11–7.
86. Chesebro JH, Fuster V, Elveback LR *et al.* Trial of combined warfarin plus dipyridamole or aspirin therapy in prosthetic heart valve replacement: danger of aspirin compared with dipyridamole. *Am J Cardiol* 1983; **51:**1537–41.
87. Pouleur H, Boyse M. Effects of dipyridamole in combination with anticoagulant therapy on survival and thromboembolic events in patients with prosthetic heart valves. A meta-analysis of the randomised trials. *J Thorac Cardiovasc Surg* 1995; **110:**463–72.
88. Altman R, Boullon F, Rouvier J. Aspirin and prophylaxis of thromboembolic complications in patients with substitute heart valves. *J Thorac Cardiovasc Surg* 1976; **72:**127–9.
89. Dale J, Myhre E, Storstein *et al.* Prevention of arterial thromboembolism with acetylsalicylic acid: a controlled clinical study in patients with aortic ball valves. *Am Heart J* 1977; **94:**101–11.
90. Turpie AGG, Gent M, Laupacis A *et al.* A comparison of aspirin with placebo in patients treated with warfarin after heart-valve replacement. *N Engl J Med* 1993; **329:**524–9.
91. Meschengieser SS, Fondevila CG, Frontroth J, Santarelli MT, Lazzari MA. Low-intensity oral anticoagulation plus low-dose aspirin versus high-intensity oral anticoagulation alone: a randomized trial in patients with mechanical prosthetic heart valves. *J Thorac Cardiovasc Surg* 1997; **113:**910–6.
92. Turpie AGG, Gustensen J, Hirsh J. Randomised comparison of two intensities of oral anticoagulant therapy after tissue heart valve replacement. *Lancet* 1988; **1:**1242–5.
93. Heras M, Chesebro JH, Fuster V *et al.* High risk of thromboemboli early after bioprosthetic cardiac valve replacement. *J Am Coll Cardiol* 1995; **25:**1111–9.
94. Salem DN, Levine HJ, Pauker SG, Eckman MH, Daudelin DH. Antithrombotic therapy in valvular heart disease. *Chest* 1998; **114**(Suppl): 590–601.
95. Brockmeier LB, Adolph RJ, Gustin BW *et al.* Calcium emboli to the retinal artery in calcific aortic stenosis. *Am Heart J* 1981; **101:**32–7.
96. Rancurel G, Marelle L, Vincent D *et al.* Spontaneous calcific cerebral embolus from a calcific aortic stenosis in a middle cerebral artery infarct. *Stroke* 1989; **20:**691–3.
97. Davidson CJ, Skelton TN, Kisslo KB *et al.* The risk of systemic embolization associated with percutaneous balloon valvuloplasty in adults. *Ann Intern Med* 1988; **108:**557–60.
98. Di Pasquale G, Ribani MA, Andreoli A, Zampa GA, Pinelli G. Cardioembolic stroke in primary oxalosis with cardiac involvement. *Stroke* 1989; **20:**1403–6.
99. Boon A, Lodder J, Cheriex E, Kessels F. Risk of stroke in a cohort of 815 patients with calcification of the aortic valve with or without stenosis. *Stroke* 1996; **27:**847–51.
100. Gottdiener JS, Gay JA, Van Voorhees L, Di Bianco R, Flercher RD. Frequency and embolic potential of left ventricular thrombus in dilated cardiomyopathy: assessment by 2-dimensional echocardiography. *Am J Cardiol* 1983; **52:**1281–5.
101. Ciaccheri M, Castelli Q, Cecchi F *et al.* Lack of correlation between intracavitary thrombosis detected by cross-sectional echocardiography and systemic emboli in patients with dilated cardiomyopathy. *Br Heart J* 1989; **62:**26–9.
102. Yokota Y, Kawanishi H, Hayakawa M *et al.* Cardiac thrombus in dilated cardiomyopathy. Relationship between left ventricular patho-

physiology and left ventricular thrombus. *Jpn Heart J* 1989; **30:**1–11.

103. Falk RH, Foster E, Coats MH. Ventricular thrombi and thromboembolism in dilated cardiomyopathy: a prospective follow-up study. *Am Heart J* 1992; **123:**136–42.
104. Fuster V, Gersh BJ, Giuliani ER, Tajik AJ, Brandenburg RO, Frye RL. The natural history of idiopathic dilated cardiomyopathy. *Am J Cardiol* 1981; **47:**525–31.
105. Halperin JL. Thrombosis in the left ventricle in patients with dilated cardiomyopathy. *G Ital Cardiol* 1994; **24:**281–9.
106. Kyrle P, Korninger C, Gossinger H *et al.* Prevention of arterial and pulmonary embolism by oral anticoagulants in patients with dilated cardiomyopathy. *Thromb Haemost* 1985; **54:**521–3.
107. Keogh AM, Freund J, Baron DW, Hickie JB. Timing of cardiac transplantation in idiopathic dilated cardiomyopathy. *Am J Cardiol* 1988; **61:**418–22.
108. Ciaccheri M, Castelli G, Nannini M, Santoro G, Troiani V, Dolara A. Oral anticoagulant therapy in dilated cardiomyopathy. Results of treatment with warfarin in groups of patients at risk of embolic complications. *G Ital Cardiol* 1995; **25:**689–94.
109. Koniaris LS, Goldhaber SZ. Anticoagulation in dilated cardiomyopathy. *J Am Coll Cardiol* 1998; **31:**745–8.
110. Di Pasquale G, Andreoli A, Lusa AM *et al.* Cerebral embolic risk in hypertrophic cardiomyopathy. In: *Advances in Cardiomyopathies* (Baroldi G, Camerini F, Goodwin JF, eds.), pp. 90–6. Berlin; Springer-Verlag: 1990.
111. Furlan AJ, Craciun AR, Raju NR, Hart N. Cerebrovascular complications associated with idiopathic hypertrophic subaortic stenosis. *Stroke* 1984; **15:**282–4.
112. Kogure S, Yanamoto Y, Tomono S, Hasegawa A, Suzuki T, Murata K. High risk of systemic embolism in hypertrophic cardiomyopathy. *Jpn Heart J* 1986; **27:**475–80.
113. Baker DW, Wright RF. Management of heart failure: anticoagulation for patients with heart failure due to left ventricular systolic dysfunction. *J Am Med Assoc* 1994; **272:**1614–8.
114. Di Pasquale G, Passarelli P, Ribani MA, Borgatti ML, Urbinati S, Pinelli G. Prophylaxis of thromboembolic events in congestive heart failure. *Arch Gerontol Geriatr* 1996; **23:**329–36.
115. Cohn JN, Benedict CR, LeJemtel TH *et al.* Risk of thromboembolism in left ventricular dysfunction: SOLVD. *Circulation* 1992; **86**(Suppl I):1252.
116. Salgado AV, Furlan AJ, Keys TF *et al.* Neurologic complications of endocarditis: a 12-year experience. *Neurology* 1989; **39:**173–8.
117. Hart RG, Foster JW, Luther MF, Kanter MC. Stroke in infective endocarditis. *Stroke* 1990; **21:**695–700.
118. Paschalis C, Pugsley W, John R, Harrison MJG. Rate of cerebral embolic events in relation to antibiotic and anticoagulant therapy in patients with bacterial endocarditis. *Eur Neurol* 1991; **30:**87–9.
119. Horng RG, Yip PK, Chen WJ, Chen RC. Cerebrovascular complications of infective endocarditis. *J Stroke Cerebrovasc Dis* 1993; **3:**222–7.
120. Delahaye JP, Poncet P, Malquarti V *et al.* Cerebrovascular accidents in infective endocarditis: role of anticoagulation. *Eur Heart J* 1990; **11:**1074–8.
121. Gallet B, Malergue MC, Adams C *et al.* Atrial septal aneurysm: a potential cause of systemic embolism. An echocardiographic study. *Br Heart J* 1985; **53:**292–7.
122. Di Pasquale G, Andreoli A, Grazi P, Dominici P, Pinelli G. Cardioembolic stroke from atrial septal aneurysm. *Stroke* 1988; **19:**640–3.
123. Pearson AC, Nagelhout D, Castello R *et al.* Atrial septal aneurysm and stroke: a transesophageal echocardiographic study. *J Am Coll Cardiol* 1991; **18:**1223–9.
124. Zagalboita-Reys M, Herrera C, Gandhi DK *et al.* A possible mechanism for neurologic ischemic events in patients with atrial septal aneurysm. *Am J Cardiol* 1990; **66:**761–4.
125. Agmon Y, Khanderia BK, Meissner I *et al.* Frequency of atrial septal aneurysms in patients with cerebral ischemic events. *Circulation* 1999; **99:**1942–4.
126. Mugge A, Daniel WG, Angermann C *et al.* Atrial septal aneurysm in adult patients: a multicenter study using transthoracic and transesophageal echocardiography. *Circulation* 1995; **91:**2785–92.
127. Schneider B, Hofmann T, Justen MH, Meinertz T. Chiari's network: normal anatomic variant or risk factor for arterial embolic events? *J Am Coll Cardiol* 1995; **26:**203–10.
128. Schneider B, Hanrath P, Vogel P *et al.* Improved morphologic characterization of atrial septal aneurysm by transesophageal echocardiography: relation to cerebral events. *J Am Coll*

Cardiol 1990; **16:**1000–9.
129. Albers WG, Comess KA, Albers GW, Popp RL. Transesophageal echocardiography findings in stroke subtypes. *Stroke* 1994; **25:**23–38.
130. Lechat PH, Mas JL, Lascault G *et al.* Prevalence of patent foramen ovale in patients with stroke. *N Engl J Med* 1988; **318:**1148–52.
131. Webster MWI, Chancellor AM, Smith HJ *et al.* Patent foramen ovale in young stroke patients. *Lancet* 1988; **ii:**11–2.
132. Cabanes L, Mas JL, Cohen A *et al.* Atrial septal aneurysm and patent foramen ovale as risk factors for cryptogenic stroke in patients less than 55 years of age. A study using transesophageal echocardiography. *Stroke* 1993; **24:**1865–73.
133. Di Tullio M, Sacco RL, Gopal A *et al.* Patent foramen ovale as a risk factor for cryptogenic stroke. *Ann Intern Med* 1992; **117:**461–5.
134. Louie EK, Konstadt SN, Rao TL, Scanlon PJ. Transesophageal echocardiographic diagnosis of right to left shunting across the foramen ovale in adults without prior stroke. *J Am Coll Cardiol* 1993; **21:**1231–7.
135. Hausmann D, Mugge A, Becht I, Daniel WG. Diagnosis of patent foramen ovale by transesophageal echocardiography and association with cerebral and peripheral embolic events. *Am J Cardiol* 1992; **70:**1668–72.
136. Schminke U, Ries S, Daffertshafer M *et al.* Patent foramen ovale: a potential source of cerebral embolism? *Cerebrovasc Dis* 1995; **5:**133–8.
137. Ranoux D, Cohen A, Cabanes L *et al.* Patent foramen ovale: is stroke due to paradoxical embolism? *Stroke* 1993; **24:**31–4.
138. De Belder MA, Tourikis L, Leech G, Gamm AJ. Risk of patent foramen ovale for thromboembolic events in all age groups. *Am J Cardiol* 1996; **69:**1316–20.
139. Nendaz MR, Sarasin FP, Junod AF, Bogousslavsky J. Preventing stroke recurrence in patients with patent foramen ovale: antithrombotic therapy, foramen closure, or therapeutic abstension? A decision analytic perspective. *Am Heart J* 1998; **135:**532–41.
140. Biller J, Johnson MR, Adams HP *et al.* Further observations on cerebral or retinal ischemia with right–left intracardiac shunts. *Arch Neurol* 1987; **44:**740–3.
141. Pniewski J, Kwiecinski H, Mieszkowski J *et al.* Stroke patterns within patent foramen ovale [Abstract]. *Cerebrovasc Dis* 1995; **5:**231.
142. Hanna JP, Sun JP, Furlan AJ *et al.* Patent foramen ovale and brain infarct. *Stroke* 1994; **25:**782–6.
143. Stone D, Godard J, Hawke MW *et al.* Patent foramen ovale: the degree of shunting by contrast echocardiography predicts future events [Abstract]. *Circulation* 1994; **90**(Suppl): I-237.
144. Bogousslavski J, Garazi S, Jeanrenaud X, Aebischer N, Van Melle G. Stroke recurrence in patients with patent foramen ovale: the Lausanne study. *Neurology* 1996; **46:**1301–5.
145. Dearani JA, Morris JJ, Click RJ, Petty GW, Bailey KR, Khandheria BK. PFO closure to prevent recurrent stroke or TIA in young adults. *J Am Coll Cardiol* 1996; **27**(Suppl A):409A.
146. Ende DJ, Chopra PS, Rao PS. Transcatheter closure of atrial septal defect or patent foramen ovale with the buttoned device for prevention of recurrence of paradoxic embolism. *Am J Cardiol* 1996; **78:**233–6.
147. Bridges ND, Hellenbrand W, Latson L, Filiano J, Newburger JW, Lock JE. Transcatheter closure of patent foramen ovale after presumed paradoxical embolization. *Circulation* 1992; **86:**1902–8.
148. Ruchat P, Bogousslavsky J, Hurni M, Fischer AP, Jeanrenaud X, Von Segesser LK. Systematic surgical closure of patent foramen ovale in selected patients with cerebrovascular events due to paradoxical embolism. Early results of a preliminary study. *Eur J Cardiothorac Surg* 1997; **11:**824–7.
149. Cujec B, Mainra R, Johnson DH. Prevention of recurrent cerebral ischemic events in patients with patent foramen ovale and cryptogenic strokes or transient ischemic attacks. *Can J Cardiol* 1999; **15:**57–64.
150. Homma S, Di Tullio MR, Sacco RL, Sciacca RR, Smith C, Mohr JP. Surgical closure of patent foramen ovale in cryptogenic stroke patients. *Stroke* 1997; **28:**2376–81.
151. Barnett HCM, Jones MW, Boughner DR, Kostuk WJ. Cerebral ischemic events associated with prolapsing mitral valve. *Arch Neurol* 1976; **33:**777–82.
152. Hart RG, Easton DJ. Mitral valve prolapse and cerebral infarction. *Stroke* 1982; **13:**429–30.
153. Nishimura RA, McGoon MD, Shub C, Miller FA, Ilstrup DM, Taijk AJ. Echocardiographically documented mitral valve prolapse. Long-term follow-up of 237 patients. *N Engl J Med* 1985; **313:**1305–9.
154. Devereux RB, Hawkins I, Kramer-Fox R *et al.*

Complications of mitral valve prolapse. *Am J Med* 1986; **81:**751–8.
155. Marks AR, Choong CY, Sanfilippo AJ, Ferry M, Weyman AE. Identification of high-risk and low-risk subgroups of patients with mitral valve prolapse. *N Engl J Med* 1989; **313:**1305–9.
156. Sharf RE, Hennerici M, Blutschke V, Lueck J, Kladetzky RG. Cerebral ischemia in young adults: is it associated with mitral valve prolapse and abnormal platelet activity in vivo? *Stroke* 1982; **13:**454–8.
157. Fisher M, Weiner BH, Ockene IS, Forsberg A, Duffy CP, Levine PH. Platelet activation and mitral valve prolapse. *Neurology* 1983; **33:**384–6.
158. The Antiphospholipid Antibodies in Stroke Study Group. Clinical and laboratory findings in patients with antiphospholipid antibodies in cerebral ischemia. *Stroke* 1990; **21:**1268–73.
159. de Bono DP, Warlow CP. Mitral annulus calcification and cerebral or retinal ischemia. *Lancet* 1979; **ii:**383–5.
160. Nair CK, Thomson W, Ryschon K *et al.* Long-term follow-up of patients with echocardiographically detected mitral annular calcium and comparison with age- and sex-matched control subjects. *Am J Cardiol* 1989; **63:**465–70.
161. Aronow WS, Koenigsberg M, Kronzon I, Gutstein H. Association of mitral annular calcium with new thromboembolic stroke and cardiac events at 39-month follow-up in elderly patients. *Am J Cardiol* 1990; **65:**1511–12.
162. Aronow WS, Schoenfeld MR, Gutstein H. Frequency of thromboembolic stroke in persons ⩾60 years of age with extracranial carotid arterial disease and/or mitral annular calcium. *Am J Cardiol* 1992; **70:**123–4.
163. Benjamin EJ, Plehn JF, D'Agostino RB *et al.* Mitral annular calcification and the risk of stroke in an elderly cohort. *N Engl J Med* 1992; **327:**374–9.
164. Freedberg RS, Goodkin GM, Perez JL, Tunick PA, Kronzon L. Valve strands are strongly associated with systemic embolization: a transesophageal echocardiographic study. *J Am Coll Cardiol* 1995; **26:**1709–12.
165. Orsinelli DA, Pearson AC. Detection of prosthetic valve strands by transesophageal echocardiography: clinical significance in patients with suspected cardiac source of embolism. *J Am Coll Cardiol* 1995; **26:**1713–8.
166. Tice FD, Slivka AP, Walls ET, Orsinelli DA, Pearson AC. Mitral valve strands in patients with focal cerebral ischemia. *Stroke* 1996; **27:**1183–6.
167. Roberts JK, Omarali I, Di Tullio MR, Sciacca RR, Sacco RL, Homma S. Valvular strands and cerebral ischemia: effects of demographics and strand characteristics. *Stroke* 1997; **28:**2185–8.
168. Reynen K. Cardiac myxoma. *N Engl J Med* 1995; **333:**1610–6.
169. Knepper LE, Biller J, Adams HP, Bruno A. Neurologic manifestations of myxoma. *Stroke* 1988; **19:**1435–40.
170. Tunick PA, Kronzon I. Protruding atherosclerotic plaque in the aortic arch of patients with systemic embolization: a new finding seen by transesophageal echocardiography. *Am Heart J* 1990; **120:**658–60.
171. Katz E, Tunick PA, Rusinek H *et al.* The prevalence of ulcerated plaques in the aortic arch in patients with stroke. *N Engl J Med* 1992; **336:**221–5.
172. Amarenco P, Cohen A, Tzourco C *et al.* Atherosclerotic disease of the aortic arch and the risk of ischemic stroke. *N Engl J Med* 1994; **331:**1474–9.
173. Mitusch R, Doherti C, Wucherpfennig H *et al.* Vascular events during follow-up in patients with aortic arch atherosclerosis. *Stroke* 1997; **28:**36–9.
174. The French Study of Aortic Plaques in Stroke Group. Atherosclerotic disease of the aortic arch as a risk factor for recurrent ischemic stroke. *N Engl J Med* 1996; **334:**1216–21.
175. Blackshear JL, Pearche LA, Hart RG *et al.*, for the SPAF Investigators Committee on Echocardiography. Aortic plaque in atrial fibrillation: prevalence, predictors and thromboembolic implications. *Stroke* 1999; **30:**834–40.
176. Bruns FJ, Segel DP, Adler S. Case report, control of cholesterol embolization by discontinuation of anticoagulant therapy. *Am J Med Sci* 1978; **1:**105–8.
177. Hilton TC, Menke D, Blackshear JL. Variable effect of anticoagulation in the treatment of severe protruding atherosclerotic aortic debris. *Am Heart J* 1994; **127:**1645–7.
178. Hyman BT, Landas SK, Ashman RF, Schelper RL, Robinson RA. Warfarin-related purple toes syndrome and cholesterol microembolization. *Am J Med* 1987; **82:**1233–7.
179. Freedberg RS, Tunick PA, Culliford AT, Tatelbaum RJ, Kronzon I. Disappearance of a large intraaortic mass in a patient with prior systemic embolization. *Am Heart J* 1983; **125:**1445–7.
180. Dressler FA, William RC, Castello R *et al.*

Mobile aortic atheroma and systemic emboli: efficacy of anticoagulation and influence of plaque morphology on recurrent stroke. *J Am Coll Cardiol* 1998; **31:**134–8.
181. Ferrari E, Vidal R, Chevallier T, Baudouy M. Atherosclerosis of the thoracic aorta and aortic debris as a marker of poor prognosis: benefit of oral anticoagulants. *J Am Coll Cardiol* 1999; **33:**1317–22.
182. Heyden S, Heiss G, Heyman A *et al.* Cardiovascular mortality in transient ischemic attacks. *Stroke* 1980; **11:**252–5.
183. Kannel WB, Wolf PA, Verter J. Manifestations of coronary artery disease predisposing to stroke. The Framingham Study. *J Am Med Assoc* 1983; **250:**2942–6.
184. Cartlidge NEF, Whisnant JP, Elveback LR. Carotid and vertebral basilar transient ischemic attacks. *Mayo Clin Proc* 1977; **52:**117–21.
185. Toole JF, Juson CPP, Janeway R. Transient ischemic attacks. A prospective study of 225 patients. *Neurology* 1978; **28:**746–8.
186. Canadian Cooperative Study Group. A randomized trial of aspirin and sulfinpyrazone in threatened stroke. *N Engl J Med* 1978; **299:**53–9.
187. Chambers BR, Norris JW. Outcome in patients with asymptomatic neck bruits. *N Engl J Med* 1986; **315:**860–5.
188. Eagle KA, Rihal CS, Foster ED *et al.*, for the CASS Investigators. Long-term survival in patients with coronary artery disease: importance of peripheral vascular disease. *J Am Coll Cardiol* 1994; **23:**1091–5.
189. Stuart Lee K, Courtland Davis H. Stroke, myocardial infarction and survival during long-term follow-up after carotid endarterectomy. *Surg Neurol* 1989; **31:**113–9.
190. Salonen JT, Salonen R. Ultrasonographically assessed carotid morphology and the risk of coronary heart disease. *Arterioscler Thromb* 1991; **11:**1245–9.
191. Bots ML, Hoes AW, Koudstaal PJ, Hofman A, Grobbee DE. Common carotid intima–media thickness and risk of stroke and myocardial infarction: the Rotterdam Study. *Circulation* 1997; **96:**1432–7.
192. Chambless LE, Heiss G, Folsom AR *et al.* Association of coronary heart disease incidence with carotid arterial wall thickness and major risk factors: the Atherosclerosis Risk in Communities (ARIC) Study 1987–1993. *Am J Epidemiol* 1997; **146:**483–94.
193. Hodis HN, Mack WJ, LaBree L *et al.* The role of carotid artery intima–media thickness in predicting clinical coronary events. *Ann Intern Med* 1998; **128:**262–9.
194. O'Leary DH, Polak JF, Kronmal RA *et al.*, for the Cardiovascular Health Study Collaborative Research Group. Carotid artery intima and media thickness as a risk factor for myocardial infarction and stroke in older adults. *N Engl J Med* 1999; **340:**14–22.
195. Adams HP, Kassel NK, Mazuz H. The patient with transient ischemic attacks: is this the time for a new therapeutic approach? *Stroke* 1984; **15:**371–5.
196. Hertzer RN, Young JR, Beven EG *et al.* Coronary angiography in 506 patients with extracranial cerebrovascular disease. *Arch Intern Med* 1985; **145:**849–52.
197. Stratmann HG, Kennedy HL. Evaluation of coronary artery disease in the patients unable to exercise: alternatives to exercise stress testing. *Am Heart J* 1989; **117:**1344–64.
198. Iskandrian A, Heo J, Askenase A, Segal B, Auerbach N. Dipyridamole cardiac imaging. *Am Heart J* 1988; **115:**432–43.
199. Lette J, Carini GC, Tatum JL *et al.* Safety of dipyridamole testing in patients with cerebrovascular disease. *Am J Cardiol* 1995; **75:**535–7.
200. Boucher CA, Brewster DC, Darling RC *et al.* Determination of cardiac risk by dipyridamole Thallium imaging before peripheral vascular surgery. *N Engl J Med* 1985; **312:**269–76.
201. Mangano DT, London MJ, Tubau JF *et al.*, for the Study of Perioperative Ischemia research group. Dipyridamole Thallium 201 scintigraphy as a preoperative screening test. A reexamination of its predictive potential. *Circulation* 1991; **84:**493–502.
202. Baron JF, Mundler O, Bertrand M *et al.* Dipyridamole Thallium scintigraphy and gated radionuclide angiography to assess cardiac risk before abdominal aortic surgery. *N Engl J Med* 1994; **330:**663–9.
203. Sicari R, Lusa AM, Salustri A *et al.* on behalf of the EPIC study-subproject risk stratification before major vascular surgery. The value of dipyridamole echocardiography in risk stratification before vascular surgery: a multicenter study. *Eur Heart J* 1995; **16:**842–7.
204. Davila Roman VG, Waggoner AD, Sicard GA, Geltman EM, Schechtman KB, Perez JE. Dobutamine stress echocardiography predicts surgical outcome in patients with an aortic

aneurysm and peripheral vascular disease. *J Am Coll Cardiol* 1993; **21:**957–63.

205. Poldermans D, Fioretti PM, Forster T *et al.* Dobutamine stress echocardiography for assessment of perioperative cardiac risk in patients undergoing major vascular surgery. *Circulation* 1993; **87:**1506–12.
206. Rokey R, Rolak LA, Harati Y *et al.* Coronary artery disease and cardiac events in patients with cerebrovascular disease: a prospective study. *Ann Neurol* 1984; **16:**50–3.
207. Di Pasquale G, Andreoli A, Pinelli G *et al.* Cerebral ischemia and asymptomatic coronary artery disease: a prospective study of 83 patients. *Stroke* 1986; **17:**1098–1101.
208. Urbinati S, Di Pasquale G, Andreoli A *et al.* Frequency and prognostic significance of silent coronary artery disease in patients with cerebral ischemia undergoing carotid endarterectomy. *Am J Cardiol* 1992; **69:**1166–70.
209. Love BB, Grover McKay M, Biller J *et al.* Coronary artery disease and cardiac events in patients with asymptomatic and symptomatic cerebrovascular disease. *Stroke* 1992; **23:**939–45.
210. Di Pasquale G, Andreoli A, Carini GC *et al.* Noninvasive screening for silent ischemic heart disease in patients with cerebral ischemia unable to exercise. *Cerebrovasc Dis* 1991; **1:**31–7.
211. Rihal CS, Gersh BJ, Whisnanti JP *et al.* Influence of coronary heart disease on morbidity and mortality after carotid endarterectomy: a population-based study in Olmsted County, Minnesota 1970–1988. *J Am Coll Cardiol* 1992; **69:**1166–70.
212. Urbinati S, Di Pasquale G, Andreoli A *et al.* Preoperative noninvasive coronary risk stratification in patients candidates to carotid endarterectomy. *Stroke* 1994; **25:**2022–7.
213. Landesberg G, Wolf Y, Schechter D *et al.* Preoperative Thallium scanning, selective coronary revascularization and long-term survival after carotid endarterectomy. *Stroke* 1998; **29:**2541–2548.
214. Marinelli G, Turinetto B, Cazzato M, Pierangeli A. Surgical strategy in patients with associated carotid and coronary artery lesions: staged or combined operations? In: *Heart–Brain Interactions* (Di Pasquale G, Pinelli G, eds.), pp. 221–4. Heidelberg; Springer-Verlag: 1992.
215. Graor RA, Hertzer NR. Management of coexistent carotid and coronary artery disease. *Stroke* 1988; **19:**1441–4.
216. Salasidis GC, Latter DA, Steinmetz OK, Balir JF, Graham AM. Carotid artery duplex scanning in preoperative assessment for coronary artery revascularization: the association between peripheral vascular disease, carotid artery stenosis and stroke. *J Vasc Surg* 1995; **21:**154–62.
217. Duda AM, Letwin LB, Sutter FP, Golmand SM. Does routine use of aortic ultrasonography decrease the stroke rate in coronary artery bypass surgery? *J Vasc Surg* 1995; **21:**98–109.
218. Chimowitz MI, Weiss DG, Cohen SL *et al.* Cardiac prognosis of patients with carotid stenosis and no history of coronary artery disease. *Stroke* 1994; **25:**759–65.

4

Hematological evaluation of stroke risk

Richard C Becker and Frederick A Spencer

CONTENTS • **Introduction** • **Platelets: their role in arterial thrombosis** • **Vascular thromboresistance** • **Congenital (inherited) thrombophilias** • **Acquired thrombophilias** • **Summary**

INTRODUCTION

The pathobiology of acute ischemic stroke, although complex and varied in origin, is mediated most often by intra-arterial thrombosis that can develop either in situ or embolize from one or more sites of origin, including the left-sided heart chambers, aortic arch and great vessels that serve the brain. In more rare circumstances, paradoxical emboli originating either within the deep venous system of the upper or lower extremities or right-sided heart chambers, and thrombosis of the cerebral veins can substantially compromise the dynamics of nutritive blood flow and precipitate stroke.

The development of thrombi within the arterial and venous circulatory systems represents, from a teleological perspective, a vital adaptive response to vessel wall injury that prevents excessive blood loss following injury and also facilitates local repair. Considering vascular biology and hemostatic potential in the context of acute ischemic stroke, one could postulate that thromboembolic occlusion, irrespective of the stimulus, represents a poorly regulated or 'excess' response to vessel wall injury or a pathological 'shift' in the normal balance between procoagulation and anticoagulation within the vasculture that, under normal conditions, allows blood to remain in a 'liquid' state, while at the same time having the capacity for prompt clotting should hemostasis be needed.

The hematological approach to stroke risk must consider the pathobiology of intravascular thrombosis and the potential sites for abnormalities (congenital, acquired) within existing mechanisms designed to prevent unwanted or non-physiological clotting. Clinicians involved in the management of patients with acute ischemic stroke must understand the basis for, and the availability of, tests that can be used to assess the integrity of thrombotic regulation and normal vascular thromboresistance.

PLATELETS: THEIR ROLE IN ARTERIAL THROMBOSIS

Platelets, under physiological conditions, circulate freely within the vasculture. It has become increasingly clear, however, that many of the recognized risk factors for atherosclerosis and thrombosis, in essence, 'prime' circulating platelets for future cell–cell and cell–vessel wall interactions. Thus early in the evolution of atherosclerotic vascular disease and other prothrombotic states, there is a 'shift' in the delicate balance between coagulation, developed for the purpose of hemostatic defense, and anticoagulation, limiting the thrombotic process to a well-localized area of vessel wall injury, that favors the former.

The participation of platelets in arterial thrombosis can be divided conceptually into five steps: (1) platelet adhesion, (2) activation, (3) secretion, (4) aggregation, and (5) support of coagulation.

Platelet adhesion

Platelets quickly recognize abnormalities within the vascular system and adhere by means of adhesive proteins that interact with specific platelet membrane glycoproteins (receptors). To date, nine of the predominant and physiologically important platelet membrane glycoproteins have been characterized[1–4] (Table 4.1). Most platelet membrane receptors consist of non-covalent complexes of individual glycoproteins or heterodimers (integrins) derived from α and β subunits. Platelets express at least two β subunits (β_1 and β_2) and five α subunits, which in varying combinations, identify distinct surface receptors.[5]

The initial events in adhesion are contact and binding, accomplished predominantly by an interaction between the platelet glycoprotein (GP) Ib-IX complex and vonWillebrand factor.[6] interactions between GPIIb/IIIa and vonWillebrand factor also facilitate platelet adhesion, particularly in high shear stress conditions.

Platelet activation

Platelets can be activated by a wide variety of biochemical and mechanical stimuli (in addition to platelet adhesion). Many of the biochemical agonists are produced or released by platelets themselves after vessel wall adhesion, initiating a positive feedback loop that amplifies the response to a given stimulus. The list of biochemical agonists is extensive, numbering 100 or more; however, the most physiologically relevant agonists are summarized in Table 4.2

Platelets agonists bind surface glycoprotein receptors and provoke both conformational changes and signal transduction ('outside-in

Table 4.1 Surface membrane glycoprotein receptors and their physiological ligands

Receptor	*Ligand*	*Integrin components*	*Biological action*
GP Ia/IIa	Collagen	$\alpha_2\beta_1$	Adhesion
GP Ib/IX	vonWillebrand factor	–	Adhesion
GP Ic/IIa	Fibronectin	$\alpha_5\beta_1$	Adhesion
GP IIb/IIIa	Collagen	$\alpha_{IIb}\beta_3$	Aggregation
	Fibrinogen		(secondary role in adhesion)
	Fibronectin		
	Vitronectin		
	vonWillebrand factor		
GP IV	Thrombospondin	–	Adhesion
(GP IIIb)	Collagen		
Vitronectin receptor	Vitronectin	$\alpha_v\beta_3$	Adhesion
	Thrombospondin		
VLA-6	Laminin	$\alpha_6\beta_1$	Adhesion

Table 4.2 Physiological agonists for platelet activation and their surface receptors

Agonist	*Source*	*Receptor(s)*
Thrombin	End product of coagulation cascade	Seven-transmembrane domain receptor
Adenosine diphosphate (ADP)	Platelet dense body	Aggregin
Collagen	Subendothelium component	GP Ia/IIa GP IIb/IIIa GP IV
Serotonin	Platelet dense body	$5HT_2$ receptor
Thromboxane A_2	Produced by platelets after initial stimulation	PGH_2/TXA_2 receptor
Platelet activating factor	Lipid mediator produced by other cells	PAF receptor

phenomenon') via a messenger protein that, in turn, triggers several intracellular pathways. The phosphoinositide pathway is initiated with activation of phospholipase C. Phosphatidylinositol 4-5-biphosphate (PIP_2) is cleaved to form two secondary messengers, inositol 1,4,5 triphosphate (IP_3) and diacylglycerol. IP_3 stimulates calcium mobilization from the dense tubular system. Increased cellular CA^{2+} concentrations are required for the activation of other intracellular enzymes responsible for physiological platelet responses. Diacylglycerol activates protein C, causing protein phosphorylation, granule secretion and fibrinogen receptor expression.

The second activation pathway (phosphatidylcholine) is mediated by phospholipase A_2 which liberates arachidonate from cell membranes. Arachidonate is subsequently converted to thromboxane A_2 (TXA_2) by the platelet's cyclo-oxygenase enzyme system. TXA_2 is a potent platelet agonist in its own right, thus providing yet another positive feedback mechanism that facilitates platelet-dependent thrombotic events.

Platelet conformational (shape) change is a pivotal component in the thrombotic process for several reasons. First, it provides a large phospholipid surface area on which clotting can proceed. Second, it exposes a large number of surface receptors, including GPIIb/IIIa, that are critical for platelet aggregation and thrombus growth, and third, it stimulates the release of activating substances from intracellular storage pools.

Platelet secretion

Platelet activation, as previously described, stimulates the secretion of contents from within three different types of platelet storage granules: lysosomes, α-granules, and dense bodies. The precise mechanism for granule secretion has not been determined fully, but the available evidence suggests that an energy-dependent contractile process, resulting in the extrusion of granule contents is directly involved. Fusion of α granules with each other and with deep invaginations of the plasma membrane (the open canalicular system) followed by an 'emptying' of contents (ADP, epinephrine, thrombin) to the exterior has since been demonstrated.[7,8] It is unclear if other platelet granules use a similar mechanism to release their contents externally.

The process of platelet secretion, in addition to the release of calcium, coagulation proteins, and biochemical agonists, also includes phospholipid-rich microparticle formation. Emerging information derived from flow cytometry and electron microscopy suggests that microparticles are, in fact, small procoagulant vesicles that can support the entire coagulation cascade. Thus, in addition to conformational shape change, platelets can further extend the surface area for thrombosis through microparticle release.

Platelet aggregation

The physiological goal of platelet activation, in fact, is platelet aggregation which provides the 'template' or 'scaffold' for subsequent thrombus growth. One of the most important responses to platelet activation is a conformational change in the GPIIb/IIIa membrane receptor, facilitating the binding of fibrinogen, fibronectin and vonWillebrand factor, and promoting platelet–platelet and platelet–leukocyte interactions. Because the GPIIb/IIIa receptor represents the only means for platelets to aggregate with one another, it is considered the 'final common pathway' for platelet aggregation (Fig. 4.1).

Platelet support of coagulation

The phospholipid membrane of activated platelets, platelet aggregates, and microparticles, forms an ideal template for coagulation processes that facilitate thrombus growth. The prothrombinase complex, responsible for the conversion of prothrombin to thrombin, consists of factor Va (predominantly derived from activated platelets), factor Xa, phospholipid and calcium. Factor Xa, the pivotal coagulation protein in the prothrombinase complex, can be derived from either the intrinsic (factors XII, XI, IX, VII) or extrinsic (factor VII, tissue factor) coagulation pathways. Because tissue factor (thromboplastin) is available in high concentrations within the vascular system, particularly in atherosclerotic vessels, it is felt to be the 'driving force' in pathological thrombosis.

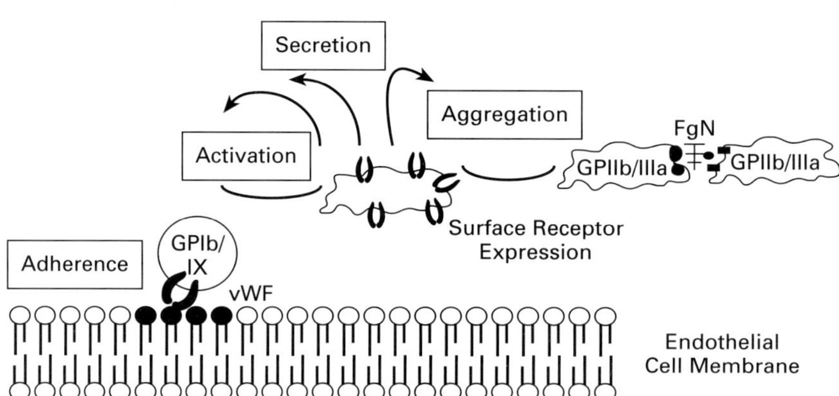

Figure 4.1 Critical steps in physiological hemostasis and arterial thrombosis. Platelets adhere to areas of vessel wall injury and, soon thereafter, are activated by both mechanical and biochemical mediators, producing conformational (shape) change, expression of surface receptors, and further release of platelet activating substances. The latter process is referred to as secretion. Activated platelets, possessing a large number of GPIIb/IIIa receptors on their surface, subsequently aggregate via the binding of fibrinogen—the 'linker' molecule between platelets.

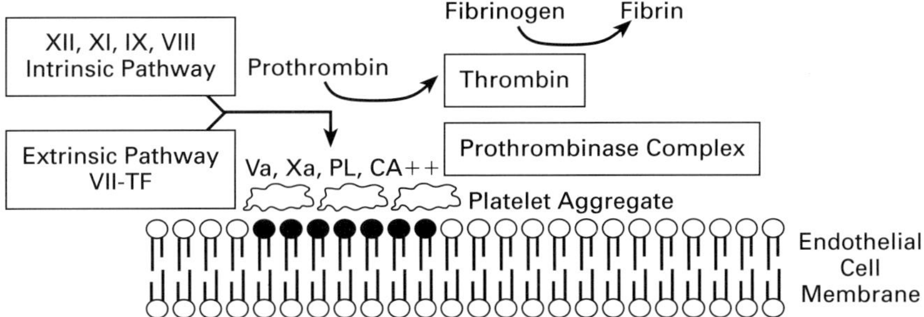

Figure 4.2 Platelet aggregates provide a template for coagulation that is facilitated by assembly of the prothrombinase complex (factors Va, Xa, PL, and CA^{2+}). The pivotal coagulation protein, factor Xa, is generated largely by tissue factor (TF) in the presence of factor VIIa. Ultimately, prothrombin is converted to thrombin which enzymatically drives the conversion of fibrinogen to fibrin—a key structural protein.

Thrombin, in turn, converts fibrinogen to fibrin that is responsible for the stabilization of the platelet-rich thrombus (Fig. 4.2). It is very important to recognize that although platelets are the predominant source of phospholipids in both physiological hemostasis and pathological thrombosis, prothrombinase assembly can occur on dysfunctional vascular endothelial cells and factor Xa can be generated through tissue factor that is present in high concentrations within atheromatous plaques and on the surface of activated monocytes.[9,10]

VASCULAR THROMBORESISTANCE

As an active site of protein synthesis, endothelial cells synthesize, secrete, modify, and regulate connective tissue components, vasodilators, vasoconstrictors, anticoagulants, procoagulants, fibrinolytic proteins, and prostanoids. Possibly the most important function of the vascular endothelium is to prevent the initiation and development of thrombus where it is not needed (i.e., not required for hemostasis).

Prostacyclin

Prostacyclin (PGI_2) is a potent vasodilating substance released locally in response to biochemical and mechanical stimuli. PGI_2, by increasing intracellular cyclic adenosine monophosphate (cAMP), also inhibits platelet aggregation. Furthermore, there is evidence that PGI_2 increases the rate of smooth-muscle-cell cholesterol ester metabolism, suppresses lipid metabolism within macrophages, and inhibits the release of growth factors, thus limiting proliferative responses to shear stress and vascular injury.

Nitric oxide

Endothelium-derived relaxing factor (EDRF), recently identified as nitric oxide, is an L-arginine derivative that relaxes smooth muscles by increasing intracellular cyclic guanosine monophosphate (cGMP). It is released locally in response to a number of biochemical mediators, including thrombin, bradykinin, thromboxane A_2, histamine, adenine nucleotides, shear stress and aggregating platelets. In addition to its vasoactive properties, nitric oxide is also a potent inhibitor of platelet adhesion and

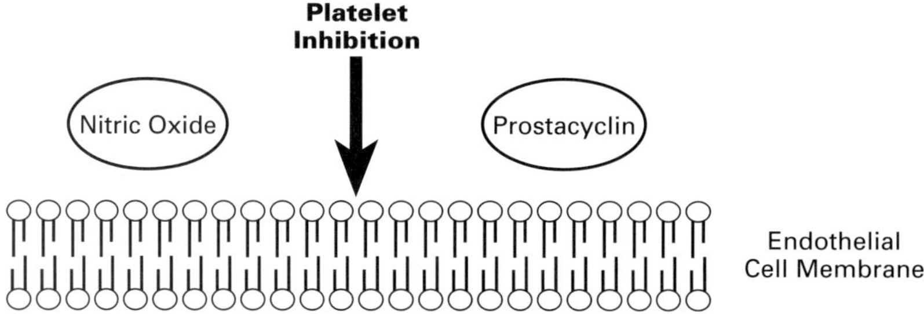

Figure 4.3 The modulation of platelet aggregation is a vital component of normal vascular thromboresistance. Nitric oxide and prostacyclin (PGI_2) are particularly important.

aggregation. Moreover, nitric oxide and PGI_2 appear to have synergistic antiaggregatory properties (Fig. 4.3).

Plasminogen activators

Vascular endothelial cells synthesize and release activators that are capable of converting plasminogen to the serine protease plasmin, an enzyme that proteolytically degrades fibrin (and fibrinogen). Tissue plasminogen activator (tPA) and urokinase-type plasminogen activator (UPA) generate plasmin locally; therefore, fibrinolysis is limited to the immediate area. Stimuli for the release of vascular plasminogen activators include epinephrine, thrombin, heparin, interleukin 1, venous occlusion, aggregating platelets, and desamino-8-D-arginine vasopressin (DDAVP) (Fig. 4.4).

Heparin-like species

Endothelial cells are capable of synthesizing heparin-like molecules with anticoagulant properties. As a result, it is currently accepted that vascular thromboresistance is mediated, at least in part, through the interaction of heparin-like substances with antithrombin and heparin

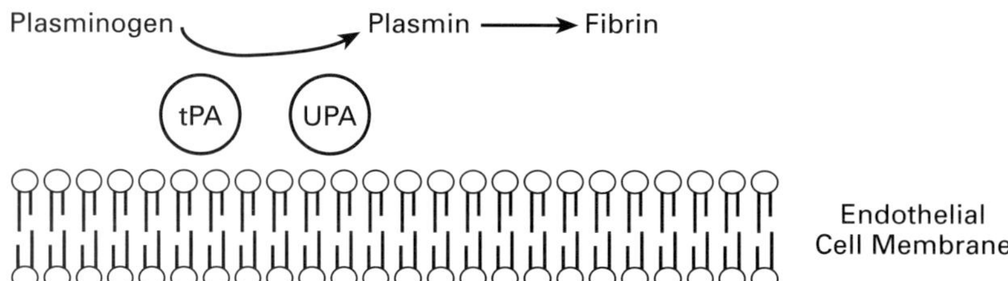

Figure 4.4 The intrinsic fibrinolytic system, consisting of tissue plasminogen activator (tPA) and urokinase-type plasminogen activator (UPA), regulates thrombus growth on vascular endothelial surfaces. Both serine proteases can rapidly and efficiently convert plasminogen (an inactive precursor protein) to plasmin (an active enzyme). Plasmin degrades fibrin—the predominant structural protein in arterial thrombi.

cofactor II (both located on the endothelial surface), accelerating the neutralization of hemostatic (procoagulant) proteins.

Heparin cofactor II, a potent inhibitor of thrombin, is secreted by the liver into circulating blood where it is present at a concentration of 1.0–2.0 μm/l. Unlike antithrombin, heparin cofactor II activity is augmented predominantly by dermatan sulfate; however, under high shear stress heparan sulfate can stimulate its inhibitory action as well. In vivo, thrombin inhibition by heparin cofactor II appears to be mediated by the interaction of dermatan sulfate with the vessel wall, predominantly in the extracellular matrix.[11,12] At least four distinct subspecies have been identified in endothelial cells: two high molecular weight complexes, a heterodimeric form bound to fibronectin, and two small molecules referred to as decorin and biglycan.[13]

Antithrombin

Antithrombin is a 58 kd glycoprotein that circulates at a concentration of 2.3 mmol/l and is capable of neutralizing the coagulation proteins, thrombin and factors IXa, Xa, XIa and XIIa, through covalent binding at their active sites. Antithrombin is a major component of the vascular endothelium's thromboresistant mechanism.

Protein C and protein S

Protein C is synthesized in the liver and secreted into plasma as a two-chain disulfide-bonded glycoprotein. It acts as an important anticoagulant (activated protein C) (APC) by preferentially neutralizing the activated forms of factor V and factor VIII (principally by cleaving their heavy chains). Protein S supports the anticoagulant function of activated protein C by promoting its interaction with factors Va and VIIIa. Because protein S enhances activated protein C-mediated factor Va inactivation only two-fold, it has been suggested that there may be an APC-independent anticoagulant effect.[14] Indeed protein S is able to inhibit both the prothrombinase complex and the intrinsic tenase complex. Protein S can also interact directly with factor Va and factor VIIIa.

Both protein C and protein S are found on the vascular endothelial surface. Thrombomodulin, an integral membrane protein located on the luminal surface of most endothelial cells, forms a 1:1 complex with thrombin. In this complex, thrombin activates protein C (while at the same time thrombin is neutralized). Accordingly, thrombomodulin is able to inhibit thrombin-catalyzed fibrinogen clotting, factor V activation, and platelet activation.

Tissue factor pathway inhibitor

Tissue factor pathway inhibitor (TFPI)-I is also located on the endothelial surface. It acts against the combined action of tissue factor and factor VII in the presence of factor Xa. The proposed mechanism for inhibition of tissue factor–factor VIIa involves the formation of a quaternary complex with TFPI and factor X in a two-step reaction: factor Xa generated by tissue factor–factor VIIa binds reversibly with TFPI and the formed binary complex binds, in a calcium-dependent manner, to membrane bound tissue factor–factor VII.[15] In essence, TFPI prevents the extrinsic coagulation cascade from activating the prothrombinase complex; however, it has also been recognized that TFPI inhibits the intrinsic coagulation cascade, supporting the role of tissue factor on factor VIIIa and factor IX-mediated clotting (cross-over phenomenon).[16] The presence of factor IX also impairs TFPI-mediated inhibition of tissue factor VIIa.

In the presence of glycosaminoglycans, including heparin (unfractionated, fractionated), heparin sulfate, and dextran sulfate, the inhibiting activity of TFPI is increased.[17]

Tissue factor pathway inhibitor-2

A second human TFPI has recently been identified and characterized.[18] TFPI-2 is found within human umbilical vein endothelial cells, the liver and the placenta and has been shown to inhibit tissue factor VIIa, kallikrein, factor XIa, and factor X activation by factor IXa.[19] It does not (in the absence of heparin) independently inactivate factor Xa or thrombin.

Annexin V

Annexins are an interesting family of non-glycosylated proteins that bind to negatively charged phospholipids, including phosphatidylserine and phosphatidylethanolamine.[20] One of the 13 recognized annexins, annexin V, is recognized as a potent endothelial surface anticoagulant based on its ability to displace phospholipid-dependent coagulation factors. It also reduces platelet adhesion (Fig. 4.5).

Disorders of heightened thrombotic potential

The term 'thrombophilia' is applied to patients with a defined congenital (inherited) or acquired disorder of either vascular thromboresistance or hemostatic regulation which predisposes to thrombosis. While most have been extensively characterized in the context of venous thromboembolism, the contribution of thrombophilias to arterial thrombosis and atherosclerosis is becoming more widely appreciated. Ischemic stroke is most commonly the result of arterial thromboembolism; however, the occasional case of paradoxical thromboembolism and venous thrombosis in the central venous system must not be overlooked (Table 4.3).

CONGENITAL (INHERITED) THROMBOPHILIAS

Antithrombin deficiency

Antithrombin (AT) is a single chain glycoprotein belonging to the serine protease inhibitor (serpin) superfamily. It binds and inactivates thrombin and other coagulation enzymes including factors Xa, IXa, XIa and XIIa. The inhibition of coagulation factors achieved by AT is markedly enhanced (upwards of 1000-fold) by heparin (unfractionated, fractionated) and endogenous heparan sulfate found on the endothelial surface.[21]

In accordance with an accepted classification scheme, AT deficiency characterized by a reduction in functional activity and protein antigen is termed type I deficiency. In type II deficiency, low AT activity occurs in the

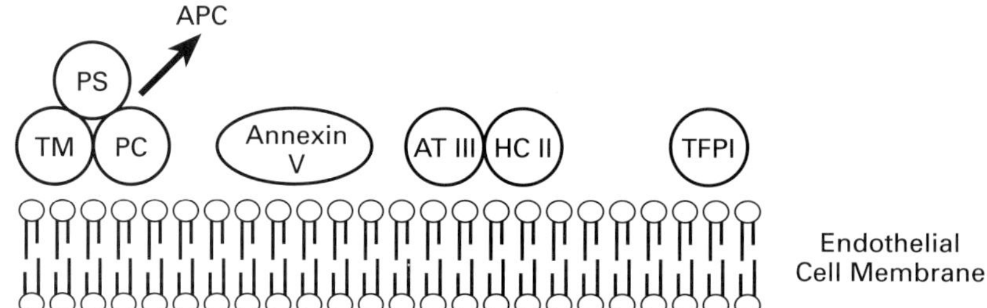

Figure 4.5 The modulation of coagulation is a vital component of normal vascular thromboresistance. Protein C (PC) binds to surface thrombomodulin (TM) and, in the presence of protein S (PS), forms activated protein C (APC), which then neutralizes two coagulation proteins—factor V and factor VIII. Tissue factor pathway inhibitor (TFPI), antithrombin (AT), heparin cofactor II (HCII), and annexin V are also important constituents of thromboresistance.

Table 4.3 Congenital and acquired thrombophilias

Congenital abnormalities predisposing to thrombosis
- Antithrombin defect
- Protein C defect
- Protein S defect
- Activated protein C resistance (factor V Leiden)
- Prothrombin variant G20210A
- Thrombomodulin defect
- Dysfibinogenemia
- Hyperhomocysteinemia
- Plasminogen defects
- Plasminogen activator inhibitor (PAI) excess
- Factor XII defects
- Platelet hyperaggregability (sticky platelet, TXA_2 excess, impaired nitric oxide responsiveness)

Acquired abnormalities predisposing to thrombosis
- Antiphospholipid antibodies
- Lupus anticoagulants
- Malignancy
- Hyperhomocysteinemia

presence of normal antigen levels, indicating a functional impairment of the protein. Over 100 different genetic mutations resulting in AT deficiency have been identified.[22] Both type I and type II AT deficiencies are associated with an increased risk of venous thrombosis and, on rare occasions, arterial thrombosis including stroke; however, the overall risk within a given kindred (family members with the defect) will vary with a given mutation. Variance in expression is probably the result of differing AT levels (and activity), concomitant defects (combined thrombophilias) and coexistent risk factors for thrombosis (pregnancy, inactivity, trauma).[23] Congenital AT deficiency is transmitted in an autosomal dominant pattern. A vast majority of affected patients are heterozygotes with AT levels ranging from 40 to 70% of normal. Most homozygotes die in utero or early in life from widespread intravascular thrombosis.

The prevalence of type I AT deficiency has been estimated at approximately 1/2000 to 1/5000[24–26] while the prevalence of type II AT deficiency may be much greater (~1/600 to 1/700).[27] In unselected patients with venous thromboembolism, the frequency of AT deficiency is 1.1%,[28] while in selected patients it is 2.4% (range 0.5–4.9%)[29–32] (Table 4.4).

Protein C deficiency

Protein C is a vitamin K-dependent glycoprotein synthesized by the liver. Thrombin complexed to endothelium-bound thrombomodulin cleaves an arginine–leucine bond within protein C, causing activation. In turn, activated protein C inactivates factors Va and XIIIa, thus affecting both the intrinsic and extrinsic coagulation pathways. Activated protein C also neutralizes plasminogen activator inhibitor-1 (PAI-1), thus enhancing fibrinolytic activity.[33,34]

A large number of genetic mutations (>160) causing protein C deficiency have been identified. The overwhelming majority of defects produce a quantitative (type I) deficiency, but

Table 4.4 Frequency (%) of congenital thrombophilias in the general population and in patients with venous thrombosis. (Reproduced with permission from De Stefano et al[24])

Syndrome	*General population*	*Unselected patients with venous thrombosis*	*Selected patients with venous thrombosis**
AT deficiency	0.02–0.17	1.1	0.5–4.9
Protein C deficiency	0.14–0.5	3.2	1.4–8.6
Protein S deficiency	–	2.2	1.4–7.5
Activated protein C resistance	3.6–6.0	21	10–64

* *Age <45 years and/or recurrent thrombosis (without obvious precipitant).*

qualitative (type II) protein C deficiency is recognized as well.[35–37]. In almost all cases these defects are transmitted via an autosomal dominant pattern of inheritance.

The frequency of protein C deficiency is 3.2% in unselected patients with venous thrombosis and 3.8% (range 1.4–8.6%) in selected patients. Both type I and type II protein C deficiency predispose to venous thromboembolism and it has been reported that up to 50% of heterozygotes suffer a thrombotic event by the age of 50. Among severely affected individuals, at least 75–80% experience one or more events by the age of 60.[38] Arterial thromboembolism is a rare occurrence in patients with protein C deficiency.

A recent analysis of nearly 10 000 healthy blood donors determined that protein C deficiency occurs with a frequency of 1/500–1/700.[39] Although the prevalence may be overestimated, it remains clear that, in many cases, heterozygous protein C deficiency alone does not increase thrombotic risk substantially (to the degree observed with AT deficiency). Differing mutations result in widely different clinical phenotypes and combined defects in vascular thromboresistance probably influence the expression of disease as well.[40]

Protein S deficiency

Protein S, like protein C, is a vitamin K-dependent glycoprotein. Approximately 40% of protein S circulates in an active, or free form; the remaining 60% is inactive and circulates bound to C4b-binding protein. Free protein S acts as the principal cofactor for APC and increases the protein's affinity for negatively charged phospholipids. The resulting membrane bound APC–protein S complex has enhanced factor Va and VIIIa neutralizing potential.

Relatively few mutations of the protein S gene have been identified, perhaps because of its large size, the existence of many exons, and the presence of a homologous pseudogene.[41] Both type I and type II deficiencies have been described. Type 1 protein S deficiency can be further divided into two distinct phenotypes: type 1a—characterized by a normal level of total protein S antigen but a low level of free protein S; and type Ib—characterized by low levels of both total and free protein S. It is important to acknowledge that C4b-binding protein is an acute phase reactant whose concentration is increased in association with a wide variety of inflammatory states. This causes an increased proportion of protein S in the bound state which, in turn, lowers the level of free protein S (and protein S activity). Indeed, up to 20% of hospitalized patients have low levels of free protein S.[42] The overall clinical relevance of this common transformation is unclear, but it may contribute to the procoagulant state associated with many serious medical and surgical illnesses.

The prevalence of protein S deficiency in the general population has been difficult to establish. A frequency of 2.2% for unselected patients with venous thromboembolism has been reported, while for selected patients there is a slightly higher prevalence (3.0%). As with AT and protein C deficiencies, most patients with protein S deficiency are at increased risk for venous thromboembolism and up to 50% of affected individuals may suffer a first thrombotic event by the age of 25.[43] Although arterial thrombosis has been reported, a cause–effect relationship, with the exception of paradoxical embolism,[44] has been questioned.

Activated protein C resistance

As previously summarized, thrombin bound to the endothelial cell protein, thrombomodulin, cleaves protein C causing activation. Activated protein C, through its inactivation of factors Va and VIIIa, is a critical inhibitor of coagulation. In 1993 Dahlback and colleagues[45] introduced the term 'APC resistance' to describe a patient with recurrent thrombosis whose activated partial thromboplastin time (aPTT) failed to prolong with the addition of APC. Subsequent investigators found that between 20% and 60% of patients with recurrent venous thrombosis displayed the same resistance to APC on laboratory testing.[46,47] Furthermore, a familial tendency with an autosomal dominant pattern of inheritance was established.

In 1994 the underlying molecular defect responsible for approximately 90–95% of cases of APC resistance was identified as a single base pair mutation in the factor V gene resulting in an Arg^{506} to Gln substitution at one of the APC cleavage sites.[48,49] The mutated factor V molecule (factor V Leiden) resists inactivation by APC but can still participate in coagulation. The cause(s) of APC resistance in the remaining 5–10% of cases have not yet been clearly delineated. There have been reports of patients with severely reduced APC-sensitivity ratios consistent with presumed homozygosity for factor V Leiden, who are in fact compound heterozygotes for factor V Leiden and a type I quantitative deficiency of factor V. Several investigators have also demonstrated the inhibition of APC by antiphospholipid antibodies, suggesting a possible etiology for the increased thrombogenicity seen in patients with antiphospholipid antibody syndrome by virtue of 'acquired APC resistance'.[50–52] It is possible that other congenital and acquired causes of APC resistance will be uncovered as work in this area continues.

The factor V Leiden mutation is present in approximately 4–6% of the general population.[53] It is the most prevalent hereditary thrombophilia known, occurring in 6–33% of consecutive unselected patients with prior venous thromboembolism.[54,55] Up to 66% of women who experience venous thromboembolic events during oral contraceptive use are APC resistant.[56] The available evidence suggests that heterozygosity for factor V Leiden is associated with a three- to seven-fold increased risk for venous thrombosis and approximately 30% of patients experience an event by 60 years of age. Interestingly, although patients who are homozygous for factor V Leiden are at even greater risk for thromboembolsim, a full 40% remain thrombosis-free at the age of 60, strongly suggesting that additional risk factors are necessary to provoke events in patients with APC resistance.

A proposed link between factor V Leiden and arterial thrombosis remains controversial. The prevalence of heterozygosity was similar among men in the Physicians Health Study who went on to have myocardial infarctions (6.1%) and strokes (4.3%), to those who remained free of vascular disease (6.0%).[53] However, a recent case–control study of young women with myocardial infarction (18–44 years of age) reported a four-fold increased risk for those who carried the factor V Leiden mutation.[57] The association was confined largely to a subset of women who were active smokers. The possibility that subtle functional abnormalities in APC predispose to arterial thrombotic events requires further investigation.

Factor II (prothrombin) G20210A

A mutation involving Gly to Arg substitution within nucleotide 20210 of the factor II (prothrombin) gene leading to increased plasma prothrombin concentrations has recently been identified. This defect may be present in 18% of selected patients and 6.2% of unselected patients with venous thromboembolism. The calculated relative risk for venous thrombosis associated with the 20210A mutation is 2.8 (95% CI, 1.4–5.6).[58] Arterial thrombosis, although much less common, has been reported.[59,60]

Thrombomodulin defects

Thrombomodulin, an endothelial cell surface receptor, is responsible for thrombin's activation of protein C and ultimately the neutralization of factors V and VIII. Several mutations of the thrombomodulin gene have been described in patients with venous thromboembolism.[61,62] More recently a ^{127}G to A mutation was reported in patients with arterial thrombosis.[63]

Dysfibrinogenemias

Plasma fibrinogen is cleaved by thrombin to form fibrin which, in turn, spontaneously polymerizes to form a stable, non-soluble fibrin clot. Dysfibrinogenemia, by definition, is a structurally or functionally abnormal fibrinogen that can occur with hemorrhage, thrombosis, or both. Data derived from a meta-analysis of nine studies including a total of 2376 patients with venous thromboembolism revealed a low (0.8%) prevalence of dysfibrinogenemia;[64] however, from a total of 250 cases of congenital dysfibrinogenemia, 20% experienced thromboembolic events. A total of 25 distinct mutations of the fibrinogen molecule have been described, but not all have been linked to an increased thrombotic tendency. For those that have, the risk is not solely fibrinogen-mediated; decreased binding of tPA,[65] increased resistance to plasmin[66] and an increased capacity to aggregate platelets[67] may also be contributory factors.

Dysplasminogenemias/abnormal plasminogen activation/PAI-1 excess

The fibrinolytic system is a proteolytic enzyme system with a diversity of physiological functions, of which degradation of fibrin deposits in the cardiovascular system is the most well known and widely investigated. Plasminogen variants have been identified in patients with thromboembolic disease, including deep venous thrombosis, pulmonary embolism, mesenteric vein thrombosis, cerebral vein thrombosis, and less commonly, stroke, and myocardial infarction (MI). To date, 12 reported variants have been described.[68–70] Congenital dysplasminogenemias are characterized by decreased plasminogen functional activity. In contrast, familial hypoplasminogenemia exhibits a proportional decrease in both antigenic and functional activity.

Large epidemiological studies, including middle-aged men and other patient populations at risk for atherosclerotic coronary artery disease, have failed to demonstrate a clear relationship between deficient fibrinolytic activity and cardiovascular events;[71] however, in patients with typical angina pectoris, or those with a previous MI, a number of cross-sectional studies have identified an association between impaired fibrinolytic potential and major cardiac events, including recurrent infarction and death.[72] Fibrinolytic impairment, secondary to either decreased vascular tissue plasminogen activator release or increased circulating plasminogen activator inhibitor (PAI-1) concentrations, has been commonly observed, particularly in young survivors of MI.[73] Prospective studies will be required, however, to define more clearly the role of impaired fibrinolysis in predicting thrombotic cardiovascular events.

Hyperhomocysteinemia

Homocysteine, a sulfhydryl amino acid derived from the metabolism of methionine, is produced through one of three specific enzymatic pathways (Fig. 4.6).

1. Remethylation to methionine catalyzed by methionine synthase; the methyl group is donated by methyltetrahydrofolate; cobalamin (vitamin B_{12}) serves as cofactor.
2. Remethylation to methionine catalyzed by betaine–homocysteine methyltransferase; betaine is the methyl donor.
3. Transsulfuration by cystathionine β-synthase into cystathionine; pyridoxal 5′ phosphate (vitamin B_6) is the cofactor.

Several congenital or acquired conditions affecting these pathways can yield varying degrees of hyperhomocysteinemia; severe (>100 μmol/l), moderate (30–100 μmol/l), and mild (15–30 μmol/l).

Severe homocysteinemia is quite rare and caused by either a homozygous deficiency of cystathionine β-synthase (90–95% of cases) or inherited defects in the remethylation pathway (5–10% of cases). Affected individuals experience a variety of neurological and developmental abnormalities as well as premature vascular disease and thromboembolism.[74]

Mild to moderate homocysteinemia can also be caused by a variety of genetic defects. Heterozygous cystathionine β-synthase deficiency has a frequency of 0.4–1.5% within the general population[75] and homozygosity for a thermolabile mutant of methylenetetrahydrofolate reductase is found in ~5% of the general population; both abnormalities are associated with a 50% reduction in enzymatic activity. Phenotypic expression is influenced by other factors; conversely genetically 'normal' individuals may have mild to moderately increased levels of homocysteine from one or more acquired abnormalities.

The most common causes of acquired hyperhomocysteinemia are nutritional deficiencies of cobalamin (vitamin B_{12}), folate, and/or pyridoxine (vitamin B_6) (cofactors for homocysteine metabolism).[76–78] Chronic renal failure and

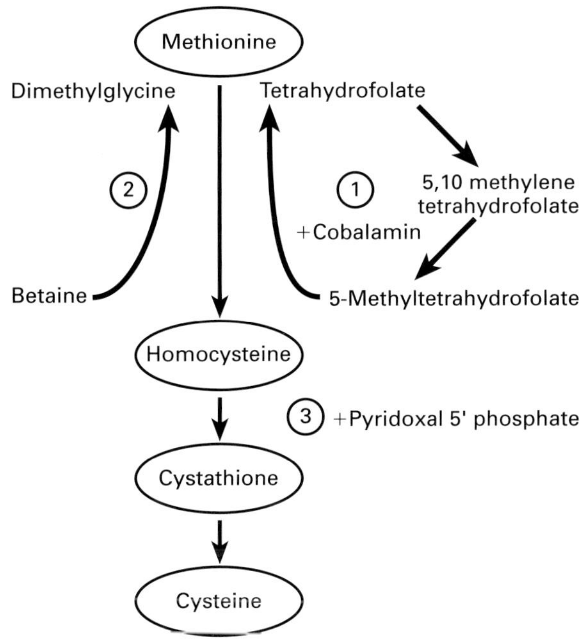

Figure 4.6 Metabolic pathways for methionine and hemocysteine. Cobalamin acts as a cofactor in the reaction catalyzed by methionine synthesis. Pyridoxal 5′ phosphate acts as a cofactor in the reaction catalyzed by cystathionine β synthase.

drugs that interfere with folate metabolism (methotrexate, anticonvulsants), cobalamin metabolism (nitrous oxide), or pyridoxine metabolism (theophylline) can cause hyperhomocysteinemia.[79] Other factors which may influence homocysteine levels include gender, age, smoking, hypertension, and hypercholesterolemia.

Due to the relatively large number of potential enzymatic defects, the variable phenotypic expression, and the influence of acquired factors, the risk of arterial and venous thromboembolism directly attributable to hyperhomocysteinemia has been difficult to ascertain.

None the less, in vitro and ex vivo studies have provided important information concerning the potential mechanisms for increased thrombogenicity that include: activation of factor V; interference with protein C activation and thrombomodulin expression; inhibition of tissue plasminogen activator binding; impaired generation of nitric oxide and prostacyclin; induction of tissue factor activity; and suppression of vessel wall heparan sulfate. In vivo studies performed in non-human primates have provided evidence that homocysteine causes endothelial cell injury, smooth muscle cell proliferation, and intimal thickening.[80,81]

Epidemiological studies have identified mild to moderate homocysteinemia as an independent risk factor for peripheral vascular disease, extracranial carotid artery disease,[82] coronary artery disease and acute myocardial infarction.[83] Mild to moderate homocysteinemia has also been associated with an increased risk of venous thromboembolism.[84] The thrombotic manifestations of hyperhomocysteinemia do not differ substantially from those of other thrombophilic disorders. In a series of 67 patients with hyperhomocysteinemia,[24] most thrombotic events were associated with other risk factors (e.g. oral contraceptives, pregnancy, and immobilization).

ACQUIRED THROMBOPHILIAS

Among the most commonly acquired disorders that predispose individuals to thrombosis are antiphospholipid antibody syndrome and malignancy. Other less common (but not rare) causes include myeloproliferative disorders, the nephrotic syndrome, and paroxysmal nocturnal hemoglobinuria.[85] Iatrogenic etiologies include prolonged periods of inactivity, chemotherapy for cancer, oral contraceptives and hormone replacement, and, perhaps the most commonly acquired thrombophilia, major surgical procedures, particularly those involving bone and soft tissue manipulation.[86]

Antiphospholipid antibody syndrome

Antiphospholipid antibodies (aPLs) are a heterogeneous group of circulating serum polyclonal immunoglobulins (IgG, IgM, IgA, or mixed) directed against negatively charged or neutral phospholipids. Within this group, the lupus anticoagulant (LA) and anticardiolipin antibodies (aCLs) are the most commonly acquired blood protein defects associated with arterial and venous thrombosis.[87,88]

Anticardiolipin antibody thrombosis syndrome

The aCL antibodies are directed primarily against the phospholipids, phosphatidyl serine and phosphatidyl inositol. Unlike the LA they do not prolong any of the phospholipid-dependent anticoagulation tests, (i.e. aPTT, dRVVT (diluted Russell's viper venom test) and/or KCT (kaolin clotting time)). Three idiotypes (IgG, IgA and IgM) are currently identified with the solid-phase ELISA anticardiolipin assay. This assay is dependent on a plasma cofactor, β_2 glycoprotein I.

The mechanism(s) responsible for aCL antibodies, provocation of intravascular thrombosis, have not been fully elucidated but there is little doubt that their high affinity for phospholipid substrate is involved. Several prothrombotic abnormalities have been identified.[89,90]

1. Inhibition of endothelial cell prostacyclin release.
2. Inhibition of protein C activation and protein S activity.
3. Interference with antithrombin activity.
4. Platelet activation.
5. Inhibition of pre-kallikrein activation (impaired fibrinolysis).
6. Inhibition of plasminogen activator release.

The overall prevalence of aCL antibodies in the general population has not been established; however, a recent study of 1014 hospitalized patients identified 72 (7.1%) with at least one idiotype,[90] while another study of 552 healthy blood donors identified 64 (15.9%) with either IgG or IgM idiotypes.[91] The prevalence is higher among patients with a prior arterial or venous thromboembolic event. Several studies have reported that an increased proportion of young (less than 50 years of age) survivors of acute MI have circulating aCL antibodies,[92] and that they are at increased risk for recurrent events. The association of aPLs (including aCLs) and cerebrovascular events is even more impressive with an incidence varying from 20% to 40% (depending on the study design and patient selection).[93,94] In the Antiphospholipid Antibodies in Stroke Study registry the prevalence was ~10%[95] and the risk of stroke recurrence was eight-fold higher for those with aPLs compared to those without aPLs.

Anticardiolipin antibodies are also associated with venous thromboembolism, most commonly deep venous thrombosis and pulmonary embolism. Thrombosis involving unusual sites has also been reported, including the venous system of the brain, inferior vena cava, superior vena cava, and the hepatic and portal veins.[96]

Lupus anticoagulant thrombosis syndrome

The LA was originally described in two patients with systemic lupus erythematosus and prolongation of the prothrombin time and whole blood clotting time.[97] An antiphospholipid antibody with the ability to prolong phospholipid-dependent coagulation tests was subsequently identified.[98,99] The term LA is, in fact, a misnomer since patients are at risk for thrombosis, not hemorrhage. Although occasionally associated with arterial thrombosis including stroke, the LA more commonly predisposes to venous thromboembolism that can develop in a wide variety of vascular beds.[100] The overall prevalence of the LA in the general population has not been clearly defined; however, it has been estimated that 6–8% of otherwise healthy patients with the LA will experience thromboembolism.

Malignancy

It has long been recognized that patients with malignancy are at risk for thromboembolic complications. The overall incidence ranges from 1% to 15% in clinical series and even higher rates have emerged from autopsy studies.[101,102] Malignancies with the highest rates of thromboembolism include mucin-producing adenocarcinomas of the gastrointestinal tract followed by lung, breast, ovarian and brain tumors.

There is increasing evidence for the existence of circulating 'procoagulant factors' in patients with malignancy. A variety of solid tumors and leukemic cells have been found to express tissue factor, an activator of the extrinsic coagulation cascade.[103,104] A new protein labeled 'cancer procoagulant', capable of directly activating factor X, has been found in extracts of numerous malignant tissues.[105,106] Interestingly, a sialic acid moiety from mucin (found in adenocarcinomas) has direct factor X-activating properties as well.

In addition to tumor-derived procoagulant factors, host cells can express procoagulant activity.[102] Monocytes, probably stimulated by tumor-derived chemokines, express tissue factor, direct factor X activators, fibrinogen, and coagulation protein binding sites. Similarly, platelets and endothelial cells become increasingly procoagulant under the influence of tumor-derived cytokines.[107]

Myeloproliferative disorders

The myeloproliferative disorders include polycythemia vera, essential thrombasthenia, myelofibrosis, chronic myelogenous leukemia, and myeloid metaplasia. Hemorrhagic and thrombotic events occur, the latter typified by recurrent venous thrombosis, pulmonary embolism, stroke, MI and microvascular thrombi. Although increased plasma and/or whole blood viscosity may be a contributory feature, particularly in polycythemia vera and essential thromblasthemia, qualitative platelet abnormalities with increased adhesion, aggregation, and activation are centrally involved in the observed thrombotic tendency.[108,109] Abnormal vascular fibrinolytic activity stemming from PAI-1 excess may also contribute (L Pechet, personal communication).

Paroxysmal nocturnal hemoglobinuria

Paroxysmal nocturnal hemoglobinuria is an acquired hemolytic disorder characterized by the proliferation of an abnormal clone of stem cells that are susceptible to complement-mediated cellular membrane damage. Microcirculatory thrombosis is common, as is recurrent venous thrombosis involving the hepatic, splenic, portal, cerebral, and deep peripheral veins. Arterial thrombosis occurs rarely.

Platelet (prothrombotic) abnormalities

Despite the fact that platelets represent the true 'gatekeeper' for arterial thrombosis, by providing a template for prothrombinase assembly and activation, there is a relative paucity of information linking heightened platelet activity to clinical events. Instead, much of the investigation pertaining to platelets that has been conducted to date has focused on platelet dysfunction, hemostatic defects, and hemorrhagic tendencies. It is likely that the platelet will serve as a major target for thrombophilia research in the years to come.

The Wein–Penzing defect[110] is characterized by a deficiency in the lipoxygenase metabolic pathway with concomitant increases in byproducts of the cyclo-oxygenase pathway, including TXA_2. Arterial thrombotic events can occur at a young age.

The 'sticky platelet syndrome' was first described by Mammen and colleagues[111] during a report at the 9th International Joint Conference on Stroke and Cerebral Circulation. Since that time, several hundred families have been identified with the defect which is apparently transmitted in an autosomal dominant pattern. Although both venous and arterial thrombotic events can occur, the majority of cases described in the medical literature have consisted of strokes (50%), myocardial infarction (21%) and transient ischemic attacks (15%).

A diagnosis of sticky platelet syndrome is supported by platelet hyperaggregability to one or more agonists (e.g. epinephrine, adenosine diphosphate). A repetitively excessive response to at least two concentrations of one or both agonists is considered strong evidence for the abnormality.

Although rare, stroke has been reported in children who exhibit decreased platelet inhibition by nitric oxide. In the original description by Loscalzo and colleagues,[112] two brothers who experienced neurological events before 15 months of age were found to have impaired metabolism of reactive oxygen species in their plasma, reducing the bioavailability of nitric oxide and defective thromboresistance.

Platelet glycoprotein III polymorphisms

Platelet membrane glycoproteins are highly polymorphic and can be recognized as alloantigens and autoantigens. Within the past several years a high prevalence of the PI^{A2} polymorphism (proline at position 33 of glycoprotein IIIa) has been reported in patients with acute coronary syndromes.[113] In patients younger than 60 years of age, the odds ratio for the genetic abnormality was 6.2. Although a cause–effect relationship has not been established, it is possible that increased platelet aggregation as well as facilitated, platelet–leukocyte and platelet–endothelial cell interactions explain the prothrombotic tendency. Further investigation is needed.

Essential thrombasthenia

Essential thrombasthenia, also referred to as primary thrombocytosis, is a myeloproliferative disorder that has been associated with thromboembolic complications, bleeding tendency and both quantitative and qualitative platelet abnormalities. Although the likelihood of arterial thrombotic events, including stroke, increases with platelet counts exceeding $600\,000/mm^3$, the correlation between the absolute number of platelets and thrombotic risk is weak, suggesting that other factors (yet to be defined) are involved.

Heparin-induced thrombocytopenia

Heparin-induced thrombocytopenia (HIT) is an underestimated and clinically significant complication of heparin therapy that is important for three reasons. First, it is a drug-related immunohematological reaction. Second, it can be complicated by stroke and limb-threatening thrombotic complications. Third, the optimal treatment approach, although uncertain, is steadily being defined.

The syndrome is due to the development of an antibody, usually IgG, which binds to and activates platelets in the presence of heparin. The pathogenic antibody is directed toward an immunogenic complex formed by heparin (or other mucopolysaccharides) and a basic protein, most commonly platelet factor 4 (PF4). The immune complex formed by IgG, heparin and protein then binds to and clusters the platelet F*cy*IIa receptor, initiating platelet activation and clearance in the reticuloendothelial system. Rarely, HIT can be caused by alternative mechanisms, including IgA and/or IgM anti-PF4/heparin antibodies or antibodies directed against PF4-related chemokines. Platelet activation is associated with the generation of procoagulant platelet microparticles and there is additional evidence that the antibody can also bind vascular endothelial cells (or PF4 located on their surface) leading to endothelial cell damage or activation with expression of tissue factor (stimulating the extrinsic coagulation pathway). In this situation, the intense surge of procoagulant activity overwhelms heparin's anticoagulant effects, leading to intravascular thrombosis that can be life-threatening.[114–117]

The true incidence of HIT is uncertain, predominantly because the criteria for its diagnosis are lacking. Well-designed prospective studies suggest that the incidence varies from less than 1% to about 3% of patients exposed to unfractionated heparin, while the incidence is significantly lower in patients only exposed to low molecular weight heparin. Assays used to detect heparin antibodies vary widely in their sensitivity. Widescale screening demonstrated an incidence as low as 8% and as high as 50% when very sensitive immunoassays were used to detect the presence of antibody directed at the PF4 heparin complex in selected patients with clinical conditions, such as cardiopulmonary bypass surgery. This recent finding indicates that there is a clinical spectrum in the expression of HIT, ranging from asymptomatic antibody formation to antibody formation associated with thrombocytopenia and thrombosis. The clinical significance of heparin antibodies without thrombocytopenia remains unclear and is a subject that warrants further investigation.

The major clinical manifestations of HIT are thrombocytopenia and thrombosis. The onset of thrombocytopenia and/or thrombosis (venous or arterial) usually occurs 5–12 (range 4–20) days after treatment is initiated in patients who are exposed to the drug for the first time. Symptoms may occur more rapidly (within hours) in patients who have had previous exposure to heparin, particularly if the exposure occurred within the last 3 months. Rarely, the onset of thrombocytopenia and/or thrombosis may be delayed. Patients with HIT usually develop mild to moderate thrombocytopenia with the nadir ranging from 20 to 150×10^9/l. However, HIT should be suspected whenever an unexplained decrease of >50% from the baseline platelet count occurs during heparin therapy, even if the platelet count remains in the reference page, or if the platelet count falls below 100×10^9/l.

Initial assessment of patients with ischemic stroke and suspected thrombophilia

All patients with venous or arterial thromboembolism should have a complete history (including a family history of thrombotic events) and physical examination with special attention to concomitant clinical disorders that may predispose to a 'procoagulant state' or be associated with mural thrombosis of the cardiac chambers (atrial fibrillation, prior MI, cardiomyopathy). A medication history should be conducted with particular emphasis on comprehensive oral contraceptives, hormone-replacement therapy and illicit drugs including cocaine, amphetamines and anabolic steroids. An initial laboratory investigation should include a complete blood count (with platelets), peripheral smear (with review), and an activated partial thromboplastin time (aPTT).

Screening tests for thrombophilia

In the event that the initial evaluation fails to reveal an obvious direct cause for thrombosis, one must consider a more detailed laboratory investigation (Tables 4.5 and 4.6). Although there is some support for a global screening test (Acticlot®, Universal, Pro® C Global), its clinical utility has not been established.

Three types of assay are available for the evaluation of patients with suspected thrombophilia: (1) functional assays that employ either synthetic substrates or clotting methodology to assess the enzymatic activity of the coagulation cascade; (2) clotting factor antigen concentration, measured by immunological methods including enzyme immunoassays (EIA) and enzyme-linked immunoabsorbent assays (ELISA); and (3) genetic tests. The laboratory diagnosis of thrombophilia can be divided into several stages. The first is typically functional in nature and if an abnormality is uncovered a second series of tests to determine specific protein concentrations are performed.

Patients with an unexplained thromboembolic event who are <45 years of age should be screened for the following congenital abnormalities: APC resistance/factor V Leiden, AT deficiency, protein C deficiency and protein S deficiency. An antiphospholipid antibody screen should also be performed. Patients older than 45 years of age with unexplained thromboembolism are less likely to have AT, protein C or protein S deficiency; however, screening for factor V Leiden and antiphospholipid antibody syndrome is recommended. The most accurate results are obtained when testing is performed prior to the initiation of anticoagulant therapy. Heparin (unfractionated, low molecular weight) reduces AT antigen and activity by approximately 10–15%. Warfarin reduces both protein C and protein S levels by 30%. Accordingly, these tests should be performed prior to, or at least 2 weeks after, completion of warfarin therapy to allow for the resynthesis of coagulation proteins. Both heparin and warfarin influence LA assays but do not affect antiphospholipid antibody screening tests.

If the initial screening tests are unremarkable, a second tier of tests should be considered (Table 4.7). These are best performed through a specialized laboratory.

Table 4.5 Initial laboratory testing for suspected thrombophilia

- AT activity
- Protein C activity
- Protein S antigen level
- Activated protein C resistance functional assay or factor V Leiden genetic analysis
- Lupus anticoagulant screen
- Anticardiolipin antibody assay

APC resistance

The most commonly used functional assay for determining APC resistance is an aPTT calculated in the presence and absence of a known concentration of APC. The ratio of the two clotting times normalized against the APC resistance ratios of pooled plasma provides an accurate means of identifying patients with APC resistance. Ninety per cent of all patients with a 'positive' functional APC resistance test will have factor V Leiden; the remainder will probably have one or more alternative mutations of the factor V gene. Modification of the functional APC resistance test using factor V deficient plasma increases the sensitivity and specificity for factor V Leiden to nearly 100%.[118,119] This modification also allows for the analysis of samples from patients receiving anticoagulant therapy.

The mutation responsible for factor V Leiden can be identified directly by genetic analysis

Table 4.6 Screening for thrombophilic conditions

Investigation	*Type of assay*	*Indication*	*Ideal timing of assays*	*Causes of acquired deficiencies*	*Comments*
AT activity	Chromogenic (functional)	Venous thromboembolism	Prior to heparinization*,‡	Heparin, sepsis, acute thrombosis/DIC liver disease nephrotic syndrome, estrogens, chemotherapeutic agents (asparaginase)	Detects both types I and II defects
Protein C activity	Chromogenic (functional)	Venous thromboembolism	Prior to initiation of warfarin*,†	Warfarin, sepsis, acute thrombosis/DIC liver disease chemotherapeutic agents (asparaginase)	Detects both types I and II defects
Protein S antigen	ELISA total antigen ELISA free antigen	Venous thromboembolism	Prior initiation of warfarin*,†	Warfarin, acute thrombosis/DIC liver disease, pregnancy, estrogens, chemotherapeutic agents (asparaginase), inflammation (C4b-BP), vitamin K deficiency	Functional assays give false (+) results in presence of factor V Leiden
Activated protein C resistance	aPTT assay	Venous thromboembolism—consider in older patients with idiopathic event	Prior to heparinization*,†,‡	Warfarin acute thrombosis/DIC	90–95% patients with (+) APC resistance have factor V Leiden
Factor V Leiden	Genetic analysis	Venous thromboembolism—consider in older patients with idiopathic event	Anytime	None	
Anticardiolipin antibodies	ELISA IgG aCL ELISA IgM aCL	Venous thromboembolism, Arterial thromboembolism, Pregnancy loss, Thrombocytopenia	Anytime	See text	
Lupus anticoagulant	• Sensitive PTT • RVVT (dilute) • Kaolin clotting time	Venous thromboembolism, Arterial thromboembolism, Pregnancy loss, Thrombocytopenia	Prior to warfarin/heparin*,†,‡	See text	Heparin and warfarin can prolong clotting assays causing false-positives
Homocysteine	Plasma chromatography	Arterial thromboembolism, Venous thromboembolism—consider screening if other causes ruled out	Improved sensitivity performed after methionine load	Folate deficiency B_{12} deficiency Medications interfering with folate/B_{12} metabolism	

* Positive test performed at time of acute presentation should be repeated as out-patient.
† Must be performed prior to, or 2 weeks after, completion of warfarin therapy.
‡ Presence of heparin does not interfere with some assays; check with laboratory.

Table 4.7 Second tier of laboratory evaluation for suspected thrombophilias

- Prothrombin levels ± genetic analysis for prothrombin G20210A
- Evaluation for dysfibrinogenemia
- Plasminogen/plasminogen activator/plasminogen activator inhibitor levels*
- Heparin cofactor II levels*
- Evaluation for thrombomodulin abnormalities*
- Evaluation for the impaired response of 'sticky platelets' to nitric oxide and excess thromboxane A_2 production.

*only available in speciality laboratories.

(genomic amplification followed by nucleotide sequencing, DNA hybridization, or restriction enzyme fragment analysis). This method of diagnosis has the advantage of not being affected by concomitant coagulation abnormalities or anticoagulant therapy, but is more costly. Genetic testing will also miss the small percentage of patients with APC resistance who do not have factor V Leiden.

Antiphospholipid antibodies

Individual idiotypes of aCL antibodies can be identified by specific enzyme linked immunosorbent assays (ELISAs). It is now recognized that the aCL antibodies associated with an increased risk of thrombosis require β_2 glycoprotein I (a natural anticoagulant) for binding in vitro.[120,121] The role of this cofactor in vivo is still unclear. Non-autoimmune aCL antibodies can develop in the setting of infection; however, they are not dependent on β_2 glycoprotein 1 for binding, and carry little risk of thrombosis.[122]

The presence of a circulating LA can be identified by the prolongation of various in vitro clotting tests. Initially the standard aPTT was used as a screening tool but it was subsequently found to lack sensitivity. Therefore, a diluted Russell's Viper venom test (dRVVT) is usually performed regardless of the aPTT result.[123] Prolongation of thc dRVVT will not correct with the addition of normal plasma in the presence of LA (in contrast to the clotting factor deficiency). For confirmation, a platelet neutralization procedure, to show the dependence of phospholipid inhibitors, should be performed. A third assay, the kaolin clotting time test, has also been used to detect LA; however, it is not as sensitive as the dRVVT.

Individual laboratory evaluations

AT deficiency

Initial screening for a suspected AT deficiency is commonly based on the inhibition of factor Xa or thrombin using patient plasma. A chromogenic assay is preferred because it can distinguish between several qualitative deficiency subtypes. The AT protein concentration can be quantified using immunochemical methods.

Protein C deficiency

Functional methods to determine protein C abnormalities are based on the protein's separation from plasma, its activation, and the measurement of activated protein C activity. A chromogenic assay is preferred over an aPTT-based determination; however, many laboratories recommend that an immunoassay be performed in parallel to increase the overall precision.

Protein S deficiency

Immunoassays of total and free protein S, most often enzyme immunoassays using monoclonal or polyclonal antibodies, are employed as screening tests. Functional assays, although requiring special reagents that are not available in most clinical laboratories, are necessary to exclude qualitative defects.

Hyperhomocysteinemia

Homocysteine levels are measured by high performance liquid chromatography under fasting conditions. It has been suggested that quantification be performed both before and after methionine loading to detect mild defects and to distinguish variants of the inherited condition.

Prothrombin G20210A
Clotting and chromogenic assays are available in both clinical and reference laboratories to determine factor II concentrations. Specialized laboratories currently use specific genetic tests to confirm the diagnosis.

Heparin-induced antibodies

Specific testing for heparin-induced antibodies (HIT) can be grouped into two types of assays: (1) platelet-based or functional assays; and (2) antibody recognition of the heparin–PF4 complex. Platelet-based assays depend on the activation or lysis of platelets in the presence of a test sample and heparin. Washed normal platelets provide a sensitive test system when either ^{14}C-serotonin release or platelet aggregation is used as an endpoint. The ^{14}C-serotonin release assay has been evaluated in a prospective clinical study and a positive assay was strongly associated with HIT (odds ratio, 78.2; 95% CI, 12.0–818.8; $P < 0.001$) with a specificity of 96%. The specificity of these assays may be improved by performing the assay at low (0.1–0.3 U/ml) and high 10–100 U/ml) concentrations of heparin. High concentrations of heparin dissociate the heparin–PF4 complexes from the platelet surface and interfere with HIT antibody interaction with platelet Fc*y*RIIa and subsequent platelet activation. Thus platelet activation or lysis, manifested by platelet aggregation or ^{14}C-serotonin release, at low, but not high, concentrations of heparin is regarded as diagnostic of HIT. Experience with these test systems has also confirmed the need for careful selection of platelet donors, washed platelets and the use of weakly positive HIT control samples. Substantial variation in the sensitivity of Fc*y*RIIa-mediated platelet activation may be found among normal donors. Thus, it is essential to use donor platelets known to be responsive to HIT samples.

The second laboratory approach to the diagnosis of HIT uses assays which detect antibodies to the PF4–heparin macromolecular complex. Enzyme-linked immunoabsorbent assays (ELISAs) have been developed which permit identification of antibodies reacting with PF4–heparin. Microtiter plate wells are coated with PF4–heparin and allowed to incubate with a patient sample. Bound antibody is then detected by appropriate antisera to IgG, IgA or IgM by standard techniques. Although the concordance between platelet-based activation and ELISA is high, the results are discordant in approximately 10–20% of cases. Several factors may contribute to this discordance. First, the ELISA may detect IgA and IgM antibodies that are incapable of mediating Fc*y*RIIa-induced platelet activation. Second, some antibodies appear to be directed at complexes of heparin and other proteins, such as interleukin 8 and neutrophil activating peptide 2. Third, the ELISA method may detect low titer (or avidity) antibodies that are not associated with clinical manifestations. To date there are no data from prospective clinical trials delineating the performance of these two approaches to the laboratory confirmation of HIT. Therefore, it is difficult to recommend one technique over another, although, as previously mentioned, there is level 1 evidence correlating the serotonin release assay with clinical HIT. Both assays should be available at reference laboratories.[124,125]

SUMMARY

The hematological evaluation of stroke risk begins with the knowledge of normal hemostasis and the underlying mechanisms of pathological intravascular thrombosis, followed by a comprehensive evaluation of prothrombotic risk including associated medical illness, family history and medication. Based on clinical suspicion, carefully selected laboratory studies should be performed in experienced laboratories and interpreted by a team of clinicians and scientists well-versed in the field of congenital and acquired thrombophilias.

REFERENCES

1. George JN. Studies on platelet plasma membranes: IV–Quantitative analysis of platelet membrane glycoproteins by (^{125}I)-diazotized diiodosulfanilic acid labeling and SDS-polyacrylamide gel electrophoresis. *J Lab Clin Med* 1978; **92:**430–6.
2. Nurden AT, Caen JP. Membrane glycoproteins and human platelet function. *Br J Haematol* 1978; **38:**155–60.
3. Phillips DR, Agin PP. Platelet membrane defects in Glanzmann's thrombasthenia. Evidence for decreased amounts of two major glycoproteins. *J Clin Invest* 1977; **60:**535–45.
4. Phillips DR, Agin PP. Platelet plasma membrane glycoproteins. Evidence for the presence of nonequivalent disulfide bonds using nonreduced–reduced two-dimensional gel electrophoresis. *J Biol Chem* 1977; **252:**2121–6.
5. Plow EF, Ginsberg MH. The molecular basis of platelet function. In: *Hematology. Basic Principles and Practice* (Hoffman R, Benz EJ, Shaltil SJ, Furie B, Cohen HJ, eds), p. 1165. New York; Churchill Livingston: 1991.
6. Fauvel F, Grant ME, Legrand YJ *et al.* Interaction of blood platelets with a microfibrillar extract from adult bovine aorta: requirement for von Willebrand factor. *Proc Natl Acad Sci USA* 1983; **80:**551–4.
7. Stenberg PE, Shuman MA, Levine SP, Bainton DF. Redistribution of alpha-granules and their contents in thrombin-stimulated platelets. *J Cell Biol* 1984; **98:**748–60.
8. Ginsberg MH, Taylor L, Painter RG. The mechanism of thrombin-induced platelet factor 4 secretion. *Blood* 1980; **55:**661–8.
9. Van't Veer C, Hackeng TM, Delahaye C, Sixma JJ, Booma BN. Activated factor X and thrombin formation triggered by tissue factor on endothelial cell matrix in a flow model. *Blood* 1994; **84:**1132–9.
10. Gupta M, Doellgast GJ, Cheng T, Lewis JC. Expression and localization of tissue factor-based procoagulant activity in pigeon monocyte derived macrophages. *Thromb Haemost* 1993; **70:**963–9.
11. Vogel KG, Peterson DW. Extracellular, surface and intracellular proteoglycans produced by human embryo lung fibroblasts in culture. *J Biol Chem* 1981; **256:**13235–40.
12. Jarvelainen HT, Kinsella MG, Wight TN, Sandell LJ. Differential expression of small chondroitin/dermatan sulfate proteoglycans, PG-I/biglycan and PG-II/decorin, by vascular smooth muscle and endothelial cells in culture. *J Biol Chem* 1991; **266:**23274–9.
13. Kresse H, Hausser H, Schonherr E, Bittner K. Biosynthesis and interactions of small chondroitin/dermatan sulfate proteoglycans. *Eur J Clin Chem Clin Biochem* 1994; **32:**259–66.
14. Heeb MJ, Mesters RM, Tans G, Rosing J, Griffin JH. Binding of protein S to factor Va associated with inhibition of prothrombinase that is independent of activated protein C. *J Biol Chem* 1993; **268:**2872–7.
15. Broze GJJR, Warren LA, Novotny WF, Higuchi DA, Girard TJ, Miletich JP. The lipoprotein-associated coagulation inhibitor that inhibits factor VII-tissue factor complex also inhibits factor Xa: insight into its possible mechanism of action. *Blood* 1994; **84:**1132–9.
16. van't Veer C, Hackeng TM, Delahye C, Sixma JJ, Bouma BN. Activated factor X and thrombin formation triggered by tissue factor on endothelial cell matrix in a flow model: effect of the tissue factor pathway inhibitor. *Blood* 1994; **84:**1132–9.
17. Kaider B, Hoppensteadt DA, Jeske W, Wun TC, Fareed J. Inhibitory effects of TFPI of thrombin and factor Xa generation in vitro—modulatory action of glycosaminoglycans. *Thromb Res* 1994; **75:**609–19.
18. Sprecher CA, Kisiel W, Mathewes S, Foster DC. Molecular cloning, expression, and partial characterization of a second human tissue-factor-pathway inhibitor. *Proc Natl Acad Sci USA* 1994; **91:**3353–7.
20. Tait JF, Gibson D, Fukikawa K. Phospholipid binding properties of human placental anticoagulant protein-1, a member of the lipocortin family. *J Biol Chem* 1989; **264:**7944–51.
21. Marcum JA, McKenney JB, Rosenberg RD. Acceleration of thrombin–antithrombin complex formation in rat hindquarters via heparin-like molecules bound to the endothelium. *J Clin Invest* 1984; **74:**341–50.
22. Cooper DN, Blajchman M, Perry D, Emmerich J, Aiach M. Antithrombin III mutation database: first update. *Thromb Haemost* 1993; **70:**361.
23. Demers C, Ginsburg JS, Hirsh J, Henderson P, Blajchman MA. Thrombosis in antithrombin-III-deficient persons. Report of a large kindred and literature review. *Ann Intern Med* 1992; **116:**754–61.
24. De Stefano V, Finazzi G, Mannuccio Mannucci

P. Inherited thrombophilia: pathogenesis, clinical syndromes, and management. *Blood* 1996; **87:**3531–44.
25. Abildgaard U. Antithrombin and related inhibitors of coagulation. In: *Recent Advances in Blood Coagulation* (Poller L, ed.), pp. 151–73. Edinburgh; Churchill Livingstone: 1981.
26. Odegard OR, Abildgaard U. Antithrombin III: critical review of assay methods: significance of variations in health and disease. *Haemostasis* 1978; **7:**127–34.
27. Tait RC, Walker ID, Perry DJ *et al.* Prevalence of antithrombin III deficiency in the healthy population. *Br J Haem* 1994; **87:**106–12.
28. Heijboer H, Brandjes DPM, Buller HR, Sturk A, ten Cate JW. Deficiencies of coagulation-inhibiting and fibrinolytic proteins in outpatients with deep-vein thrombosis. *N Engl J Med* 1990; **323:**1512–6.
29. Tabernero MD, Tomas JF, Alberca I, Orfao A, Borrasca AL, Vicente V. Incidence and clinical characteristics of hereditary disorders associated with venous thrombosis. *Am J Hematol* 1991; **36:**249–54.
30. Malm J, Laurell M, Nilsson IM, Dahlbäck B. Thromboembolic disease. Critical evaluation of laboratory investigation. *Thromb Haemost* 1992; **68:**7–13.
31. Pabinger I, Brucker S, Kyrle PA *et al.* Hereditary deficiency of antithrombin III, protein C and protein S: prevalence in patients with a history of venous thrombosis and criteria for rational patient screening. *Blood Coag Fibrinol* 1992; **3:**547–53.
32. Melissari E, Monte G, Lindo VS *et al.* Congenital thrombophilia among patients with venous thromboembolism. *Blood Coag Fibrinol* 1992; **36:**749–58.
33. Stenflo J. The biochemistry of protein C. In: *Protein C and Related Proteins* (Bertina RM, ed.), pp. 21–54. Edinburgh; Churchill Livingstone: 1988.
34. deFouw NJ, de Jong YF, Haverkate K, Bertina RM. Activated protein C increases fibrin clot lysis by neutralization of plasminogen activator inhibitor: no evidence for a cofactor role of protein S. *Thromb Haemost* 1988; **60:**328–33.
35. Romeo G, Hassan HJ, Staempfli S *et al.* Hereditary thrombophilia: identification of nonsense and missense mutations in the protein C gene. *Proc Natl Acad Sci USA* 1987; **84:**2829–32.
36. Reitsma PH, Poort SR, Allaart CF, Briët E, Bertina RM. The spectrum of genetic defects in a panel of 40 Dutch families with symptomatic protein C deficiency type 1: heterogeneity and founder effects. *Blood* 1991; **78:**890–4.
37. Bertina RM, Broekmans AW, Krommenhoek van Es C, van Wijngaarden A. The use of a functional and immunologic assay for plasma protein C deficiency. *Thromb Haemost* 1984; **51:**1–5.
38. Allaart CF, Poort SR, Rosendaal FR, Reitsma PH, Bertina RM, Briët E. Increased risk of venous thrombosis in carriers of hereditary protein C deficiency defect. *Lancet* 1993; **341:**134–8.
39. Tait RC, Walker ID, Reitsma PH. Prevalence of protein C deficiency in the healthy population. *Thromb Haemost* 1995; **73:**87–93.
40. Miletich JM, Prescott SM, White R, Majerus PW, Bovill EG. Inherited predisposition to thrombosis. *Cell* 1993; **72:**477–80.
41. Aiach M, Grandrille S, Emmerich J. A review of mutations causing deficiencies of antithrombin, protein C and protein S. *Thromb Haemost* 1995; **74:**81–9.
42. Cavenagh JD, Colvin BT. Guidelines for the management of thrombophilia. *Postgrad Med J* 1996; **72:**87–94.
43. Bick RL, Ancypa D. Blood protein defects associated with thrombosis. Thrombosis and hemostasis for the clinical laboratory. *Med Clin N Am* 1995; **15:**125–63.
44. Sie P, Boneu B, Bierme R, Wiesel ML, Grunebaum L, Cazenave JP. Arterial thrombosis and protein S deficiency. *Thromb Haemost* 1989; **61:**144–7.
45. Dahlback B, Carlsson M, Svensson PJ. Familial thrombophilia due to a previously unrecognized mechanism characterized by poor anticoagulant response to activated protein C: prediction of a cofactor to activated protein C. *Proc Natl Acad Sci USA* 1993; **90:**1004–8.
46. Koster T, Rosendaal FR, de Ronde H, Briet E, Vandenbroucke JP, Bertina RM. Venous thrombosis due to poor anticoagulant response to activated-protein C: Leiden Thrombophilia Study. *Lancet* 1993; **342:**1503–6.
47. Svensson PJ, Dahlback B. Resistance to activated protein C as a basis for venous thrombosis. *N Engl J Med* 1994; **330:**517–22.
48. Bertina R, Koeleman BPC, Koster T *et al.* Mutation in blood coagulation factor V associated with resistance to activated protein C. *Nature* 1994; **369:**64–7.

49. Voorberg J, Roelse J, Koopman R *et al.* Association of idiopathic venous thromboembolism with single point mutation at Arg[506] of factor V. *Lancet* 1994; **343:**1535–6.
50. Marciniak E, Romond EH. Impaired catalytic function of activated protein C: a new in vitro manifestation of lupus anticoagulant. *Blood* 1989; **74:**2426–32.
51. Malia RG, Kitchen S, Greaves M, Preston FE. Inhibition of activated protein C and its cofactor protein S by antiphospholipid antibodies. *Br J Haematol* 1990; **76:**101–7.
52. Griffin JH, Heeb MJ, Kojima Y. Activated protein C resistance: molecular mechanisms. *Thromb Haemost* 1995; **74:**444–8.
53. Ridker PM, Hennekens CH, Lindpaintner K, Stampfer MJ, Eisenberg PR, Miletich JP. Mutation in the gene coding for coagulation factor V and the risk of myocardial infarction, stroke, and venous thrombosis in apparently healthy men. *N Engl J Med* 1995; **332:**912–7.
54. Greengard JS, Eichinger S, Griffin JH, Bauer KA. Brief report: variability of thrombosis among homozygous siblings with resistance to activated protein C due to an Arg–Gln mutation in the gene for factor V. *N Engl J Med* 1994; **331:**1559–62.
55. Pickering W, Dixit M, Campbell P, Cohen H. Prevalence of activated protein C resistance and other thrombophilic defects in patients with venous thromboembolism. *Br J Haematol* 1994; **86**(Suppl 1):68.
56. Cumming AM, Fildes S, Pylypczwk CC *et al.* Low incidence of resistance to activated protein C in patients with venous thrombosis. *Br J Haematol* 1994; **86**(Suppl 1):34.
57. Rosendaal FR, Siscovick DS, Schwartz SM *et al.* Factor V Leiden (resistance to activated protein C) increases the risk of myocardial infarction in young women. *Blood* 1997; **89:** 2817–21.
58. Hillarp A, Zöller B, Svensson PJ, Dahlbáck B. The 20210A allele of the prothrombin gene is a common risk factor among Swedish outpatients with verified deep venous thrombosis. *Thromb Haemost* 1997; **78:**990–2.
59. Rosendal FR, Siscovick DS, Schwartz SM, Psaty BM, Raghuhathan TE, Vos HL. A common prothrombin variant (20210G to A) increases the risk of myocardial infarction in young women. *Blood* 1997; **90:**1747–50.
60. Doggen CJM, Manger Cats V, Bertina RM, Rosendaal FR. Interaction of coagulation defects and cardiovascular risk factors: increased risk of myocardial infarction associated with factor V Leiden or prothrombin 20210A. *Circulation* 1998; **97:**1037–41.
61. Norlund L, Zöller B, Ohlin AK. A novel thrombomodulin gene mutation in a patient suffering from sagittal sinus thrombosis. *Thromb Haemost* 1997; **78:**1164–6.
62. Ohlin A, Norlund L, Marlar RA. Thrombomodulin gene variations and thromboembolic disease. *Thromb Haemost* 1997; **78:**396–400.
63. Doggen CJM, Kunz G, Rosendaal FR *et al.* A mutation in the thrombomodulin gene. [127]G to A coding for Ala25Thr, and the risk of myocardial infarction in men. *Throm Haemost* 1998; **80:**743–8.
64. Haverkate F, Samama M. Familial dysfibrinogenemia and thrombophilia. Report on a study of the SSC subcommittee on fibrinogen. *Thromb Haemost* 1995; **73:**151–61.
65. Engesser L, Koopman J, de Munk G. Fibrinogen Nijmegen: congenital dysfibrinogenemia associated with impaired t-PA mediated plasminogen activation and decreased binding of t-PA. *Thromb Haemost* 1988; **60:**113–20.
66. Beckmann R. Plasminogen activation by tissue plasminogen activator in the presence of stimulating CNBr fragment FCB-2 of fibrinogen is a two-phase reaction. *J Biol Chem* 1988; **263:**7167–80.
67. Galanakis DK. Inherited dysfibrinogenemia: emerging abnormal structure associations with pathologic and nonpathologic dysfunctions. *Sem Thromb Hemost* 1993; **19:** 386–95.
68. Aoki N, Moroi M, Sakata Y *et al.* Abnormal plasminogen. A hereditary molecular abnormality found in a patient with recurrent thrombosis. *J Clin Invest* 1978; **61:**1186–95.
69. Wohl RC, Summaria L, Robbins KC. Physiologic activation of the human fibrinolytic system. Isolation and the characterization of human plasminogen variants, Chicago I and Chicago II. *J Biol Chem* 1979; **254:**9063–9.
70. Liu Y, Lyons RM, McDonah J. Plasminogen San Antonio: an abnormal plasminogen with a more cathodic migration, decreased activation and associated thrombosis. *Thromb Haemost* 1988; **59:**49–53.
71. Meade TW, North WRS, Chakrabarti RR *et al.* Hemostatic function and cardiovascular death: early results of a prospective study. *Lancet* 1980; **i:**1050–4.

72. Hamsten A, Blomback M, Wimam B *et al.* Hemostatic function in myocardial infarction. *Br Med J* 1986; **55:**58–66.
73. Hamsten A, Winmam B, Faire UD *et al.* Increased plasma levels of a rapid inhibitor of tissue plasminogen activator in young survivors of myocardial infarction. *N Engl J Med* 1985; **313:**1557–63.
74. Mudd SH, Levy HL, Skovby F. Disorders of transsulfuration. In: *The Metabolic Basis of Inherited Disease* (Scriver CR, Beaudet AL, Sly WS, Valle D, eds), p. 693. New York, NY; McGraw-Hill: 1989.
75. Rees MW, Rodgers GM. Homocysteinemia: association of a metabolic disorder with vascular disease and thrombosis. *Thrombos Res* 1993; **71:**337–59
76. Selhub J, Jacques PF, Wilson PWF, Rush D, Rosenberg JH. Vitamin status and intake as primary determinants of Homocysteinemia in an elderly population. *J Am Med Assoc* 1993; **270:**2693–8.
77. Ubbink JB, van der Merwe A, Delport R *et al.* The effect of a subnormal vitamin B-6 status on homocysteine metabolism. *J Clin Invest* 1996; **98:**177–84.
78. Joosten E, van den Berg A, Riezler R *et al.* Metabolic evidence that deficiencies of vitamin B-12 (cobalamin), folate, and vitamin B-6 occur commonly in elderly people. *Am J Clin Nutr* 1993; **58:**468–76.
79. McCully KS. Homocysteine and vascular disease. *Nature Med* 1996; **2:**386–9.
80. Nishinaga M, Ozawa T, Shimada K. Homocysteine, a thrombogenic agent, suppresses anticoagulant heparan sulfate expression in cultured porcine aortic endothelial cells. *J Clin Invest* 1993; **92:**1381–6.
81. Harker LA, Ross R, Slichter SJ, Scott CR. Homocystine-induced arteriosclerosis: the role of endothelial cell injury and platelet response in its genesis. *J Clin Invest* 1976; **58:** 731–41.
82. Selhub J, Jaques PF, Bostom AG *et al.* Association between plasma homocysteine concentrations and extracranial carotid-artery stenosis. *N Engl J Med* 1995; **332:**286–91.
83. Kang SS, Wong PW, Susmano A, Sora J, Norusis M, Ruggie N. Thermolabile methylenetetrahydrofolate reductase: an inherited risk factor for coronary artery dsiease. *Am J Hum Genet* 1991; **48:**536–45.
84. Den Heijer M, Koster T, Blom HJ *et al.* Hyperhomocystinemia as a risk factor for deep vein thrombosis. *N Engl J Med* 1996; **334:**759–62.
85. Hirsh J, Hoak J. Management of deep vein thrombosis and pulmonary embolism. A statement for healthcare professionals from the Council on Thrombosis (in consultation with the Council on Cardiovascular Radiology), American Heart Association. *Circulation* 1996; **93:**2212–45.
86. Prins MH, Hirsh J. A critical review of the evidence supporting a relationship between impaired fibrinolytic activity and venous thromboembolism. *Arch Intern Med* 1991; **151:**1721–31.
87. Bick RL, Baker WF. Anticardiolipin antibodies and thrombosis. *Hematol Oncol Clin North Am* 1992; **6:**1287–300.
88. Bick RL. Lupus anticoagulants and anticardiolipin antibodies. *Biomed Prog* 1993; **6:**35–9.
89. Khamashta MA, Harris EN, Gharavi AE. Immune mediated mechanism for thrombosis: antiphospholipid antibody binding to platelet membranes. *Ann Rheum Dis* 1988; **47:** 849–53.
90. Schved JF, Dupuy-Fios C, Biron C. A perspective epidemiological study on the occurrence of antiphospholipid antibody: the Montpellier Antiphospholipid (MAP) Study. *Haemostasis* 1994; **24:**175–82.
91. Vila P, Hernandez MC, Lopez-Fernandez MF. Prevalence, follow-up and clinical significance of the anticardiolipin antibodies in normal subjects. *Thromb Haemost* 1994; **72:** 209–13.
92. Hamsten A, Norberg R, Bjorkholm M. Antibodies to cardiolipin in young survivors of myocardial infarction: an association with recurrent cardiovascular events. *Lancet* 1986; **i:**113–6.
93. Montalban J, Khamashta M, Davalos A *et al.* value of immunologic testing in stroke patients. A prospective multicenter study. *Stroke* 1994; **25:**2412–5.
94. Brey RL, Hart RG, Sherman DG, Tegeler CH. Antiphospholipid antibodies and cerebral ischemia in young people. *Neurology* 1990; **40:**1190–6.
95. APASS (The Antiphospholipid Antibodies in Stroke Study) Group. Anticardiolipin antibodies are an independent risk factor for first ischemic stroke. *Neurology* 1993; **43:** 2069–73.
96. Bick RL. Antiphospholipid thrombosis syndromes: etiology, pathophysiology, diagnosis and management. *Int J Hematol* 1997; **65:** 193–213.

97. Conley CL, Hartmann RC. A hemorrhagic disorder caused by circulating anticoagulant in patients with disseminated lupus erythematosus. *J Clin Invest* 1952; **31:**621–2.
98. Criel A, Collen D, Masson PL. A case of IgM antibodies which inhibit the contact activation of blood coagulation. *Thromb Res* 1978; **12:**883–92.
99. Kunkel L. Acquired circulating anticoagulants. *Hematol Oncol Clin North Am* 1992; **6:**1341–58.
100. Bick RL. Hypercoagulability and thrombosis. *Med Clin North Am* 1994; **78:**635–66.
101. Minna JD, Bunn PA Jr. Paraneoplastic syndromes. In: *Cancer: Principles and Practice of Oncology* (De Vita VT Jr, Hellman S, Rosenberg SA, eds), 3rd end, pp. 1920–40. Philadelphia; JB Lippincott: 1989.
102. Green KB, Silverstein RL. Hypercoagulability in cancer. *Hematol/Oncol Clin N Am* 1996; **10:**499–530.
103. Rao LV. Tissue factor as a tumor procoagulant. *Cancer Metast Rev* 1992; **11:**249–66.
104. Semeraro N. Differential expression of procoagulant activity in macrophages associated with experimental and human tumors. *Haemostasis* 1988; **18:**47–54.
105. Falanga A, Alessio MG, Donati MB. A new procoagulant in acute leukemia. *Blood* 1988; **71:**870–5.
106. Donati MB, Gambacorti PC, Casali B *et al.* Cancer procoagulant activity in human tumor cells: evidence from melanoma patients. *Cancer Res* 1986; **46:**6471–4.
107. Jaffe EA. Biochemistry, immunology, and cell biology of endothelium. In: *Hemostasis and Thrombosis: Basic Principles and Clinical Practice* (Colman RW, Hirsh J, Marder VJ, Salzman EW, eds), 3rd edn. Philadelphia; JB Lippincott: 1994.
108. Murphy S. Thrombocytosis and thrombocythemia. *Clin Haematol* 1983; **12:**89.
109. Maldonado JE, Pinaido T, Pherre RV. Dysplastic platelets and circulating megakaryocytes in chronic myeloproliferative disease. 1. The platelets: ultrastructure and peroxidase reaction. *Blood* 1974; **43:** 797–809.
110. Sinzlinger H, Kaliman J, O'Grady J. Platelet lipoxygenase defect (Wein–Penzing Defect) in two patients with myocardial infarction. *Am J Hematol* 1991; **36:**202–5.
111. Mammen EF. Ten year's experience with the sticky platelet syndrome. *Clin Appl Thromb Hemost* 1995; **1:**66.
112. Freedman JE, Loscalzo J, Benoit SE *et al.* Decreased platelet inhibition by nitric oxide in two brothers with a history of arterial thrombosis. *J Clin Invest* 1996; **97:**979–87.
113. Weis EJ, Bray PF, Tayback DR *et al.* A polymorphism of a platelet glycoprotein receptor as an inherited risk factor for coronary thrombosis. *N Engl J Med* 1996; **334:**1090–4.
114. Hong BH. Heparin-induced thrombocytopenia. *Br J Haematol* 1995; **89:**431–9.
115. Amiral J, Bridey F, Dreyfus M *et al.* Platelet factor 4 complexed to heparin is the target for antibodies generated in heparin-induced thrombocytopenia. *Thromb Haemost* 1992; **68:**95–6.
116. Warkentin TE, Hayward CPM, Boshkov LK *et al.* Sera from patients with heparin-induced thrombocytopenia generate platelet-derived microparticles with procoagulant activity; an explanation for the thrombotic complications of heparin-induced thrombocytopenia. *Blood* 1994; **84:**3691–9.
117. Cines DB, Tomaski A, Tasnnebaum S. Immune endothelial-cell injury in heparin-associated thrombocytopenia. *N Engl J Med* 1987; **316:**581–9.
118. Jorquera JI, Montoro JM, Ferández MA *et al.* Modified test for activated protein C resistance. *Lancet* 1994; **344:**1162–3.
119. Trossaërt M, Conard J, Horellou MH *et al.* Modified APC resistance assay for patients on oral anticoagulants. *Lancet* 1994; **344:** 1162–3.
120. Matsuura E, Igarashi Y, Fujimoto M *et al.* Anticardiolipin cofactor(s) and differential diagnosis of autoimmune disease. *Lancet* 1990; **i:**177–8.
121. McNeil HP, Simpson RJ, Chesterman CN *et al.* Antiphospholipid antibodies are directed against a complex antigen that includes a lipid-binding inhibitor: β_2-glycoprotein 1 (apolipoprotein H). *Proc Natl Acad Sci USA* 1990; **87:**4120–4.
122. Triplett DA, Brandt JT, Musgrave KA *et al.* The relationship between lupus anticoagulants and antibodies to phospholipid. *J Am Med Assoc* 1988; **259:**550–4.
123. Petri M, Nelson L, Weimer F *et al.* The automated modified Russell viper venom time test for the lupus anticoagulant. *J Rheumatol* 1991; **18:**1823–5.
124. Warkentin TE, Hayward CPM, Smith CA, Kelly PM, Kelto JG. Determinants of donor platelet variability when testing for heparin-induced thrombocytopenia. *J Lab Clin Med* 1992; **120:**371–9.

125. Visentin DP, Ford SE, Scott JP, Aster RH. Antibodies from patients with heparin-induced thrombocytopenia/thrombosis are aspecific for platelet factor 4 complex with heparin or bound to endothelial cells. *J Clin Invest* 1994; **93:**81–8.

5

Epidemiology and etiology of stroke in the young: new therapeutic perspectives for prevention

José Biller, Bhuwan P Garg and Maurizia Rasura

CONTENTS • **Introduction** • **Cardiac embolism** • **Non-atherosclerotic cerebral vasculopathies** • **Cervicocephalic arterial dissections** • **Traumatic cerebrovascular disease** • **Moyamoya** • **Fibromuscular dysplasia** • **Cerebral vasculitis** • **Migrainous infarction and other vasospastic disorders** • **Hypercoagulable disorders** • **Primary hypercoagulable states** • **Secondary hypercoagulable states** • **Metabolic disorders** • **Genetic disorders** • **Miscellaneous disorders**

INTRODUCTION

In the elderly, atherosclerotic cerebrovascular disease is the most common cause of ischemic stroke, while the etiology of ischemic stroke in the young is more diverse and challenging. Although over 70 different causes or potential risk factors for childhood stroke have been described, ischemic stroke in children and young adults frequently results from non-atherosclerotic vasculopathies, cardiac embolism, or prothrombotic states.[1–5] Yet, the etiology or the underlying disorder of approximately one-third of ischemic strokes in children and young adults remains undetermined.

CARDIAC EMBOLISM

Although non-valvular atrial fibrillation and ischemic heart disease are the most common causes of cardioembolic stroke in older people, the causes in infants and children are more diverse, and more unusual disorders need to be more seriously considered. It is estimated that 25–30% of children with stroke have congenital heart disease.[6] Congenital heart disease, rheumatic heart disease, and infective endocarditis are among the most common cardiac disorders leading to embolic ischemic strokes in children (Fig. 5.1).

Among young patients with cerebral ischemia, one-fifth to one-third are presumed to be due to emboli of cardiac origin.[7] Cardiac emboli may be composed of platelet, fibrin, platelet–fibrin, calcium, micro-organisms, or neoplastic fragments. Cerebral ischemia may result from systemic or paradoxical emboli, emboli occurring during cardiopulmonary bypass, or arterial or venous thromboses. Children with congenital heart disease and a low hemoglobin concentration are at special risk for arterial strokes; those with a high hematocrit are more likely to experience cerebral venous thrombosis.[8] Aortic coarctation increases the risk for intracranial aneurysms. Subarachnoid hemorrhage due to a ruptured intracranial aneurysm usually occurs in the

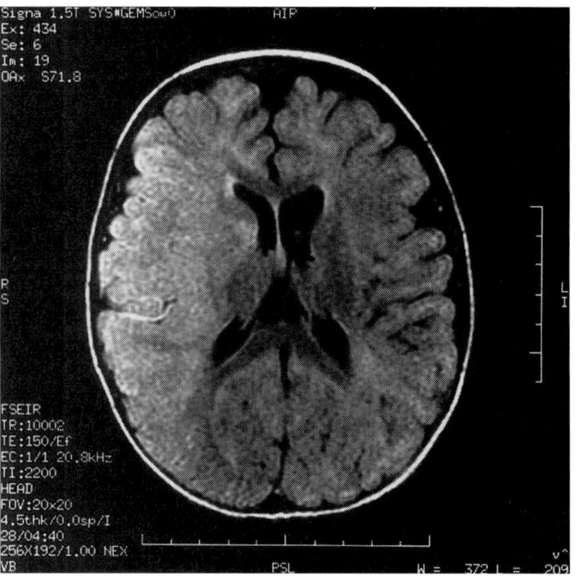

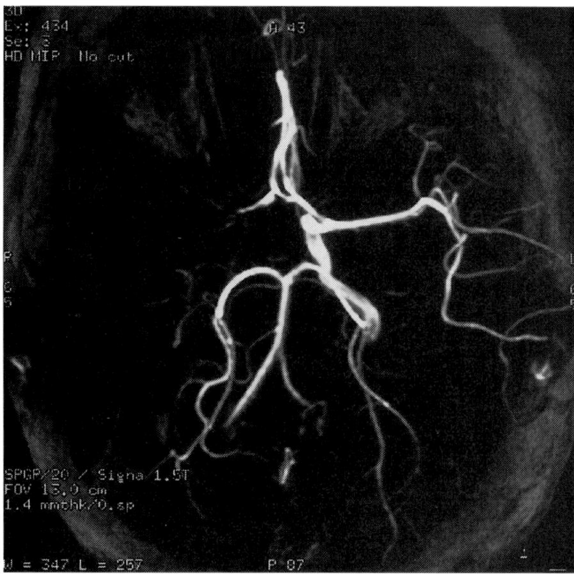

Figure 5.1 (a) Axial FLAIR image of the brain demonstrates an area of a large right middle cerebral artery infarction in a 10-month-old male following surgical correction of a complex congenital heart disease. (b) 3-D time of flight MRA demonstrates a complete occlusion of the right M1 segment of the middle cerebral artery consistent with an embolic occlusion (same patient).

second or third decade of life; multiple aneurysms are common. Patients with aortic coarctation may also suffer intracerebral hemorrhage as a result of arterial hypertension. Spinal cord ischemia may complicate surgery for aortic coarction, and aortic coarction may also complicate Turner's syndrome.[9]

Right-to-left shunts can occur at the atrial level (e.g., atrial septal defect, ASD, with pulmonary hypertension), ventricular level (ventricular septal defect with pulmonary hypertension), or at the arterial level (e.g., pulmonary arteriovenous fistula). ASD is one of the more common congenital heart diseases found in adults. They are classified as secundum ASD, primum ASD, or sinus venosus defect according to their location relative to the fossa ovalis. During right-to-left shunting, there is an opportunity for the passage of thrombi leading to paradoxical embolism.

Ventricular septal defect (VSD) is the most common defect in patients with congenital heart disease. Patients with VSD usually have a left-to-right shunt. However, in patients with Eisenmenger's syndrome there is a right-to-left shunt across the VSD.[8] The most common cardiac abnormalities associated with Down's syndrome include VSD (Roger defect), atrioventricular septal defects, tetralogy of Fallot, and patent ductus arteriosus. Patients with tetralogy of Fallot are cyanotic due to a right-to-left shunt.

Polycythemia and high hematocrit predispose to thrombotic complications, especially during common childhood illnesses with dehydration.[9] Pulmonary arteriovenous fistulae are commonly found in patients with hereditary hemorrhagic telangiectasia (Rendu–Osler–Weber disease), an autosomal dominant vascular dysplasia associated with a genetic defect at a locus on chromosome 9q34.[10] Paradoxical embolism to the brain is also a potential complication of the intrapulmonary right-to-left shunt. Other central nervous system manifestations include intracranial hemorrhage and septic embolism leading to brain abscess. Common central nervous system lesions include arteriovenous malformations and fistulae, telangiectasias, and aneurysms.

The Fontan operation is one of the most common cardiac operations for children with congenital heart disease after the first year of life. Thromboembolic complications account both for morbidity and mortality after a modified Fontan procedure and may even occur months or years after surgery. In one of the largest series, of 645 patients who had the Fontan operation over a 15-year period, a total of 17 patients (2.6%) had a stroke following surgery. The risk period extended from the first postoperative day to 32 months after surgery.[11]

Patients may develop paradoxical cerebral embolism from clots forming on the sutures crossing the fenestration; formation of right atrial thrombus is also a known complication.[12] The use of purse-string sutures around the fenestration and platelet antiaggregant drugs can probably minimize the occurrence of paradoxical embolism.[13] In a review of 68 consecutive Fontan procedures performed from 1978 to 1993, six surviving patients had strokes. Collectively, patients with neurological symptoms had normal hematological and coagulation parameters at the onset of the neurological symptoms. Two patients were on platelet antiaggregants, and one patient was on warfarin.[14] Strokes may also result from transposition of the great vessels or from their surgical repair. A subclavian steal may complicate a Blalock–Taussig shunt for the repair of a tetralogy of Fallot and may also occur during an extracorporeal membrane oxygenation (ECMO) procedure.[8]

Cardiac valvular heart disease may result from rheumatic, prosthetic, myxomatous, inflammatory, infective, marantic, traumatic, degenerative, or congenital etiologies. Rheumatic fever is a common cause of acquired heart disease in children and young adults worldwide, and the most common cause of mitral valve stenosis. Rheumatic atrial fibrillation increases the risk of stroke about 17-fold.[15] Thromboembolism may be the first manifestation of mitral stenosis. The lifetime risk of systemic thromboembolism with rheumatic mitral stenosis is 20%; atrial fibrillation increases the risk of systemic thromboembolism.[16] Approximately 4% of patients with congenital heart disease have aortic valve stenosis.[17] A bicuspid aortic valve is a common congenital heart malformation and may remain asymptomatic throughout life unless associated with coarction of the aorta, or it may only be discovered when a young person without an apparent history of structural heart disease has infective endocarditis. Men are more commonly affected. Cerebral embolism is a rare occurrence.

There are two major types of prosthetic heart valves: mechanical and bioprosthetic. Mechanical valves have a substantial risk of thromboembolism, and therefore require lifetime anticoagulation. Bioprosthetic heart valves have a reduced risk of thromboembolism in comparison to mechanical heart valves, but are less durable. The rate of systemic thromboembolism in patients with mechanical heart valves receiving anticoagulant therapy is 4% per year in the mitral position, and 2% per year in the aortic position. The frequency of thromboembolic complications is greater if there is associated atrial fibrillation. The risk of embolization is less in patients with bioprosthetic valves.[18] Mitral valve prolapse (MVP) is inherited in an autosomal dominant fashion and is frequently associated with a number of heritable disorders of connective tissue. Despite the high prevalence of MVP in the general population, it is an extremely rare cause of embolic stroke. Most young adults with MVP and cerebral infarction have another cause for cerebral infarction.

Infective endocarditis is often a complication in patients with congenital or rheumatic heart disease. A distinction must be made between native valve endocarditis, early or late prosthetic valve endorcarditis, and infective endocarditis among intravenous drug users. Involvement of the central nervous system is possibly the most serious complication of infective endocarditis. Neurological complications are common with infective endocarditis involving the left side of the heart. Mechanical valves are at greater risk for early endocarditis, while bioprosthetic heart valves are at greater risk for late endocarditis. Almost half of the neurological complications are ischemic or hemorrhagic cerebrovascular events. The diagnosis should be suspected in any febrile stroke patient with an organic heart murmur. The presence of petechiae, splinter hemorrhages, Osler nodes, Janeway lesions, Roth spots on funduscopic examination, splenomegaly, and hematuria are helpful diagnostic clues. Laboratory data frequently show anemia, leukocytosis, elevated erythrocyte sedimentation rate, and positive blood cultures. Atypical presentations are not uncommon. The pathophysiological mechanisms include septic embolization, mycotic aneurysm formation, and vasculitis. Infective endocarditis poses an embolic stroke risk of approximately 20%.[19] The importance of appropriate stratification of infective endocarditis risk (i.e., low or no risk, moderate risk, or high risk) must be emphasized. Arteriography may be necessary to exclude mycotic aneurysms in patients who develop focal neurological signs.

Libman–Sacks endocarditis may be associated with stroke; findings resembling verrucous endocarditis of the mitral and aortic valves have been described in patients with the antiphospholipid antibody syndrome.[20]

Atrial fibrillation is rare in the pediatric population while the prevalence of AF increases with advancing age. The Framingham study found an incidence of 0.26% among men, and 0.22% among women, aged 25–34 years.[21]

Sick sinus syndrome (SSS) is rare in young adults. The 'bradycardia–tachycardia' syndrome, especially when complicated by atrial fibrillation, has the greatest risk of embolization. Patients with SSS may experience systemic embolism, even after pacemaker insertion, and the syndrome may occur in the presence of a variety of neuromuscular disorders. Complete heart block is frequently seen in patients with Kearns–Sayre syndrome. Initially, there is a left anterior fascicular block and occasionally a right bundle branch block. Strokes may result from cardiac emboli.[22]

Strokes may complicate the course of cardiomyopathies. Primary cardiomyopathies (unrelated to valvular, ischemic, hypertensive, or inflammatory heart disease) may be dilated, restrictive, hypertrophic, or obliterative. Most patients with dilated cardiomyopathies present with symptoms of pulmonary venous congestion or cardiac arrhythmia. Some patients present with neurological symptoms related to systemic embolization. Cardiomyopathy may also be present in several genetic, neurological and neurometabolic disorders such as neonatal and early infantile mitochondrial disorders, Duchenne and Becker muscular dystrophy, myotonic dystrophy, carnitine-palmitoyltransferase II deficiency, tyrosinemia type I, Friedreich ataxia, Refsum disease, Pompe disease, and the mucopolysaccharidoses. Cardiomyopathy may also be seen with hemochromatosis, endocardial fibroelastosis, and Löffler hypereosinophilic syndrome.

Mitochondrial disorders are seldom associated with dilated cardiomyopathies; in most instances, patients have hypertrophic cardiomyopathies. Apical aneurysms may complicate Chagas cardiomyopathy; emboli may arise from the left or right heart chambers.[1,16] Also myocardial infarction is rare in young adults. Myocardial infarction may occur in the presence of congenital anomalies of the origin of the coronary arteries, calcific coronary arteriopathy of infancy, coronary artery dissection, ostial stenosis from primary disease of the aorta, medial calcification with fibroplastic proliferation of the intima, coronary emboli, childhood polyarteritis nodosa, mucocutaneous lymph node syndrome (Kawasaki's syndrome), and Fabry disease. Acute myocardial infarction is complicated by cerebral embolism in 1–3% of cases.[23]

Atrial myxomas, rare in children, are the most common primary cardiac tumors, they are often in the region of the fossa ovalis, and most protrude into the left atrium. They are sometimes familial and are more common in women. Most atrial myxomas are single, but multiple cardiac myxomas have been described, and may be associated with lentiginosis, myxoid fibroadenomas of the breast, and cutaneous myxomas. Cardiac rhabdomyomas are closely associated with tuberous sclerosis.[24–26]

Patent foramen ovale (PFO) is present in 35% of people between the ages of 1 and 29 years, and in 25% of people aged 30–79 years.[27] A PFO provides opportunity for right-to-left shunting during transient increases in the right atrial pressure above the left atrial pressure, reversing the interatrial gradient. Patients with PFO are more likely to have an unknown cause of stroke. Lechat *et al.* studied the prevalence of PFO as detected by contrast echocardiography in 60 adults younger than 55 years of age, with ischemic strokes and normal cardiac examination. PFO was present in 40% of patients with stroke, compared with 10% in a control group. In patients with no identifiable cause of stroke, the prevalence was 54%.[28] Stroke recurrence is uncommon in these patients.[29–31]

Atrial septal aneurysm (ASA) is an occult embolic cardiac source of cerebral ischemia. ASAs occur more often as an isolated abnormality than in association with other cardiac malformations. In a series of 36 patients with ASA, reported by Belkin *et al.*, 28% had cerebrovascular events and 90% had interatrial shunting, suggesting paradoxical embolism as the mechanism for cerebral ischemia.[32] Initial studies failed to correlate morphology and extent of ASA with embolic risk. More recently, however, it has been shown that patients with ASA, especially those with a greater than 10 mm excursion, are at greater risk of stroke.[33] PFO and ASA have also been associated with mitral valve prolapse.

Thromboembolism can complicate cardiac surgery using cardiopulmonary bypass with deep hypothermia and cardiac arrest. Patients undergoing cardiac catheterization and a variety of cardiac surgical procedures including coronary artery bypass, percutaneous transluminal valvuloplasty and coronary angioplasty, intra-aortic balloon pump, ventricular assist devices, and cardiac transplantation, are at risk for cerebral embolization. Strokes may also follow the use of the extracorporeal membrane oxygenator. Air embolism may complicate cardiopulmonary bypass surgery. Fat and air embolism may also follow manipulation of the heart and chest during surgery.[34,35] Advanced age, prior stroke, severe atherosclerosis of the ascending aorta, history of congestive heart failure, postoperative atrial fibrillation, and cardiopulmonary bypass time greater than 2 h increase the risk of perioperative stroke.[36–38]

Prolonged parenteral bactericidal antibiotics are the mainstay of treatment of infective endocarditis; cardiac surgery may be required in selected instances. Endocarditis prophylaxis is recommended for patients with MVP and associated mitral regurgitation. Prompt surgical resection is indicated for patients with atrial myxomas. Selective surgical repair is indicated for major ASDs. Transcatheter techniques for closure of these defects have been proposed. Optimal treatment of paradoxical embolism associated with PFO or ASA is currently unknown.[39–43]

NON-ATHEROSCLEROTIC CEREBRAL VASCULOPATHIES

Many non-atherosclerotic cerebral vasculopathies may produce cerebral infarction in young adults. The leading non-atherosclerotic vasculopathies are discussed.

Bilateral agenesis or aplasia of the carotid arteries is uncommon. In these cases the basilar artery supplies the anterior circulation via large posterior communicating arteries. Unilateral absence of the carotid artery may similarly be compensated by a large ipsilateral posterior communicating artery. Sometimes, in cases of unilateral absence of the carotid artery, the contralateral carotid artery may supply all major cerebral vessels including both posterior cerebral arteries. Hypoplastic vertebral arteries are more commonly seen. The vertebral arteries are often asymmetric in size and the right vertebral is usually hypoplastic. In some cases of bilateral vertebral artery hypoplasia, the basilar artery may receive most of the blood supply from the carotid artery via an enlarged persistent trigeminal artery. Some authors speculate that cerebral arterial anomalies may be an important association in cerebral malformations.[44–47]

Kinks, coils, and other forms of tortuosity of the carotid artery result from its redundant length with an estimated 16% incidence in the general population. Kink is an angulation of one or more segments of the internal carotid artery associated with a stenosis of the affected segment. Coiling of the internal carotid artery is due to elongation and redundancy and results in an exaggerated S-shaped curve or circular configuration. Cerebral ischemia may be due to a combination of factors such as obstruction, neck rotation, and microembolization. These anomalies may become pronounced with aging and pose unsuspected risk to the surgeon.[48,49] Surgical treatment has been proposed in some instances.[50]

CERVICOCEPHALIC ARTERIAL DISSECTIONS

Cervicocephalic arterial dissections are an important cause of stroke in children and young adults. Most dissections involve the extracranial internal carotid artery. Vertebrobasilar and intracranial carotid artery dissections are less common. The recurrence rate of cervicocephalic dissections is approximately 1% per year. The risk of recurrent dissections is increased in younger patients and in patients with a family history of arterial dissections.[51–61]

Cervicocephalic arterial dissections have been reported after blunt or penetrating trauma and chiropractic manipulation. Although the trauma itself may be trivial, intraoral and peritonsillar trauma is an important cause of stroke in children. They have also been associated with fibromuscular dysplasia, Marfan syndrome, Ehlers–Danlos syndrome type IV, coarctation of the aorta, cystic medial necrosis, atherosclerosis, extreme vessel tortuosity, moyamoya, pharyngeal infections, syphilitic arteritis, α1-antitrypsin deficiency, sympathomimetic drug abuse, and lentiginosis. Not infrequently, they occur spontaneously. Dissection of the cervicocephalic vessels may cause transient retinal, hemispheric, or posterior fossa ischemia, Horner's syndrome, hemicrania, cranial nerve palsies, cerebral infarction, or subarachnoid hemorrhage.[62–65]

Cervicocephalic arterial dissections are often misdiagnosed and underevaluated. Dissection should be considered in the differential diagnosis of transient ischemic attacks (TIAs) or cerebral infarction in any young adult, particularly when traditional risk factors are absent. Diagnosis is based on arteriographic findings. High resolution magnetic resonance imaging (MRI) and magnetic resonance angiography (MRA) provide valuable non-invasive information and are increasingly replacing cerebral angiography in many centers.

Based on anecdotal evidence, treatment of cervicocephalic arterial dissections has included anticoagulation with intravenous unfractionated heparin followed by warfarin. However, as the value of anticoagulation therapy is unclear and controversial, platelet antiaggregants are frequently used instead by many physicians. Surgical correction has been proposed for selected patients who have failed to respond to medical therapy. Surgery used in the treatment of cervicocephalic arterial dissections includes proximal ligation, trapping procedures, and extracranial–intracranial bypass procedures. Stents have been successfully used in some patients.[62]

TRAUMATIC CEREBROVASCULAR DISEASE

Traumatic cerebrovascular disease is often overlooked. Severe shaking of an infant may result in subdural hematomas, a major cause of severe morbidity and mortality in child abuse cases.[66] Penetrating cervical injuries may cause bleeding from the carotid and vertebral arteries, as well as jugular veins. Traumatic cerebrovascular disease may also result in arterial and venous sinus thromboses, arterial tear or rupture, arterial dissection, traumatic aneurysm, or arteriovenous fistulae.[67] Children may be prone to carotid artery injuries by a lollipop or pencil in the region of the tonsillar fossa with resultant thrombosis or dissection. Vertebrobasilar artery dissection due to cervical trauma is an under-recognized etiology of stroke in children.[68] Carotid artery laceration and delayed fusiform dilation may also follow surgery for suprasellar lesions.[69] Surgical embolization or repair is required for traumatic arteriovenous fistulae.

MOYAMOYA

Moyamoya disease is a chronic, occlusive, noninflammatory arteriopathy, of largely unknown etiology. The disorder is characterized primarily by arterial narrowing of the distal internal carotid arteries and proximal portion of the anterior and middle cerebral arteries (i.e., the carotid fork), with secondary development of a fine collateral vascular network at the base of the brain. Pathologically, there is fibrocellular thickening of the intima, waving of the internal elastic lamina, and attenuation of the media.[70] Elevated levels of fibroblastic growth factor (FGF) may play a critical role in its pathogenesis. Increased levels of FGF have been found in the cerebrospinal fluid. A strong FGF receptor immunoreactivity has also been demonstrated in superficial temporal vessels in patients with moyamoya.[71–73]

The condition is most common among the Japanese, Chinese, and Korean population, but has been reported in all ethnic groups. The disease, seen in both children and adults, has a bimodal age distribution with a peak in the first and fourth decades of life, with a female to male ratio of approximately 1.8. Half of the affected patients present before 10 years of age and familial occurrence has been reported.[74] Moyamoya has been found among identical twins and has been associated with certain human leukocyte antigen (HLA) haplotypes, including the B40 HLA antigen in patients younger than 10 years of age, and with the B52 HLA antigen in those older than 10 years. Moyamoya has also been associated with the AW24, BW46, B51-DR4, and the BW54 antigens.[75]

Some moyamoya cases have been associated with neonatal anoxia, trauma, basilar meningitis, tuberculous meningitis, leptospirosis, cranial irradiation therapy for optic pathway gliomas, neurofibromatosis, tuberous sclerosis, brain tumors, fibromuscular dysplasia, polyarteritis nodosa, Marfan's syndrome, pseudoxanthoma elasticum, hypomelanosis of Ito, William's syndrome, cerebral dissecting and saccular aneurysms, sickle cell anemia, β thalassemia, Fanconi anemia, Apert's syndrome, factor XII deficiency, type I glycogenosis, NADH-coenzyme Q reductase deficiency, renal artery stenosis, Down's syndrome, and coarctation of the aorta.[70]

The following criteria have been proposed for the diagnosis of moyamoya disease: (1) stenosis or occlusion involving the region of the internal carotid artery bifurcation (CI), and proximal portions of the anterior cerebral artery (A1) and middle cerebral arteries (M1); (2) presence of unusual net-like ('puff of smoke') appearance of basal collateral arteries arising from the circle of Willis justifying the Japanese expression moyamoya); and (3) bilateral abnormalities. Occasionally, such abnormalities are found in association with a variety of other disease states as previously described and the angiographic abnormality is then termed moyamoya syndrome rather than moyamoya disease. The term probable moyamoya is used for cases when the moyamoya pattern is found on one side only, and none of the listed conditions is present.

Clinical manifestations depend upon the age of presentation. Children most often present with carotid artery territory TIAs or ischemic strokes. As the posterior half of the circle of Willis is less frequently involved, episodes of vertebrobasilar ischemia are rare, although posterior watershed ischemia leading to visual difficulties may go unnoticed by the patients or parents. Moyamoya may cause alternating hemiparesis, early morning headaches and nausea, seizures, involuntary (mostly choreiform) movements, intellectual decline, cerebral infarction, and intracranial hemorrhage. Hemodynamic paraparetic TIAs have been described in childhood moyamoya. Ischemic strokes are often multiple and recurrent, predominantly involving the carotid circulation. Infarctions may be superficial or deep and are often found in watershed territories. Ischemic symptoms may be preceded by hyperventilating activity leading to cerebral vasoconstriction and decreased cerebral blood flow. Seizures may be induced by crying. A characteristic finding on electroencephalography is a slowing of the background, 20–60 s after cessation of hyperventilation (rebuild-up phenomenon). However, as hyperventilation may also precipitate ischemic symptoms, it is best to avoid eliciting this phenomenon in patients with moyamoya. In adults, the most common symptoms are hemorrhagic, due to subarachnoid, subependymal, or intraventricular hemorrhage. Intracranial bleeding is rare among the Japanese.

Routine hematological, biochemical, and serological investigations are unrevealing, except for reports of elevated FGF in the cerebrospinal fluid. Diagnosis is based on a distinct arteriographic appearance characterized by bilateral stenosis of the distal internal carotid arteries extending to the proximal anterior, and middle cerebral arteries with frequent involvement of the circle of Willis and development of an extensive collateral network at the base of the brain fed by the supraclinoid carotid, posterior communicating, anterior choroidal, lateral and medial lenticulostriate arteries, premammillary, interpeduncular, thalamoperforators, thalamogeniculate, and medial and lateral posterior choroidal arteries. Other collaterals may arise from ethmoidal, meningeal, tentorial, and falxine vessels. Intracranial aneurysms associated with childhood moyamoya are rare. Three-dimensional computed tomographic angiography, post-contrast MRI, and MRA provide valuable information in moyamoya patients (Fig. 5.2). MRA is a useful screening tool in subjects at high risk for developing moyamoya. Transcranial Doppler sonography is valuable in the diagnosis and postoperative follow-up of these patients. SPECT, especially with acetazolamide, may be useful in selecting patients likely to benefit from surgical intervention; PET may also provide useful information.[76–79]

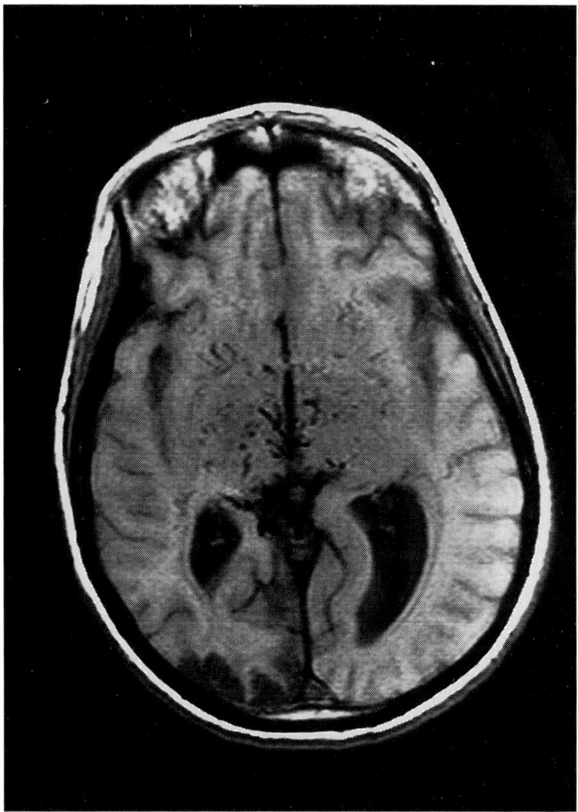

Figure 5.2 Axial T1-weighted MRI demonstrates pronounced flow voids involving the globus pallidus, putamen and thalami with evidence of marked dilatation of perforating vessels with large flow voids in a patient with moyamoya disease. Note is made of an incidental area of right occipital ischemia.

The optimal treatment for moyamoya disease has not yet been determined. Platelet antiaggregants, calcium channel blockers, corticosteroids, vasodilators, antifibrinolytics, and low-molecular weight dextran have been used. Surgical revascularization has been used in the management of the ischemic complications of childhood moyamoya. Good results have been reported with indirect and direct revascularization techniques. Surgery used in the treatment of moyamoya include encephalo-duro-arterio-synangiosis, encephalo-duro-arteriomyosynangiosis, encephalo-myosynangiosis, duro-encephalosynangiosis, durapexia, cerebro-arteriosynangiosis, pial synangiosis, intracranial omental transplantation, superficial temporal artery to middle cerebral artery anastomosis and other direct anastomoses, gracilis muscle transplantation, cervical perivascular sympathectomy and superior cervical ganglionectomy. Important preoperative, intraoperative and postoperative precautions include the avoidance of hypotension, intraoperative hypercapnia and hyperventilation.[80] Revascularization surgery is less useful in patients presenting with intracranial hemorrhage.[81]

FIBROMUSCULAR DYSPLASIA

Fibromuscular dysplasia (FMD) is a non-segmental, non-inflammatory, non-atheromatous angiopathy, usually confined to the renal arteries, and may also involve the cervicocephalic vessels. Its etiology is unknown, although smoking may be a contributing factor. An association with αl-antitrypsin deficiency has been described.[82] It is believed that FMD is usually inherited as an autosomal dominant trait. A clinical syndrome has been described in several FMD patients, characterized by headaches, tinnitus, vertigo, hypertension, ECG abnormalities, TIAs, cardiac arrhythmia, and syncope.[83,84]

Cervicocephalic FMD usually involves the extracranial internal carotid arteries at the level of the C1 and C2 vertebrae, and has also been associated with an increased frequency of intracranial aneurysms. Bilateral extracranial internal carotid artery involvement is common, while intracranial carotid or vertebrobasilar compromise is rare. Most patients are middle-aged (40–50 years old) women. Symptoms of cervicocephalic FMD are diverse and include headaches, hemicrania, carotidynia, tinnitus, vertigo, amaurosis fugax, and Horner's syndrome. Thromboembolic complications may result in TIAs or cerebral infarction. Cervicocephalic arterial dissection is a well-recognized complication. Subarachnoid hemorrhage, exceedingly rare in children, or intracerebral hematoma, may complicate the presence of an intracranial aneurysm or renovascular hypertension. Arterial hypertension may reflect concomitant renal FMD. However, most patients remain asymptomatic. The diagnosis is made by cerebral angiography, which typically shows a string of beads appearance. Less commonly, unifocal or multifocal tubular stenosis may be seen.

The optimal treatment of symptomatic cervicocephalic FMD has not been determined. Medical treatment has been attempted with platelet antiaggregants or anticoagulants. Surgical intervention is seldom warranted. Attempts have been made with a variety of techniques, including endarterectomy with balloon dilation, extracranial–intracranial bypass, excision of fibromuscular tissue with primary anastomosis, or patch grafting. Percutaneous transluminal carotid angioplasty has been successfully used in some patients.[85,86]

CEREBRAL VASCULITIS

Cerebral vasculitis should be considered when the stroke is recurrent, associated with encephalopathic changes or accompanied by fever, weight loss, fatigue, arthralgias, myalgias, palpable purpura or other skin lesions, renal disease, multifocal neurological signs, anemia, hematuria, or elevated sedimentation rate.

Cerebral vasculitis is an uncommon etiology of stroke in children and young adults. Schoenberg *et al.* found no case of vasculitis in children younger than 14 years of age reflecting the rarity of vasculitis as a cause of stroke in preteen children.[87] This inference must be tempered with the realization that infectious vasculitides are an important cause of stroke in children, especially in populations with a high incidence of infectious diseases involving the central nervous system.

Infectious cerebral vasculitides may be due to bacterial, mycobacterial, spirochetal, rickettsial, viral, fungal or protozoal infections. Brain infarcts are common among children with bacterial meningitis[88] and the acute phase of a purulent meningitis may be complicated by intracranial arteritis and thrombophlebitis. Cerebral infarction should be suspected in infants with protracted seizures and severe hypoglycorrhachia. Tuberculosis is a major health problem in developing countries. Histologically, tuberculosis angiitis is a granulomatous panarteritis. CT or MRI scan in patients with tuberculous meningitis may show basilar exudates, cerebral infarction in the distribution of the thalamoperforates and lenticulostriate arteries, and occasionally a tuberculoma. Stenosis and occlusion of the supraclinoid portion of the internal carotid artery and proximal segments of the anterior cerebral and middle cerebral arteries may be seen on cerebral angiogram.

With the resurgence of syphilis, there is an increased likelihood of diagnosing meningovascular syphilis. In some populations meningovascular syphilis may account for 10–15% of strokes in young patients. Syphilitic arteritis is an obliterative endarteritis resulting in vascular occlusion and infarction. Cerebral angiogram may show arteritic features of large and small blood vessels. Vasculitis is an infrequent occurrence in Lyme disease, caused by the spirochete *Borrelia burgdorferi.*

Viruses may induce vasculitis by direct replication within the blood vessel wall or by the presence of circulating immune complexes. Cerebral infarction may be seen in chickenpox, coxsackie-9 virus infection, herpes zoster ophthalmicus (often after a latency of 4–8 weeks), herpes zoster maxillaris (delayed occipital infarct), and acquired immune deficiency syndrome related vasculitis).[89] Hemorrhagic complications are often due to thrombocytopenia or ruptured aneurysm in addition to vasculitis. Fungal cerebral vasculitis is most often seen in patients who are immunocompromised. Candidiasis, cryptococcosis, aspergillosis, coccidiodomycosis and mucormycosis may all cause fungal arteritis and subsequent cerebral infarction. Parasitic infections may sometimes cause angiitis. Trichinosis, schistosomiasis and cysticercosis are some examples of such parasitic infections. Other infectious causes of cerebral infarct include *Mycoplasma pneumoniae* and cat-scratch disease.

Cerebral infarcts and cerebral hemorrhages are also seen in patients who abuse drugs, such as amphetamines, cocaine, heroin, phenylpropanolamine, ephedrine, lysergic acid diethylamide (LSD), phencyclidine (PCP), and glue sniffing. Stroke may also follow inadvertent intra-arterial injection of methylphenidate. Patients who intravenously inject pentazocine and tripelennamine may also suffer from stroke. In a study of an urban population, illicit drug use was found in 12.1% of young adult stroke patients and was thought to be the probable cause of stroke in 4.7% of patients. Multiple mechanisms, mostly vascular in nature, may be important in ischemic stroke associated with illicit drug use. Putative mechanisms include transient cerebral vasoconstriction, unmasking of pre-existing cardiovascular disease, vasculitis and prothrombotic tendencies. Symptoms may follow soon after drug administration or they may be delayed for 2–3 weeks after exposure to the drug.[90]

Cerebral infarcts and cerebral hemorrhage may be seen in a variety of conditions where immune abnormalities have been implicated such as Behçet's disease, sarcoidosis, malignant atrophic papulosis (Kohlmeier–Degos), Sjögren's syndrome, ulcerative colitis, hemolytic–uremic syndrome, and polyarteritis nodosa. Strokes due to true immune mediated vasculitis in systemic lupus erythematosus are uncommon. A neurological complication rate of 1.1% was observed in a large series of patients with Kawasaki's disease. Henoch–Schönlein purpura, a hypersensitivity vasculitis of childhood, may rarely be complicated by cerebral infarction and intracranial hemorrhage.

Thromboangiitis obliterans (Buerger's disease) is a rare, segmental, inflammatory, obliterative angiopathy of unknown cause. The condition involves small and medium-sized arteries and veins, and often results in amputation of digits of the upper or lower extremities. It is suspected in young male smokers with a history of superficial migratory thrombophlebitis presenting with distal limb ischemia accompanied by digital gangrene. The disorder is characterized by remissions and exacerbations. Cerebral involvement is uncommon.[91]

Takayasu arteritis, known also as 'pulseless disease' or 'aortoarteritis', is a chronic non-atherosclerotic inflammatory arteriopathy of the aorta, its major branches and the pulmonary arteries. The cause is unknown, but an immune mechanism is suspected. The inflammatory process produces a localized periarteritis with multinucleated giant cells. The disease is suspected in young women of Asian, Mexican or native American ancestry. The disease develops insidiously causing stenosis, occlusion, aneurysmal dilation, or coarctation of the involved vessels. The disease has two phases; in the acute or pre-pulseless phase, non-specific systemic manifestations are present. Months or years later, the second or occlusive phase develops and is characterized by multiple arterial occlusions. Patients may have cervical bruits, absent carotid or upper extremity pulses, asymmetric blood pressure recordings, and arterial hypertension. Neurological symptoms result from central nervous system or retinal ischemia associated with stenosis or occlusion of the aortic arch and arch vessels, or arterial hypertension due to aortic coarctation or renal artery stenosis. Laboratory findings include anemia, elevated erythrocyte sedimentation rate, and hypergammaglobulinemia.

Primary (granulomatous) CNS vasculitis, a necrotizing angiopathy of unknown etiology, is characterized by exclusive or predominant involvement of the CNS (brain and spinal cord). Arteries and veins are both involved. Patients may present with headaches, stroke-like symptoms, multifocal deficits, or with signs of a mass lesion. Cerebrospinal fluid analysis may be normal, or show a lymphocytic pleocytosis, increased protein, and normal glucose. Angiography may be normal, or show arterial beading or aneurysms. Brain and leptomeningeal biopsy is essential for diagnosis. Due to the focal nature of the vasculitis a negative biopsy does not exclude the diagnosis of isolated CNS vasculitis. Extensive evaluation is often necessary when dealing with a patient suspected of having cerebral vasculitis. Angiographic features of cerebral vasculitis are non-specific. CT, MRI, MRA and CSF studies are useful ancillary studies.

In most of the systemic vasculitides, rheumatological vasculitic syndromes, and primary CNS vasculitis, treatment involves the use of corticosteroids and cytotoxic agents. Pulse cyclophosphamide has been successfully used in the treatment of isolated angiitis of the CNS in children. Surgical intervention may be required in patients with Takayasu arteritis and severe cerebral hypoperfusion once the arteritis is no longer active.

MIGRAINOUS INFARCTION AND OTHER VASOSPASTIC DISORDERS

Migrainous infarction is a rare event considering the high prevalence of migraine in the general population.

Recent epidemiological studies suggest a non-random association of both headache and migraine with stroke, particularly among young women.[92] This rare association was limited to women below the age of 35 in a large Italian case-controlled study.[93] The possible association between migraine headache and stroke was also evaluated by the Physician's Health Study; physicians reporting migraine had increased risk of subsequent total stroke and ischemic stroke compared with those not reporting migraines.[94] Migraine may also increase the risk of ischemic stroke in young women, especially if they also have other risk factors such as smoking and use of oral contraceptives.[95,96]

The new International Headache Society (IHS) classification and diagnostic criteria for headache disorders, cranial neuralgias, and facial pain, requires that one or more migrainous aura symptoms must be present and not fully reversed within 7 days from onset and/or associated with neuroimaging confirmation of ischemic infarction to establish a diagnosis of migrainous infarction.[97] The pathogenesis of migrainous infarction is controversial. Cerebral infarctions complicating migraine are mostly cortical and involve the distribution of the posterior cerebral artery. Anterior circulation infarctions may also occur. Migrainous cerebral infarctions have been classified as definite when all the IHS criteria are fulfilled, and possible when some, but not all criteria are fulfilled.[98] Patients with migrainous cerebral infarction are thought to be at increased risk for recurrent stroke.[99] Intracranial hemorrhage during a migraine attack is extremely rare.

It is probably best to discontinue and avoid beta-blocking agents in those patients in whom a possible migrainous infarct occurs during their administration for prophylaxis. Although the benefits of calcium channel blockers for patients with migrainous infarcts has not been established, we use a combination of verapamil and aspirin if there are no contraindications. Use of triptans and ergotamine is not recommended.

Cerebral autosomal dominant arteriopathy with subcortical infarcts and leukoencephalopathy (CADASIL) is a familial, non-arteriosclerotic, non-amyloid arteriopathy, characterized by recurrent subcortical ischemic strokes starting in mid-adulthood leading to pseudobulbar palsy, subcortical dementia, and early MRI abnormalities. Individuals with CADASIL typically have strokes in their 30s or 40s. The disease has been mapped to chromosome 19q12 and mutations have been found in the Notch 3 gene. A subtype of migraine, known as familial hemiplegic migraine, has also been mapped close to the CADASIL locus.[100,101] Familial hemiplegic migraine has an age of onset between 5 and 30 years old. One gene known to cause familial hemiplegic migraine is the calcium ion gene on chromosome 19p13. The new acronym 'cerebral autosomal dominant arteriopathy with subcortical infarcts, leukoencephalopathy and migraine (CADASILM) refers to a subvariety of CADASIL characterized by the high frequency of migraine.[102] Brain or skin biopsy demonstration of osmiophilic material within the basement membrane of vascular smooth muscle cells is characteristic for this disease.[103–106]

Table 5.1 Primary (hereditary) hypercoagulable states

- Antithrombin-III deficiency
- Protein C deficiency
- Protein S deficiency
- Activated protein C resistance with or without factor V Leiden mutation
- Heparin cofactor II deficiency
- Disorders of fibrinogen
- Disorders of plasminogen
- Antiphospholipid antibodies

Table 5.2 Selective secondary (acquired) hypercoagulable states

- Malignancy
- Pregnancy/postpartum
- Oral contraceptives
- Ovarian hyperstimulation syndrome
- Other hormonal treatments
- Nephrotic syndrome
- Polycythemia vera
- Essential thrombocythemia
- Paroxysmal nocturnal thrombocytopenia
- Homocystinuria
- Hyperviscosity
- Congestive heart failure
- Sickle cell disease
- Thrombotic thrombocytopenic purpura
- Chemotherapeutic agents

HYPERCOAGULABLE DISORDERS

Alterations in hemostasis are associated with an increased risk of cerebrovascular events, particularly those of an ischemic nature. These disorders account for 1% of all stroke patients, and for 2–7% of young patients with ischemic stroke. Disruption of normal hemostasis may cause a primary (hereditary) or secondary (acquired) prothrombotic state (Tables 5.1 and 5.2). Conceptually, a hypercoagulable state may be regarded as resulting from an imbalance between prothrombotic and antithrombotic forces. These disorders may lead to recurrent episodes of deep venous thrombosis, migratory thrombophlebitis (Trousseau's syndrome), pulmonary embolism, cerebral infarction, cerebral venous thrombosis or thromboses at unusual sites. The common sites of thrombosis are the deep leg and pelvic veins. Arterial thromboses may result from endothelial damage, abnormal vascular flow, or increased platelet activation.

PRIMARY HYPERCOAGULABLE STATES

Inherited disorders predisposing to thrombosis especially affect the venous circulation. These disorders include antithrombin (AT)-III deficiency, protein C and S deficiencies, activated protein C (APC) resistance, abnormalities of fibrinogen (dysfibrinogenemia), and abnormalities of plasminogen or tissue plasminogen activator. About half of all thrombotic episodes occur spontaneously, although these patients are at greatest risk when exposed to additional risk factors such as pregnancy, trauma, or use of oral contraceptives.[107,108]

Antithrombin III deficiency

Antithrombin-III (AT-III) deficiency is inherited in an autosomal dominant fashion. There are two major categories of inherited AT-III deficiency. The majority of affected kindreds have type I (classic), characterized by decreased immunological and biological activity of AT-III. The type II (functional) is characterized by low biological activity of AT-III but essentially normal immunological activity. Thrombotic manifestations occurring in adolescence are often recurrent, and involve especially the deep veins of the lower extremities, pelvic veins, or mesenteric veins. The arterial system is less frequently involved.[109–111] Acquired AT-III deficiency has been associated with the nephrotic syndrome, liver cirrhosis, the use of oral contraceptives, L-asparaginase, tamoxifen, and heparin sodium, or it may follow an acute thrombotic event or disseminated intravascular coagulation. Antithrombin III deficient patients may be 'heparin resistant'. Acute thrombotic episodes in patients with mild AT-III deficiency often respond to heparin anticoagulation followed by long-term warfarin therapy. Adjunctive AT-III concentrates, combination of plasma and heparin, and thrombolytics have been used.

Protein C deficiency

Thrombotic manifestations associated with protein C deficiency are predominantly venous and often manifest in the young age group. Arterial strokes are uncommon.[112–114] Acquired protein C deficiency has been associated with the administration of L-asparaginase, liver disease, disseminated intravascular coagulation, postoperative care, and the adult respiratory distress syndrome. Coumarin-induced skin necrosis is a serious potential complication in heterozygous protein C deficient patients at the initiation of warfarin therapy. Homozygous protein C deficiency presents as purpura fulminans neonatalis. Thrombotic complications in heterozygous protein C deficient patients respond to heparin anticoagulation. Treatment is followed by incremental doses of warfarin, starting at a low dose which is often gradually increased.

Protein S deficiency

Homozygous protein S deficient patients present with venous thromboembolic disease. Heterozygotes are prone to recurrent venous and possibly arterial thromboses, including cerebral venous thrombosis. Thrombotic manifestations become apparent in the young age group. Acquired protein S deficiency occurs during pregnancy, in association with acute thromboembolic episodes, disseminated intravascular coagulation, nephrotic syndrome, systemic lupus erythematosus, and with the administration of oral contraceptives, and L-asparaginase. Treatment of thrombotic complications associated with protein S deficiency consists of heparin anticoagulation during the acute phase followed by chronic administration of warfarin therapy.

Activated protein C resistance

Activated protein C (APC) resistance has been reported with increasing frequency among patients with venous thromboembolism.

Precipitating factors for thrombosis are frequently encountered, in particular, pregnancy and the use of oral contraceptives. APC resistance is seen as a poor anticoagulant response of the patient's plasma to APC in an aPTT assay. This is due to a mutation in factor V that accounts for the resistance to the action of APC. The responsible mutation in most cases involves the substitution of arginine 506 to glutamine 506 (Arg506Gln). This mutation is common in the Caucasian population but not among the African-American population.[115]

Heparin cofactor II deficiency

Decreased levels of heparin cofactor II have been found in patients with disseminated intravascular coagulation and liver disease. Inherited deficiencies of heparin cofactor II have been described in several families.

Fibrinogen abnormalities

In men, the risk of stroke increases with increased fibrinogen levels. Congenital afibrinogenemia may cause central nervous system bleeding. Treatment consists of infusions of cryoprecipitate. Congenital or acquired hypofibrinogenemia and dysfibrinogenemias may be associated with hemorrhagic as well as thrombotic events. Transient dysfibrinogenemia may follow chemotherapy for acute lymphoblastic leukemia. Decreased concentrations of fibrinogen have been found in association with disseminated intravascular coagulation, liver failure, snake bite, treatment with L-asparaginase, ancrod, fibrinolytic drugs, and valproic acid.

Plasminogen abnormalities

Recent studies suggest that high plasma levels of tissue plasminogen activator (tPA) and its inhibitor (plasminogen activator inhibitor 1, PAI-1) are markers of an increased risk of ischemic stroke. Thrombotic disease has also been associated with hypoplasminogenemia, dysplasminogenemia and impaired plasminogen activator release.[116]

Antiphospholipid antibodies

Although lupus anticoagulant (LA) and anticardiolipin antibodies (aCL) are both antiphospholipid antibodies, they are distinct from one another. The lupus anticoagulant (LA) is an acquired circulating immunoglobulin, either IgG, IgM, or IgA, that interferes with the activation of prothrombin by the activator complex (factor Xa, V, calcium, and phospholipid). A high IgG antiphospholipid antibody (aPL) titer is an independent risk factor for first ischemic stroke in patients of all ages. A distinct group of patients exhibiting both venous and arterial thrombotic events has recently been defined as having a 'primary' antiphospholipid syndrome. Antiphospholipid antibodies are associated with recurrent fetal loss, thrombocytopenia, a false-positive Venereal Disease Research Laboratories (VDRL), and livedo reticularis. Multiple cerebral infarctions are common in patients with aPL; a subset of patients may present with vascular dementia. Still another group may have an acute ischemic encephalopathy or a catastrophic antiphospholipid antibody syndrome.

Pathological studies of cerebral arteries involved in association with aPL demonstrate the presence of a thrombotic vasculopathy, but no evidence of vasculitis. Patients with aPL have also been reported to have an increased frequency of cardiac valvular lesions. An association with mitral and aortic regurgitation is now recognized and findings resembling verrucous endocarditis (Libman–Sacks) have been noted. However, the pathophysiological mechanisms by which aPL causes a prothrombotic state remain unknown. The notion has evolved that the prothrombotic state associated with aPL is probably multifactorial. It may relate to inhibition of prostacyclin formation which allows thromboxane-A2 to function unopposed, decreased production of AT-III, or inhibition of protein C activation. These antibodies may also affect platelets directly by binding to phospholipids in the platelet wall, thus enhancing platelet adhesion and aggregation. Additionally, aPL may limit the production of endothelium-derived relaxing factor.

Optimal treatment of antiphospholipid antibody syndrome is unclear. Patients primarily have a thrombophilic state with venous and arterial thrombosis. Antiplatelet agents and anticoagulation treatments have been used. Long-term anticoagulation aiming for an international normalized ratio (INR) of about 3 seems an effective approach in reducing the risk of thrombotic complications.[117] Children need special precautions during anticoagulation therapy and close follow-up is necessary.[118–120] There have also been several reports of the efficacy of intravenous immunoglobulin (IVIG) therapy. This has been especially helpful in cases of recurrent pregnancy losses.[121–123]

SECONDARY HYPERCOAGULABLE STATES

Malignancy

Hypercoagulability, non-bacterial thrombotic endocarditis, non-metastatic cerebral venous thrombosis, tumor emboli, radiation-induced atherosclerosis, arterial compression by tumor, and cerebral angiitis account for a large number of cases of cerebral infarction in patients with underlying malignancies.[124] In a study of 200 pediatric patients with systemic malignancy, 25 had neurological complications, and three had cerebrovascular events.[125] Hyperviscosity syndrome complicating multiple myeloma and Waldenström's macroglobulinemia can rarely cause stroke.

Pregnancy

The risks of both cerebral infarction and intracerebral hemorrhage are increased in the 6 weeks after delivery, but not during pregnancy.[126] Characteristically, arterial causes of stroke are more common during pregnancy, whereas venous causes of stroke are more common during the puerperium. Eclampsia remains the leading cause of both intracerebral hemorrhage and non-hemorrhagic stroke. During normal pregnancy there is an increase in blood volume and in many clotting factors: increased platelet adhesion, increased fibrinogen, increased factors VII, VIII, IX, and X, and decreased fibrinolysis, with reduced levels of available plasminogen activator. The level of protein S falls, whereas the level of protein C is unmodified. During the last trimester, plasma levels of fibrinopeptide A are slightly elevated. Because warfarin-induced embryopathy is a major risk during the first trimester, therapy for thromboembolism is always with heparin, at least during the first trimester. Breast feeding is not contraindicated with either heparin or warfarin therapy.

Oral contraceptives

Early epidemiological studies demonstrate an increased risk for stroke in women who used oral contraceptives containing more than 50 μg of ethinyl estradiol. Although there appears to be a small relative risk of stroke in healthy women currently using oral contraceptives, the relative risk of stroke is increased particularly with coexistent history of arterial hypertension and cigarette smoking.[127]

Despite the advent of newer oral contraceptives with low-dose estrogen, it remains unclear whether they are safe if the women are also smokers. As part of stroke prevention, women who smoke should not use oral contraceptives.

Ovarian hyperstimulation syndrome

Cerebral infarction and venous thromboses can follow the ovarian hyperstimulation syndrome after induction of ovulation with 'fertility drugs' such as clomiphene.[128] Cerebral ischemia has also been reported with the administration of hormonal therapy to transsexuals, after the use of anabolic steroids for the treatment of hypogonadism and hypoplastic anemias, and with the use of human recombinant erythropoietin in the treatment of anemia of hemodyalized patients.

Nephrotic syndrome

Nephrotic syndrome is diagnosed when generalized edema coexists with pathological proteinuria exceeding 3 g per 24 h and hypoalbuminemia. Patients with nephrotic syndrome are prone to thrombotic complications; arterial and venous infarctions may occur. These patients often have thrombocytosis, elevated fibrinogen levels, factors V, VII, and VIII, and $\alpha 2$ macroglobulin. AT-III and protein S levels are decreased. Anticoagulant therapy is recommended for those patients with thrombotic complications.[129]

Selective myeloproliferative disorders

Primary or essential polycythemia is rare in children. Secondary polycythemia is seen in association with a variety of renal disorders, tissue hypoxia, and an array of conditions associated with non-physiological erythropoietin production. Thrombotic complications, especially large vessel cerebral thrombosis, are common. Hemorrhagic stroke and spinal cord infarction are infrequent complications. Treatment includes phlebotomy, plateletpheresis, myelosuppressive therapy, and platelet antiaggregants.[130]

Paroxysmal nocturnal hemoglobinuria

Cerebral venous, and less often, cerebral arterial thrombosis may occur in patients with paroxysmal nocturnal hemoglobulinuria (PNH). Thrombotic complications may be treated with thrombolytics or anticoagulants.

Diabetes mellitus

Diabetes mellitus increases the risk of ischemic cerebrovascular disease two- to four-fold compared with the risk in non-diabetics. In addition, diabetes mellitus increases morbidity and mortality after stroke. The mechanisms of stroke secondary to diabetes may be due to cerebrovascular atherosclerosis, cardiac embolism, or abnormalities of blood rheology. High insulin levels increase the risk for atherosclerosis, and may represent a pathogenetic factor in cerebral small-vessel disease.[131]

Heparin-induced thrombocytopenia

Patients who develop type II heparin-induced thrombocytopenia may develop venous or arterial thromboses. Treatment requires prompt discontinuation of heparin, and the administration of ancrod or the low molecular weight heparinoid ORG 10172.

Homocystinuria

High homocysteine levels have potentially deleterious effects on endothelium, platelets, and smooth muscle cells. A trend towards multiple infarctions and a higher rate of lesions typical of cerebral microangiopathy has been observed in patients with hyperhomocysteinemia. Elevated levels of homocysteine can be effectively reduced with the administration of folate, occasionally requiring the addition of pyridoxine (vitamin B_6), cobalamine (vitamin B_{12}), choline or betaine. Conversely, serum folate concentrations ≤ 9.2 nmol/l have been associated with elevated plasma levels of homocysteine and the suggestion has been made that a low folate concentration may be a risk factor for ischemic stroke, particularly among African-Americans.[132]

Sickle cell disease

Cerebrovascular disease is a major cause of morbidity and mortality in sickle cell disease. Strokes in sickle cell anemia (HbSS) patients, manifest as ischemic strokes in children and as intracerebral and subarachnoid hemorrhage in adults, but both types may be present in a single episode. Cerebral infarction is caused primarily by an occlusive arteriopathy involving the distal intracranial segments of the internal carotid artery, and proximal anterior and middle cerebral arteries. Some patients have transient ischemic attacks. Untreated patients may have a mortality as high as 20%, and 70% of those who survive have a stroke recurrence, usually within the initial 3 years.[133]

The Stroke Prevention Trial in Sickle Cell Anemia (STOP) evaluated 130 children with sickle cell anemia and no history of stroke. Sixty-seven received standard exchange blood transfusion. Eleven (10 cerebral infarctions and one cerebral hemorrhage) strokes occurred among the standard care group, while only one ischemic stroke occurred among the transfused group. Maintenance of hemoglobin S concentration at a level $<30\%$ is effective in reducing the risk of cerebral infarction in children with sickle cells anemia.[134] Meticulous hydration, adequate oxygenation, and analgesia are also necessary.

METABOLIC DISORDERS

Strokes and stroke-like manifestations have been reported in several metabolic disorders, but only those neurometabolic disorders apt to cause vasculopathies or strokes, relevant to a pediatric practice are discussed in this section. Three specific deficiencies responsible for homocystinuria have been identified: cystathionine β synthase deficiency, homocysteine methyltransferase, and 5, 10-methylene tetrahydrofolate reductase.

Fabry disease (angiokeratoma corporis diffusum) is an X-linked recessive disorder of glycosphingolipid metabolism characterized by deficient lysomal α galactosidase A activity. The gene coding for α galactosidase A activity is located at Xq22.1. As a result, deposits of ceramide trihexosidase accumulate in endothelial and smooth muscle cells especially in the corneas, blood vessels, and central, peripheral, and autonomic nervous systems. Patients have corneal opacifications and recurrent episodes of painful burning dysesthetic peripheral neuropathy, fever, abdominal pain, hypohydrosis and other manifestations of autonomic dysfunction, renal disease, arterial hypertension secondary to renal involvement, cardiac conduction abnormalities, myocardial ischemia, and cardiomegaly. Characteristic dark-red or blue lesions, that do not blanch on pressure, called angiokeratoma corporis diffusum, are found between the umbilicus and knees. Endothelial cell proliferation causing small-vessel obstruction and microaneurysm formation may lead to multiorgan ischemia, especially affecting the brain and heart. The cardiac abnormalities may also result in brain embolism. Female carriers may have mild disease or be asymptomatic.

Menkes disease (kinky hair disease, steely hair disease) is a multifocal disorder associated with a defect in the intestinal absorption of copper. Serum copper and ceruloplasmin are very low. The brain and liver copper content are reduced, while the copper content in the intestinal mucosa is increased. The disease is inherited as an X-linked trait; the mutant gene has been located on the X chromosome in the q13.3 region. Affected infants have abnormal, colorless, twisted (pili torti) and friable hair and eyebrows. Focal or generalized seizures, hypotonia, and hypothermia are often present. Menkes disease can present with subdural hematomas. Cerebral arteriography and magnetic resonance angiography usually reveal tortuous, irregular, and elongated intracranial vessels. Multiple arterial occlusions can develop.

Patients with Tangier disease develop premature atherosclerosis. Tangier disease is an autosomal recessive disorder characterized by the deficiency or absence of high density lipoprotein in plasma. Serum cholesterol is low, and triglycerides are normal or elevated. Cardiovascular involvement is thought to be related to the deposition of cholesterol esters.[135]

A mitochondrial disorder is a rare etiology of stroke in children, adolescents, or young adults. Mitochondrial encephalomyopathies should be suspected in patients with intractable seizures, recurrent strokes, lactic acidosis, or respiratory failure. The syndrome of mitochondrial encephalomyopathy, lactic acidosis, and stroke-like episodes (MELAS) is a non-mendelian maternally transmitted syndrome with multiple system involvement. Four point mutations have been found in association with MELAS, three mutations at nucleotide pairs 3243, 3250, and 3271, and one at the coding region for subunit 4 of complex 1.[136] The common MELAS mutation is at the base pair 3243. After normal development, clinical manifestations of MELAS include periods of confusion, dementia, episodic vomiting, migraine-like headaches, and progressive hearing loss. Focal neurological involvement may present as sudden, transient or partially regressive attacks of hemiparesis, aphasia, hemianopia, ataxia or cortical blindness. The episodes may be precipitated by a febrile illness. Other features include lactic acidosis, short stature, muscle weakness, ragged red fibers, and exercise intolerance. The stroke-like episodes have a propensity for the posterior brain regions and occur before the age of 40. The lesions do not always conform to arterial territories (Fig. 5.3).

GENETIC DISORDERS

Marfan's syndrome is an autosomal dominant inherited connective tissue disease associated with qualitative and quantitative defects of fibrillin. Molecular analyses have identified more than 30 mutations. This disorder is characterized by a variety of skeletal, ocular, and cardiovascular abnormalities. Patients with Marfan's syndrome may display arachnodactyly, upward displacement of the lens, extreme limb length, joint laxity, pectus excavatum or carinatum, and aortic valvular insufficiency. Marfan's syndrome is associated with a high frequency of dilatation of the aortic root. Other cardiovascular abnormalities include coarctation of the aorta, mitral valve prolapse, and mitral annulus calcification with regurgitation. Progressive dilatation of the aortic root may lead to dissection of the ascending aorta resulting in ischemia of the brain, spinal cord, or plexus or peripheral nerves. Infective endocarditis can be a complicating feature, especially in patients who have mitral and/or aortic valve regurgitation,

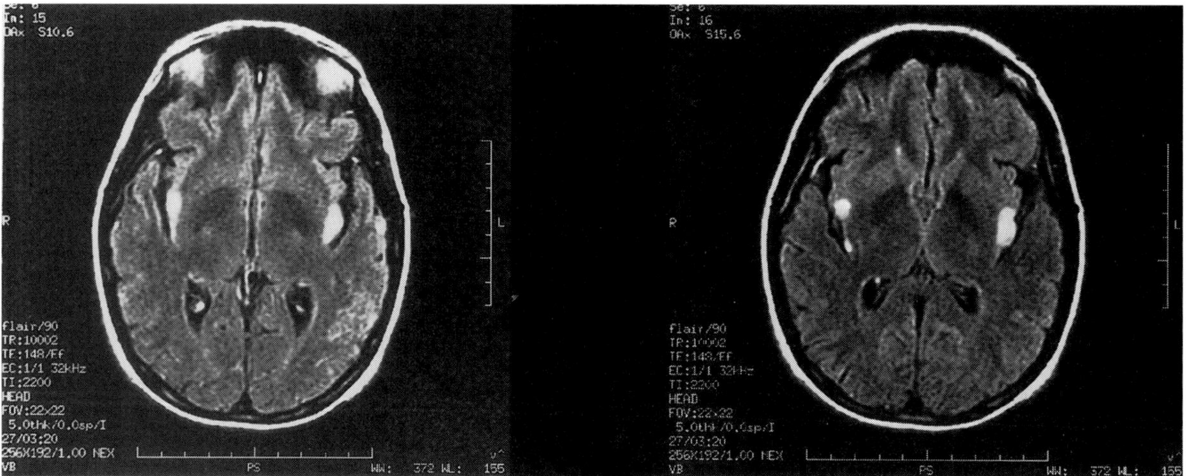

Figure 5.3 Axial FLAIR images of the brain demonstrate abnormal signal in both insular cortices in a patient with MELAS with a mutation at the base pair 3243.

and/or mitral valve prolapse. Saccular intracranial aneurysms or carotid artery dissections may also occur.

Patients with Ehlers–Danlos syndrome, an autosomal dominant defect of collagen synthesis, may display hyperextensibility of the skin, hypermobile joints, and vascular fragility leading to a bleeding diathesis.[137] Arterial complications have been reported in association with Ehlers–Danlos syndrome types I, III, and IV, and especially the latter. Diagnosis of patients with type IV Ehlers–Danlos syndrome, who usually lack the classical phenotypical manifestations, requires the demonstration of a specific defect in type III collagen synthesis. Arterial complications include dissections, arteriovenous fistulae, and intracranial aneurysms. Other cardiovascular abnormalities in patients with type IV Ehlers–Danlos syndrome include ventricular and atrial septal defects, aortic insufficiency, bicuspid aortic valve, mitral valve prolapse, and papillary muscle dysfunction. Arteriography carries special risks and should be avoided if possible.

Patients with pseudoxanthoma elasticum (PXE), often display loose skin and small, raised, orange-yellowish papules resembling 'plucked chicken skin' in intertriginous areas. Patients with PXE have a higher risk of coronary artery disease and myocardial infarction. Peripheral arterial involvement with vascular calcifications is common in patients with pseudoxanthoma elasticum; strokes are extremely rare except when there is concomitant hypertension. These patients may also have arterial hypertension, angioid streaks of the retina, retinal hemorrhages, arterial occlusive disease and arterial dissections. Intracranial aneurysms have been found in association with PXE. Women with PXE should avoid estrogens.

Neurofibromatosis type I (NF1 or von Recklinghausen's disease) is an autosomal dominant disorder with incomplete penetrance associated with a distinct chromosomal abnormality located on the long arm of chromosome 17 at locus 17q11.2. Half of the cases arise sporadically as new mutations. NF1 may be associated with occlusive cerebrovascular disease with extensive collateral channels in the basal ganglia and thalamus resembling moyamoya. Strokes in childhood due to severe hypertension associated with NF1 may occur.

Tuberous sclerosis (known also as Bourneville or Pringle's disease) is an autosomal dominant disease with cutaneous, visceral, ophthalmological, and neurological manifestations. Cerebral infarction due to cardiac rhabdomyomas, found in almost one-third of cases of tuberous sclerosis, has been reported, but hemiparesis is a rare symptom. Angiographic features resembling moyamoya and intracranial aneurysm have also been noted.

Sturge–Weber syndrome (known also as encephalotrigeminal angiomatosis or encephalo-oculoangiomatosis) is a non-hereditable disease characterized by a unilateral facial port-wine stain (nevus flammeus) over the distribution of the first and second divisions of the trigeminal nerve with contralateral hemiparesis and homonymous hemianopia, ipsilateral leptomeningeal angiomatosis, cortical calcifications, focal seizures and varying degrees of mental retardation. Facial hemihypertrophy may occur. Monocular buphthalmos (ox eye), choroidal angiomatosis, and secondary glaucoma are common.

MISCELLANEOUS DISORDERS

Susac's syndrome is an occlusive arteriolar microangiopathy involving brain, retina, and cochlea that occurs most often in young women.[138] Treatment options include antithrombotics, calcium channel blockers, corticosteroids or other immunomodulators, intravenous immunoglobulins, plasmapheresis and hyperbaric oxygen.

Eales' disease is a non-inflammatory vasoproliferative retinal perivasculitis characterized by repeated retinal and vitreous hemorrhages more prevalent in the Middle East and the Indian subcontinent. The condition predominantly affects healthy young men. Neurological complications are rare.[139]

Uncommon sources of embolism should be considered in selective cases of cerebral or multiorgan ischemia. Air embolism is a well-documented complication of cardiac surgery, neurosurgical procedures in the sitting position, hysterosalpingography, laparoscopic cholecystectomy, orthotopic liver transplantation, use of central venous catheters, hemodialysis catheters, intra-aortic balloon catheters, cerebral angiography, induced abortion, pneumothorax, undersea diving, and ingestion of hydrogen peroxide. Hyperbaric oxygen therapy is the recommended treatment of choice.[140] Fat embolism is a potentially serious complication of long bone fractures, sickle cell anemia, and autologous fat injection. Clinically, patients may exhibit neurological, pulmonary, and cutaneous manifestations.[141] Fat emboli may cause confusion, seizures and skin petechiae.

REFERENCES

1. Garg B, Durocher A, Biller J. Strokes in children and young adults. In: *Cerebrovascular Disorders* (Bogousslavsky J, Ginsberg M, eds), Vol. 2, pp. 850–73. Cambridge; Blackwell Science: 1997.
2. Walsh LE, Garg BP. Isolated acute subcortical infarctions in children. Clinical description and radiographic correlation [abstract]. *Ann Neurol* 1990; **28:**458.
3. Williams LS, Garg BP, Cohen M, Fleck JD, Biller J. Subtypes of ischemic stroke in children and young adults. *Neurology* 1997; **49:**1541–5.
4. Walsh LE, Garg BP. Ischemic strokes in children. *Indian J Pediatr* 1997; **64:**613–23.
5. Fieschi C, Rasura M, Anzini A *et al.* A diagnostic approach to ischemic stroke in young and middle-aged adults. *Eur J Neurol* 1996; **3:**324–30.
6. Riela A, Roach E. Etiology of stroke in children. *J Child Neurol* 1993; **8:**201–20.
7. Cardiogenic brain embolism. The second report of the Cerebral Embolism Task Force. *Arch Neurol* 1989; **46:**727–43.
8. Perloff JK. Neurologic disorders. In: *Congenital Heart Disease in Adults* (Perloff JK, Child JS, eds), 2nd edn, pp. 236–46. Philadelphia; WB Saunders Company: 1998.
9. Morriss MJH, McNamara DG. Coarctation of the aorta and interrupted aortic arch. In: *The Science and Practice of Pediatric Cardiology* (Garson A Jr, Bricker JT, Fisher DJ, Neish SR, eds), 2nd edn, vol. 1, pp. 1317–46. Baltimore; Williams and Wilkins: 1998.
10. Heutink P, Haitjema T, Breedveld GJ *et al.* Linkage of hereditary haemorrhagic telangiectasia to chromosome 9q34 and evidence for locus heterogeneity. *J Med Genet* 1994; **31:** 933–6.
11. du Plessis AJ, Chang AC, Wessel DL *et al.* Cerebrovascular accidents following the Fontan operation. *Pediatr Neurol* 1995; **12:**230–6.
12. Dobell A, Trusler GA, Smallhorn JF, Williams WG. Atrial thrombi after the Fontan operation. *Ann Thorac Surg* 1986; **42:**664–7.
13. Quinones JA, Deleon SY, Bell TJ *et al.* Fenestrated Fontan procedure: evolution of technique and occurrence of paradoxical embolism. *Pediatr Cardiol* 1997; **18:**218–21.
14. Day RW, Boyer RS, Tait VF, Ruttenberg HD. Factors associated with stroke following the Fontan procedure. *Pediatr Cardiol* 1995; **16:**270–5.
15. Wolf PA, Dawber TR, Thomas HE Jr, Kannel WB. Epidemiologic assessment of chronic atrial fibrillation and risk of stroke: the Framingham study. *Neurology* 1978; **28:**973–7.
16. Biller J, Love BB. Cardiac disorders and stroke in children and young adults. In: *Stroke in Children and Young Adults* (Biller J, ed.), pp. 86–101. Boston; Butterworth-Heinemann: 1994.
17. Congenital heart disease. In: *Nelson Textbook of Pediatrics* (Behrman RE, ed.), 14th edn, p. 1147. New York; Saunders: 1992.
18. Vongptanasin W, Hillis LD, Lange RA. Medical progress: prosthetic heart valves. *N Engl J Med* 1996; **345:**407–16.
19. Hart RG, Foster JW, Luther MF, Kanter MC. Stroke in infective endocarditis. *Stroke* 1990; **21:**695–700.
20. Biller J, Challa VR, Toole JF, Howard VJ. Nonbacterial thrombotic endocarditis. A neurologic perspective of clinicopathologic correlations of 99 patients. *Arch Neurol* 1982; **39:**95–8.
21. Kannel WB, Abbott RD, Savage DD, McNamara PM. Epidemiologic features of chronic atrial fibrillation—The Framingham Study. *N Engl J Med* 1982; **306:**1018–22.
22. Kanter RJ. Syncope and sudden death. In: *The Science and Practice of Pediatric Cardiology* (Garson A Jr, Bricker JT, Fisher DJ, Neish SR, eds), 2nd edn, vol. 2, pp. 2159–99. Baltimore; Williams and Wilkins: 1998.
23. Mohr JP, Albers GW, Amarenco P *et al.* American Heart Association Prevention

Conference. IV. Prevention and Rehabilitation of Stroke. Etiology of stroke. *Stroke* 1997; **28:**1501–6.

24. Tsukamoto S, Shiono M, Orime Y *et al.* Left atrial myxoma with an atrial septal defect: a case report and review of the literature. *Ann Thorac Cardiovasc Surg* 1998; **4:**133–7.
25. Bekavac I, Hanna JP, Wallace RC, Powers J, Ratliff NB, Furlan AJ. Intra-arterial thrombolysis of embolic proximal middle cerebral artery occlusion from presumed atrial myxoma. *Neurology* 1997; **49:**618–20.
26. Greeson DM, Wright JE, Zanolli MD. Cutaneous findings associated with cardiac myxomas. *Cutis* 1998; **62:**275–80.
27. Moss AJ, Adams FH Jr. Atrial septal defects. In: *Heart Disease in Infants, Children and Adolescents: Including the Fetus and Young Adults* (Emmanouilides GC, ed.), 5th edn, pp. 687–703. Baltimore; Williams and Wilkins: 1995.
28. Lechat P, Mas JL, Lascault G *et al.* Prevalence of patent foramen ovale in patients with stroke. *N Engl J Med* 1988; **318:**1148–52.
29. Hanna JP, Sun JP, Furlan AJ, Stewart WJ, Sila CA, Tan M. Patent foramen ovale and brain infarct. Echocardiographic predictors, recurrence, and prevention. *Stroke* 1994; **25:**782–6.
30. Bogousslavsky J, Garazi S, Jeanrenaud X, Aebischer N, Van Melle G. Stroke recurrence in patients with patent foramen ovale: the Lausanne Study. Lausanne Stroke with Paradoxal Embolism Study Group. *Neurology* 1996; **46:**1301–5.
31. Bogousslavsky J, Devuyst G, Nendaz M, Yamamoto H, Sarasin F. Prevention of stroke recurrence with presumed paradoxical embolism. *J Neurol* 1997; **244:**71–5.
32. Belkin RN, Hurwitz BJ, Kisslo J. Atrial septal aneurysm: association with cerebrovascular and peripheral embolic events. *Stroke* 1987; **18:**856–62.
33. Cabanes L, Mas JL, Cohen A *et al.* Atrial septal aneurysm and patent foramen ovale as risk factors for cryptogenic stroke in patients less than 55 years of age. A study using transesophageal echocardiography. *Stroke* 1993; **24:**1865–73.
34. Tuxen DV, Scheinkestel CD, Salamonson R. Air embolism—a neglected cause of stroke complicating cardiopulmonary bypass (CPB) surgery. *Aust NZ J Med* 1994; **24:**732–3.
35. Moody DM, Bell MA, Challa VR, Johnston WE, Prough DS. Brain microemboli during cardiac surgery or aortography. *Ann Neurol* 1990; **28:**477–86.
36. Adams HP Jr. Neurologic complications of cardiovascular procedures. In: *Iatrogenic Neurology* (Biller J, ed.), pp. 51–61. Boston; Butterworth-Heinemann: 1998.
37. Breuer AC, Furlan AJ, Hanson MR *et al.* Central nervous system complications of coronary artery bypass graft surgery: prospective analysis of 421 patients. *Stroke* 1983; **14:**682–7.
38. Sila CA, Furlan AJ. Neurological complications in patients with cardiovascular procedures. In: *Handbook of Cerebrovascular Diseases* (Adams HP Jr, ed.), pp. 171–89. New York; Marcel Dekker, Inc.: 1993.
39. Caplan LR. Prevention of cardioembolic stroke. *Heart Dis Stroke* 1994; **3:**297–303.
40. Cairns JA. Preventing systemic embolization in patients with atrial fibrillation. *Cardiol Clin* 1994; **12:**495–504.
41. Wilson DG, Wiseheart JD, Stuart AG. Systemic thromboembolism leading to myocardial infarction and stroke after fenestrated total cavopulmonary connection. *Br Heart J* 1995; **73:**483–5.
42. Ende DJ, Chopra RS, Rao PS. Transcatheter closure of atrial septal defect or patent foramen ovale with the buttoned device for prevention of recurrence of paradoxic embolism. *Am J Cardiol* 1996; **78:**233–6.
43. Guffi M, Bogousslavsky J, Jeanrenaud X, Devuyst G, Sadeghi H. Surgical prophylaxis of recurrent stroke in patients with patent foramen ovale: a pilot study. *J Thorac Cardiovasc Surg* 1996; **112:**260–3.
44. Lie TA. *Congenital Anomalies of the Carotid Arteries.* Amsterdam; Excerpta Medica Foundation: 1968.
45. Lhermitte F, Gautier JC, Poirier J, Tyrer JH. Hypoplasia of the internal carotid artery. *Neurology* 1968; **18:**439–46.
46. Smith RR, Kees CJ, Hogg JD. Agenesis of the internal carotid artery with an unusual primitive collateral. Case report. *J Neurosurg* 1972; **37:**460–2.
47. Vogel FS, McClehahan. Anomalies of major cerebral arteries associated with congenital malformations of the brain. *Am J Pathol* 1952; **28:**701–11.
48. Weibel J, Fields WS. Tortuosity, coiling, and kinking of the internal carotid artery. I. Etiology and radiographic anatomy. *Neurology* 1965; **15:**7–20.
49. Desai B, Toole JF. Kinks, coils, and carotids: a review. *Stroke* 1975; **6:**649–53.

50. Koskas F, Bahnini A, Walden R, Kieffer E. Stenotic coiling and kinking of the internal carotid artery. *Ann Vasc Surg* 1993; **7:** 530–40.
51. Ehrenfeld WK, Wylie EJ. Spontaneous dissection of the internal carotid artery. *Arch Surg* 1976; **111:**1294–301.
52. Fisher CM, Ojemann RG, Roberson GH. Spontaneous dissection of cervico-cerebral arteries. *Can J Neurol Sci* 1978; **5:**9–19.
53. Caplan LR, Zarins CK, Hematti M. Spontaneous dissection on the extracranial vertebral arteries. *Stroke* 1985; **16:**1030–8.
54. Mokri B, Houser OW, Sandok BA, Piepgras DG. Spontaneous dissections of the vertebral arteries. *Neurology* 1985; **38:**880–5.
55. Mokri B, Sundt TM Jr, Houser OW, Piepgras DG. Spontaneous dissection of the cervical internal carotid artery. *Ann Neurol* 1986; **19:** 126–38.
56. Biller J, Hingten WL, Adams HP Jr *et al.* Cervicocephalic arterial dissections: a ten year experience. *Arch Neurol* 1986; **43:**1234–8.
57. Bogousslavsky J, Despland PA, Regli F. Spontaneous carotid dissection with acute stroke. *Arch Neurol* 1987; **44:**137–40.
58. Mas JL, Bousser MG, Hasboun D, Laplane D. Extracranial vertebral artery dissections: a review of 13 cases. *Stroke* 1987; **18:**1037–47.
59. Caplan LR, Baquis GD, Pessin MS, D'Alton J. Dissection of the intracranial vertebral artery. *Neurology* 1988; **38:**868–77.
60. Patel H, Smith RR, Garg BP. Spontaneous extracranial carotid artery dissection in children. *Pediatr Neurol* 1995; **13:**55–60.
61. Schievink WI, Mokri B, Piepgras DG. Spontaneous dissections of cervicocephalic arteries in childhood and adolescence. *Neurology* 1994; **44:**1607–12.
62. Biller J. Non atherosclerotic vasculopathies. In: *Stroke in Children and Young Adults* (Biller J, ed.), pp. 57–81. Boston; Butterworth-Heinemann: 1994.
62. Rao TH, Schneider LB, Patel M, Libman RB. Central retinal artery occlusion from carotid dissection diagnosed by cervical computed tomography. *Stroke* 1994; **25:** 1271–2.
64. Schievink WI, Katzmann JA, Piepgras DG. Alpha-1-antitrypsin deficiency in spontaneous intracranial arterial dissections. *Cerebrovasc Dis* 1998; **8:**42–4.
65. van den Berg JS, Limburg M, Kappelle LJ, Pals G, Arwert F, Westerveld A. The role of type III collagen in spontaneous cervical arterial dissections. *Ann Neurol* 1998; **43:**494–8.
66. Duhaime AC, Christian CW, Rorke LB, Zimmerman RA. Nonaccidental head injury in infants—the 'shaken-baby syndrome'. *N Engl J Med* 1998; **338:**1822–9.
67. Komiyama M, Nakaima H, Nishikawa M, Kan M. Traumatic carotid carvernous sinus fistula: serial angiographic studies from the day of trauma. *Am J Neuroradiol* 1998; **19:**1641–4.
68. Garg BP, Ottinger CJ, Smith RR, Fishman MA. Strokes in children due to vertebral artery trauma. *Neurology* 1993; **43:**2555–8.
69. Sutton LN. Vascular complications of surgery for craniopharyngioma and hypothalamic glioma. *Pediatr Neurosurg* 1994; **21**(Suppl 1): 124–8.
70. Garg BP, Bruno A, Biller J. Moyamoya disease and cerebral ischemia. In: *Cerebrovascular Disease* (Batjer HH, ed.), pp. 489–99. Philadelphia; Lippincott-Raven Publishers: 1997.
71. Hojo M, Hoshimaru M, Miyamoto S *et al.* Role of transforming growth factor-beta 1 in the pathogenesis of moyamoya disease. *J Neurosurg* 1998; **89:**623–9.
72. Yoshimoto T, Houkin T, Takahashi A, Abe H. Angiogenic factors in moyamoya disease. *Stroke* 1996; **27:**2160–5.
72. Takahashi A, Sawamura Y, Houkin K, Kamiyama H, Abe H. The cerebropsinal fluid in patients with moyamoya disease (spontaneous occlusion of the circle of Willis) contains high level of basic fibroblast growth factor. *Neurosci Lett* 1993; **160:**214–6.
74. Hamada JI, Yoshioka S, Nakahara T, Marubayashi T, Ushio Y. Clinical features of moyamoya disease in sibling relations under 15 years of age. *Acta Neurochir* 1998; **140:**455–8.
75. Aoyagi M, Ogami K, Matsushima Y, Shikata M, Yamamoto M, Yamamoto K. Human leukocyte antigen in patients with Moyamoya disease. *Stroke* 1995; **26:**415–7.
76. Hasuo K, Mihara F, Matsushima T. MRI and MR angiography in moyamoya disease. *J Magn Reson Imag* 1998; **8:**762–6.
77. Nariai T, Senda M, Ishii K *et al.* Post-hyperventilatory steal response in chronic cerebral hemodynamic stress: a positron emission tomography study. *Stroke* 1998; **29:**1281–92.
78. Inoue Y, Momose T, Machida K, Honda N, Tsutsumi K. Cerebral vasodilatory capacity mapping using technetium-99m-DTPA-HSA SPECT and acetazolamide in moyamoya disease. *J Nucl Med* 1993; **34:**1984–6.

79. Kohno K, Oka Y, Kohno S, Ohta S, Kumon Y, Sakaki S. Cerebral blood flow measurement as an indicator for an indirect revascularization procedure for adult patients with moyamoya disease. *Neurosurgery* 1998; **42:** 752–7.
80. Sato K, Shirane R, Kato M, Yoshimoto T. Effect of inhalational anesthesia on cerebral circulation in Moyamoya disease. *J Neurosurg Anesthesiol* 1999; **11:**25–30.
81. Okada Y, Shima T, Nishida M, Yamane K, Yamada T, Yamanaka C. Effectiveness of superficial temporal artery–middle cerebral artery anastamosis in adult moyamoya disease: cerebral hemodynamics and clinical course in ischemic and hemorrhagic varieties. *Stroke* 1998; **29:**625–30.
82. Solder B, Streif W, Ellemunter H, Mayr U, Jaschke W. Fibromuscular dysplasia of the internal carotid artery in a child with alpha-1-antitrypsin deficiency. *Dev Med Child Neurol* 1997; **39:**827–9.
83. Mettinger KL, Ericson K. Fibromuscular dysplasia and the brain. I. Observations on angiographic, clinical, and genetic characteristics. *Stroke* 1982; **13:**46–52.
84. Schievink WI, Bjornsson J. Fibromuscular dysplasia of the internal carotid artery: a clinicopathological study. *Clin Neuropathol* 1996; **15:**2–6.
85. Moreau P, Albat B, Thevenet A. Fibromuscular dysplasia of the internal carotid artery: long-term surgical results. *J Cardiovasc Surg* 1993; **34:**465–72.
86. Chiche L, Bahnini A, Koskas F, Kieffer E. Occlusive fibromuscular disease of arteries supplying the brain: results of surgical treatment. *Ann Vasc Surg* 1997; **11:**496–504.
87. Schoenberg BS, Mellinger JF, Schoenberg DG. Cerebrovascular disease in infants and children: a study of incidence, clinical features, and survival. *Neurology* 1978; **28:**763–8.
88. Snyder RD, Stovring J, Cushing AH, Davis LE, Hardy TL. Cerebral infarction in childhood bacterial meningitis. *J Neurol Neurosurg Psychiatr* 1981; **44:**581–5.
89. Park YD, Belman AL, Kim TS *et al.* Stroke in pediatric acquired immunodeficiency syndrome. *Ann Neurol* 1990; **28:**303–11.
90. Sloan M, Kittner SJ, Feeser BR *et al.* Illicit drug-associated ischemic stroke in the Baltimore–Washington Young Stroke Study. *Neurology* 1998; **50:**1688–93.
91. Biller J, Asconapé J, Challa VR, Toole JF, McLean WT. A case for cerebral thromboangiitis obliterans. *Stroke* 1981; **12:**686–9.
92. Merikangas KR, Fenton BT, Cheng SH, Stolar MJ, Risch N. Association between migraine and stroke in a large-scale epidemiological study of the United States. *Arch Neurol* 1997; **54:**362–8.
93. Carolei A, Marini C, De Matteis G. History of migraine and risk of cerebral ischemia in young adults. The Italian National Research Council Study Group on Stroke in the Young. *Lancet* 1996; **347:**1503–6.
94. Buring JE, Hebert P, Romero J *et al.* Migraine and subsequent risk of stroke in the Physicians' Health Study. *Arch Neurol* 1995; **52:**129–34.
95. Tzourio C, Tehindrazanarivelo A, Iglesias S *et al.* Case–control study of migraine and risk of ischaemic stroke in young women. *Br Med J* 1995; **310:**830–3.
96. Becker WJ. Migraine and oral contraceptives. *Can J Neurol Sci* 1997; **24:**16–21.
97. Headache Classification of the International Headache Society: Classification and diagnostic criteria for headache disorders, cranial neuralgias, and facial pain. *Cephalalgia* 1998; **8**(Suppl 7):13.
98. Wober-Bingol C, Wober C, Karawauz A *et al.* Migraine and stroke in childhood and adolescence. *Cephalalgia* 1995; **15:**26–30.
99. Rothrock J, North J, Madden K, Lyden P, Fleck P, Dittrich H. Migraine and migrainous stroke: risk factors and prognosis. *Neurology* 1993; **43:**2473–6.
100. Joutel A, Bousser MG, Biousse V *et al.* A gene for familial hemiplegic migraine maps to chromosome 19. *Nature Genet* 1993; **5:**40–5.
101. Hutchinson M, O'Riordan J, Javed M *et al.* Familial hemiplegic migraine and autosomal dominant arteriopathy with leukoencephalopathy (CADASIL). *Ann Neurol* 1995; **38:**817–24.
102. Verin M, Rolland Y, Landgraf F *et al.* New phenotype of the cerebral autosomal dominant arteriopathy mapped to chromosome 19: migraine as the prominent clinical feature. *J Neurol Neurosurg Psych* 1995; **59:**579–85.
103. Chabriat H, Vahedi K, Iba-Zizen MT *et al.* Clinical spectrum of CADASIL: a study of 7 families. Cerebral autosomal dominant arteriopathy with subcortical infarcts and leukoencephalopathy. *Lancet* 1995; **346:**934–9.
104. Joutel A, Corpechot C, Ducros A *et al.* Notch3 mutations in cerebral autosomal dominant

arteriopathy with subcortical infarcts and leukoencephalopathy (CADASIL), a Mendelian condition causing stroke and vascular dementia. *Ann NY Acad Sci* 1997; **826:**213–7.

105. Desmond DW, Moroney JT, Lynch T *et al.* CADASIL in a North American family: clinical, pathologic, and radiologic findings. *Neurology* 1998; **51:**844–9.
106. Mellies JK, Bäumer T, Müller JA *et al.* SPECT study of a German CADASIL family: a phenotype with migraine and progressive dementia only. *Neurology* 1998; **50:**1715–21.
107. Bauer K. The hypercoagulable state. In: *Disorders of Hemostasis* (Ratnoff OD, Forges CD, eds), 3rd edn, pp. 269–91. Philadelphia; WB Saunders: 1996.
108. Hilgartner MW, Corrigan JJ Jr. Coagulation disorders. In: *Blood Diseases of Infancy and Childhood. In the Tradition of Carl H. Smith* (Miller DR, Baehner RL, eds), 7th edn, pp. 924–86. St Louis; Mosby: 1995.
109. Ueyama H, Hashimoto Y, Uchino M *et al.* Progressing ischemic stroke in a homozygote with variant antithrombin III. *Stroke* 1989; **20:**815–8.
110. Demers C, Ginsberg JS, Hirsh J, Henderson P, Blajchman AM. Thrombosis in antithrombin-III deficient persons. *Ann Intern Med* 1992; **116:**754–61.
111. Devilat M, Toso M, Morales M. Childhood stroke associated with protein C or S deficiency and primary antiphospholipid syndrome. *Pediatr Neurol* 1993; **9:**67–70.
112. Kohler J, Kasper J, Witt I, Von Reuthern GM. Ischemic stroke due to protein C deficiency. *Stroke* 1990; **21:**1077–80.
113. Grewal RP, Goldberg MA. Stroke in protein C deficiency. *Am J Med* 1990; **89:**538–9.
114. Camerlingo M, Finazzi G, Casto L, Laffranchi C, Barbui T, Mamoli A. Inherited protein C deficiency and nonhemorrhagic arterial stroke in young adults, *Neurology* 1991; **41:**1371–3.
115. Chaturvedi S, Dzieczkowski J. Multiple hemostatic abnormalities in young adults with activated protein C resistance and cerebral ischemia. *J Neurol Sci* 1998; **159:**209–12.
116. Nagayama T, Shinohara Y, Nagayama M, Tsuda M, Yamamura M. Congenitally abnormal plasminogen in juvenile ischemic cerebrovascular disease. *Stroke* 1993; **24:**2104–7.
117. Khamashta MA, Cuadrado MJ, Mujic F, Taub NA, Hunt BJ, Hughes GR. The management of thrombosis in the antiphospholipid-antibody syndrome. *N Engl J Med* 1995; **332:**993–7.
118. Ihara M, Tanaka H, Nishimura Y. Primary antiphospholipid syndrome with recurrent transient ischemic attacks: report of a case and its successful treatment. *Intern Med* 1998; **37:**704–7.
119. Ravelli A, Martini A. Antiphospholipid antibody syndrome in pediatric patients. *Rheum Dis Clinic North Am* 1997; **23:**657–76.
120. Bick RL. Antiphospholipid thrombosis syndromes: etiology, pathophysiology, diagnosis and management. *Int J Hematol* 1997; **65:** 193–213.
121. Parke A. The role of IVIG in the management of patients with antiphospholipid antibodies and recurrent pregnancy losses. *Clin Rev Allergy* 1992; **10:**105–18.
122. Harris EN, Pierangeli SS. Utilization of intravenous immunoglobulin therapy to treat recurrent pregnancy loss in the antiphospholipid syndrome: a review. *Scan J Rheumatol* 1998; **107**(Suppl):97–102.
123. Cowchock S. Treatment of antiphospholipid syndrome in pregnancy. *Lupus* 1998; **7** (Suppl 2): 95–7.
124. Graus F, Saiz A, Sierra J *et al.* Neurologic complications of autologous and allogeneic bone marrow transplantation in patients with leukemia: a comparative study. *Neurology* 1996; **46:**1004–9.
125. Huang LT, Hsiao CC, Weng HH, Lui CC. Neurologic complications of pediatric systemic malignancies. *J Formosa Med Assoc* 1996; **95:**209–12.
126. Kittner SJ, Stern BJ, Feeser BR *et al.* Pregnancy and the risk of stroke. *N Engl J Med* 1996; **335:**768–74.
127. Heinemann LA, Lewis MA, Spitzer WO *et al.* Thromboembolic stroke in young women. A European case–control study on oral contraceptives. *Contraception* 1998; **57:**29–37.
128. Rizk B, Meagher S, Fisher AM. Severe ovarian hyperstimulation syndrome and cerebrovascular accidents, *Hum Reprod* 1990; **5:**697–8.
129. Igarashi M, Roy S 3rd, Stapleton FB. Cerebrovascular complications in children with nephrotic syndrome. *Pediatr Neurol* 1988; **4:** 362–5.
130. Randi ML, Fabris F, Cella G, Rossi C, Girolami A. Cerebral vascular accidents in young patients with essential thrombocythemia: relation with other known cardiovascular risk

factors. *Angiology*1998; **49:**477–81.

131. Zunker P, Schick A, Buschmann HC *et al.* Hyperinsulinism and cerebral microangiopathy. *Stroke* 1996; **27:**219–23.
132. Giles WH, Kittner SJ, Anda RF, Croft JB, Casper ML. Serum folate and risk for ischemic stroke. First National Health and Nutrition Examination Survey epidemiologic follow-up study. *Stroke* 1995; **26:**1166–70.
133. Powars D, Wilson B, Imbus C, Pegelow C, Allen J. The natural history of stroke in sickle cell disease. *Am J Med* 1978; **65:**461–71.
134. Pegelow CH, Adams RJ, McKie V *et al.* Risk of recurrent stroke in patients with sickle cell disease treated with erythrocyte transfusions. *J Pediatr* 1995; **126:**896–9.
135. Shaefer EJ, Zech LA, Schwartz DE, Brewer HB Jr. Coronary heart disease prevalence and other clinical features in familial high-density lipoprotein deficiency (Tangier disease). *Ann Intern Med* 1980; **93:**261–6.
136. Lyon G, Adams RD, Kolodny EH. *Neurology of Hereditary Metabolic Diseases of Children*, 2nd edn, pp. 256–7. New York; McGraw Hill: 1996.
137. Beighton P. The Ehlers–Danlos syndromes. In: *Heritable Disorders of Connective Tissue* (Beighton P, ed.), 5th edn, pp. 189–251. St Louis; Mosby Year Book: 1993.
138. Petty GW, Engel AG, Younge BR *et al.* Retinocochleocerebral vasculopathy. *Medicine* 1998; **77:**12–40.
139. Katz B, Wheeler D, Weinreb RN, Swenson MR. Eales' disease with central nervous system infarction. *Ann Ophthalmol* 1991; **23:**460–3.
140. Dexter F, Hindman BJ. Recommendations for hyperbaric oxygen therapy of cerebral air embolism based on a mathematical model of bubble absorption. *Anesth Analg* 1997; **84:** 1203–7.
141. Bardana D, Rudan J, Cervenko F, Smith R. Fat embolism syndrome in a patient demonstrating only neurologic symptoms. *Can J Surg* 1998; **41:**398–402.

6

Cholesterol lowering and strokes: a heart/brain comparison

Michael F Oliver

CONTENTS • **Introduction** • **Cholesterol lowering and coronary heart disease** • **Regression of coronary atheroma** • **Regression of carotid atheroma** • **Effects of cholesterol-lowering in advancing age** • **Recommendations**

INTRODUCTION

The direct relationship between increased plasma total cholesterol and low density lipoprotein (LDL) cholesterol with an increased risk of coronary heart disease (CHD) is firmly established.[1] So is the inverse relationship between high density lipoprotein (HDL) cholesterol and CHD.[2] Similar relationships between these lipid moieties and stroke have not been established.[3] For cerebral hemorrhage, however, there is a strong inverse relationship with total cholesterol levels, as shown by an 18-year follow-up of 7850 Japanese-American men.[4]

There are three reasons for this weak or absent relationship. (1) Virtually all CHD can be ascribed to coronary atheroma, whereas less than half of the incidence of strokes is due to carotid or cerebral artery atheroma. Non-atheromatous causes, such as cardiac arrhythmias and small cerebral vessel disease, are responsible for most of the remainder. (2) In general, myocardial infarction and coronary deaths occur at a younger age than strokes, leading to a diminished population with elevated plasma lipids and large vessel atheroma, such as carotid artery disease, at the ages when strokes occur. (3) Plasma total and LDL cholesterol decrease with advanced age.[5]

No large randomized controlled trial to assess the effect of cholesterol-lowering specifically in stroke patients has yet been completed. Thus, we need to consider surrogate data from CHD prevention trials and atheroma-regression trials in order to consider any heart/brain analogy.

CHOLESTEROL LOWERING AND CORONARY HEART DISEASE

There are two data sets which provide evidence of the benefit of cholesterol-lowering on CHD rates. One is the effect of cholesterol-lowering in patients with existing CHD (secondary prevention) and the other is the extent to which high risk people without CHD have been benefitted (primary prevention). These data come from five large randomized controlled trials of 5 or more years duration using a statin to reduce LDL cholesterol. The results of these trials have been published in full[6–10] and it is unnecessary and inappropriate in the context of this brief review to refer to them in detail.

The three largest randomized controlled secondary prevention trials[6–8] demonstrate a degree of parallelism between the benefits for CHD and for stroke that are relevant to the question of how important it is to lower cholesterol to prevent strokes (Table 6.1). But the benefit is for non-fatal strokes and, even with

Table 6.1 CHD secondary prevention trials

	Years	LDL (%)	CHD events (incl deaths) (%)	Strokes (%) Non-fatal	Strokes (%) Deaths
4S[6] (4444) Simvastatin	5	−36	−34***	−32**	+14†
CARE[7] (4159) Pravastatin	5	−28	−24***	−31(ø)**	
LIPID[8] (9014) Lovastatin	6	−25	−24***	−17*	−18†

*$P < 0.05$; **$P < 0.03$; ***$P < 0.01$; †Numbers too small.
(ø) = risk reduction for combined non-fatal and fatal strokes.

Table 6.2 Scandinavian simvastatin survival study (4S)

Event	No. (%) of patients Placebo (N = 2223)	No. (%) of patients Simvastatin (N = 2221)	P value
Major coronary	502 (23%)	353 (16%)	<0.0001
All cerebrovascular	95 (4.3%)	61 (2.7%)	0.024
Stroke			
non-embolic	33	16	
embolic	16	13	
hemorrhagic	2	0	
unclassified	13	15	
TIA	29	19	

the large numbers of CHD patients included in these trials it was not possible to conclude that cholesterol-lowering reduced stroke mortality. The 4S trial[6] showed that the relative risk of cerebrovascular events was reduced by 37% ($P = 0.024$) but the benefit was confined to a reduction of non-embolic strokes and transient ischemic attacks (Table 6.2): embolic strokes, hemorrhagic strokes and those that could not be classified were not reduced. This emphasizes

Table 6.3 CHD primary prevention trials

Trial	*Years*	*LDL (%)*	*CHD events (incl deaths) (%)*		*Strokes (%)*	
				Non-fatal	*Deaths*	*Both*
WOSCOPS[9] (6595)	5	−26	−31	−15	+30	−10
AFCAPS/ TexCAPS[10] (6605)	5	−25	−37	−17	−40	−22

There were too few strokes in both trials to permit statistical analyses.

Table 6.4 Influence of different cholesterol-lowering regimens[12]

Intervention	*Trials*	*Risk ratios for non-fatal and fatal stroke*	*P value*
Statins	8	0.76 (CL 0.62–0.92)	0.01
Fibrates	5	1.12	NS
Resins	3	1.07	NS
Diet	10	0.98	NS

that it is strokes with a basis of large vessel atheroma that are most likely to be reduced.

Data derived from the only two large randomized primary prevention controlled trials[9,10] in people at risk for CHD provide much less convincing evidence that reduction of total and LDL cholesterol reduces strokes (Table 6.3). This is to be expected in view of the relatively low risk of strokes occurring in otherwise healthy people. But there was a trend in the right direction.

An additional relevant point is that reduction of CHD events occurred in both types of trial when LDL cholesterol was decreased by 25% and more. This can only be achieved on a long-term basis with HMG coenzyme A reductase inhibitors. Degrees of reduction of LDL of less than this have little or no benefit on CHD rates[11] (Table 6.4). Thus, the fibrates, resins or diets that do not achieve this marked reduction of LDL should not be considered for the management of stroke,[12] except possibly when there is a mixed hyperlipidemia present.

Table 6.5 Carotid ultrasound regression trials

Trial	*No. of patients*	*CCA change per year (mm)*		*P value*
		Placebo	*Statin*	
KAPS[22] Pravastatin	428	+0.03	+0.009	<0.002
PLAC II[23] Pravastatin	141	+0.45	+0.03	0.03
CAIUS[24] Pravastatin	305	+0.01	−0.008	<0.001
		CCA change after 3–4 years (mm)		
ACAPS[21] Lovastatin	461	−0.006	−0.009	<0.001
LIPID[25] Lovastatin	552	+0.48	−0.014	<0.001
Hodis *et al.*[26] Lovastatin	188	+0.046	−0.095	<0.001

REGRESSION OF CORONARY ATHEROMA

There have been five controlled trials, using serial coronary arteriography, of the effects of cholesterol-lowering on coronary pathology in patients with CHD.[13–17] The results can be summarized by stating that, when LDL cholesterol was lowered by about 20% or more by a statin or by ileal bypass surgery, there was less progression of coronary atheroma and fewer new atheromatous lesions developed. However, this took time and 4 years of treatment was necessary before a clear result was evident.[14] Interestingly, in the secondary prevention trials already described there was a significant reduction of clinical events after about 2 years suggesting that statins may have some additional and more rapid action than might be expected solely from the reduction of LDL accumulation in atheromatous lesions.

Meta-analyses of the CHD prevention trials, including the smaller regression trials, with nearly 29 000 patients involved, confirm that there has been an overall reduction of stroke risk of approximately 30%, but without reduction of stroke mortality.[18,19]

REGRESSION OF CAROTID ATHEROMA

High resolution ultrasonography conducted in nearly 6000 subjects over 65 years has clearly established that thickness of the carotid artery intima and media are risk factors for strokes.[20] Trials in asymptomatic people and in patients with known CHD using B-mode ultrasound assessment of common carotid artery lesions (CCA)[21–26] reflect the results of the coronary atheroma regression. These trials show that reduction of plasma LDL cholesterol by 25% or more, usually with a small increase in HDL cholesterol, prevented over a 4-year period any detectable progress in carotid wall thickening and reduced the development of new lesions (Table 6.5). This is particularly important in the assessment of the likely benefit of lowering cholesterol on strokes since carotid artery disease may be responsible for as much as 40% of strokes.

EFFECTS OF CHOLESTEROL-LOWERING IN ADVANCING AGE

Since strokes occur more in the elderly, the benefit of cholesterol and LDL lowering in advanced age requires some discussion. A conservative view about the need for lowering cholesterol in the elderly, which might be defined as 80 years or over, is justified for several reasons. First, plasma total cholesterol and LDL cholesterol concentrations decrease with advancing age.[5] The reasons are unclear but poor nutrition may be one: another may be occult disease, such as cancer; and another could be decreased cholesterol absorption and synthesis. Next, the positive associations between raised plasma cholesterol and LDL cholesterol with CHD—and more weakly with stroke—which exists at earlier ages, decrease in men over the age of about 70 and disappear after 80.[27–29] Thus, hypercholesterolemia is no longer a risk factor for CHD in the elderly. This may result partly from natural selection due to premature deaths of men with moderate or marked hypercholesterolemia. A weak correlation remains, however, between plasma cholesterol levels and vascular disease in elderly women.[30]

Prospective cohort studies, including the Zutphen Elderly Study,[29] suggest that low high density lipoprotein (HDL) cholesterol concentrations and low apoprotein-A1 may be a better predictor than cholesterol or LDL of CHD in advancing age, but this is not relevant to individuals and not helpful therapeutically since we do not yet know how to raise low HDL levels.

There are, as yet, no clear data to provide evidence that cholesterol-lowering is beneficial against either CHD or stroke in older patients. Nor are data likely to become available because now it is probably unethical, in view of the successful outcome of primary and secondary prevention trials in middle-age, and uneconomic to mount a controlled clinical trial in the aged to test the efficacy of statins against a placebo. The nearest answer comes from three of the trials quoted. The follow-up[31] of the 4S study suggests that male patients with CHD may benefit from a statin up to the age of 73 with the same level of risk reduction (34%) as in younger men. The LIPID trial[8] comprised 9014 patients with CHD and included 1346 patients aged between 70 and 75 years: in this subgroup the CHD risk reduction was 15% compared with 28% in those aged 65–69 years. In the AFCAPS primary prevention trial,[10] those above the median age of 57 years for men and 63 years for women also had less reduction of risk than those below these ages. Beyond the age of 75, there are no sound data. It is unwise, therefore, to extrapolate the positive trial results from middle-aged patients or otherwise healthy people and use these as an argument for treating a raised cholesterol level in the elderly.

But there has been one small controlled trial[32] in men aged 65–84 years of a diet low in cholesterol and rich in polyunsaturated fats. After 8 years, there were significantly fewer cardiovascular events due to fewer non-fatal myocardial infarcts, fewer sudden cardiac deaths and fewer cerebral infarcts. Those in the older half of this elderly population had the least benefit. To be effective dietary changes have to be stringent and permanent. The results of this trial have no practical implications for stroke patients, since advice to make a major change in food intake in the elderly, who are set in their habits, is unlikely to be heeded and might have adverse nutritional consequences.

RECOMMENDATIONS

All patients recovering from a stroke with clear-cut evidence of carotid atheroma as the cause, or with a past history of CHD, should be considered for statin treatment. This should be given indefinitely and at a dose concentration which will lower LDL cholesterol by 25% or more. Patients with concurrent diabetes mellitus or hypertension are particularly at risk.

At present, it is better to choose a natural statin, such as simvastatin, pravastatin or lovastatin, since only these have been submitted to rigorous long-term trials (see Table 6.4). Since no event data are available on the benefits of synthetic statins, such as astorvastatin or fluvastatin, it is not appropriate to assume that such drugs will be equally effective.[33]

Patients with a stroke resulting from a cardiac arrhythmia or non-atheromatous small cerebral artery disease should not be expected to benefit from cholesterol lowering.

Patients over the age of about 75 are also unlikely to benefit and screening of such patients for hypercholesterolemia is unnecessary.

REFERENCES

1. Martin MJ, Hulley SB, Browner WS, Kuller LH, Wentworth D. Serum cholesterol, blood pressure, and mortality: implications of a cohort of 361,662 men. *Lancet* 1986; **ii:**933–6.
2. Stampfer MJ, Sacks FM, Salvin S, Willet WC, Hennekens CH. A prospective study of cholesterol, apolipoproteins and the risk of myocardial infarction. *N Engl J Med* 1991; **325:**373–81.
3. Prospective Studies Collaboration. Cholesterol, diastolic blood pressure and stroke: 13,000 strokes in 450,000 people in 45 prospective cohorts. *Lancet* 1995; **346:**1647–53.
4. Yano K, Reed DM, MacLean CJ. Serum cholesterol and hemorrhagic stroke in the Honolulu Heart Program. *Stroke* 1989; **20:**1460–5.
5. Ettinger WH, Wahl PW, Kuller LH *et al.* Lipoprotein lipids in older people. *Circulation* 1992; **86:**858–69.
6. Scandinavian Simvastatin Survival Study Group. Randomised trial of cholesterol lowering in 4444 patients with coronary heart disease: the Scandinavian Simvastatin Survival Study (4 S). *Lancet* 1994; **344:**1383–9.
7. Plehn JF, Davis BR, Sacks FM *et al.* Reduction of stroke incidence after myocardial infarction with pravastatin. *Circulation* 1999; **99:**216–23.
8. The long-term intervention with pravastatin in Ischaemic Disease (LIPID) Study Group. Prevention of cardiovascular events and death with pravastatin in patients with coronary heart disease and a broad range of initial cholesterol levels. *N Engl J Med* 1998; **339:**1349–57.
9. Shepherd J, Cobbe SM, Ford I *et al.* Prevention of coronary heart disease with pravastatin in men with hypercholesterolemia. *N Engl J Med* 1995; **333:**1301–7.
10. Downs JR, Clearfield M, Weis S *et al.* Primary prevention of acute coronary events with lovastatin in men and women with average cholesterol levels. Results of AFCAPS/TexCAPS. *J Am Med Assoc* 1998; **279:**1615–22.
11. Holme I. Cholesterol reduction and its impact on coronary artery disease mortality. *Am J Cardiol* 1995; **76:**10–7.
12. Bucher HC, Griffith LE, Guyatt GH. Effect of HMGcoA Reductase inhibitors on stroke. *Ann Intern Med* 1998; **128:**89–95.
13. Brown G, Albers JJ, Fisher LD *et al.* Regression of coronary artery disease as a result of intensive lipid-lowering therapy in men with high levels of apolipoprotein-B. *N Engl J Med* 1990; **323:**1289–98.
14. MAAS Investigators. Effect of simvastatin on coronary atheroma: a multicentre antiatheroma study. *Lancet* 1994; **344:**633–8.
15. Waters D, Higginson L, Gladstone P *et al.* Effects of monotherapy with an HMGCoA reductase inhibitor on the progression of coronary atherosclerosis as assessed by serial quantitative arteriography: the Canadian Coronary Atherosclerosis Intervention Trial. *Circulation* 1994; **89:**959–68.
16. Jukema JW, Bruschke AVG, van Boven AJ *et al.* Effects of lipid lowering by pravastatin on progression and regression of coronary artery disease in symptomatic men with normal to moderately elevated serum cholesterol levels. The regression growth evaluation statin study (REGRESS). *Circulation* 1995; **91:**2528–40.
17. Buchwald H, Campos CT, Boen JR *et al.* Disease-free intervals after partial ileal bypass in patients with coronary heart disease and hypercholesterolemia: report from the program on the surgical control of the hyperlipidemias (POSCH). *J Am Coll Cardiol* 1995; **26:**351–7.
18. Hebert PR, Gaziano JM, Chan KS, Hennekens CH. Cholesterol lowering with statin drug, risk of stroke, and total mortality. *J Am Med Assoc* 1997; **278:**313–21.
19. Blauw GJ, Lagaay AM, Smelt AHM, Westendorp RGJ. Stroke, statins, and cholesterol. *Stroke* 1997; **28:**946–50.
20. O'Leary DH, Polak JF, Kronmal RA, Manolio TA, Burke GL, Wolfson SK. Carotid-artery intima and media thickness as a risk factor for

myocardial infarction and strokes in older adults. *N Engl J Med* 1999; **340:**14–22.
21. Furberg CD, Adams HP, Applegate WB *et al.* Effect of lovastatin on early carotid atherosclerosis and cardiovascular events: ACAPS. *Circulation* 1994; **90:**1679–87.
22. Salonen R, Nyyssonen K, Porkkala E *et al.* Kuopio Atherosclerosis Prevention Study (KAPS): a population-based primary preventive trial of the effect of LDL lowering on atherosclerotic progression in carotid and femoral arteries. *Circulation* 1995; **92:**1758–64.
23. Crouse JR, Byington RP, Bond MG *et al.* Pravastatin, lipids and atherosclerosis in the carotid arteries (PLAC-II). *Am J Cardiol* 1995; **75:**455–9.
24. Mercuri M, Bond MG, Sirtori CR *et al.* Pravastatin reduces carotid intima–media thickness progression in an asymptomatic hypercholesterolaemia Mediterranean population: the Carotid Atherosclerosis Italian Ultrasound Study. *Am J Med* 1996; **101:**627–34.
25. MacMahon S, Sharpe N, Gamble G *et al.* Effects of lowering average or below-average cholesterol levels on the progression of carotid atherosclerosis. *Circulation* 1998; **97:**1784–90.
26. Hodis HN, Mack WJ, LaBree L *et al.* Reduction of carotid wall thickness using lovastatin and dietary therapy. *Ann Intern Med* 1996; **124:**548–56.
27. Weverling-Rijnsburger AWE, Blauw GJ, Lagaay AM, Knook DL, Meinders AE, Westendorp RGJ. Total cholesterol and risk of mortality in the oldest old. *Lancet* 1997; **350:**1119–23.
28. Weijenberg MP, Feskens EJM, Bowles CH, Kromhout D. Serum total cholesterol and systolic blood pressure as risk factors for mortality from ischaemic heart disease among elderly men and women. *J Clin Epidemiol* 1994; **2:**197–205.
29. Weijenberg MP, Feskens EJM, Kromhout D. Total and high density lipoprotein cholesterol as risk factors for coronary heart disease in elderly men during 5 years of follow-up. The Zutphen Elderly Study. *Am J Epidemiol* 1996; **143:**151–8.
30. Räihä I, Marniemi J, Puukka P, Tikka T, Ehnholm C, Sourander L. Effect of serum lipids, lipoproteins, and apolipoprotein on vascular and nonvascular mortality in the elderly. *Arterioscler Thromb Vasc Biol* 1997; **17:**1224–32.
31. Miettinen TA, Pyörälä K, Olsson AG *et al.* Cholesterol-lowering therapy in women and elderly patients with myocardial infarction and angina. *Circulation* 1997; **96:**4211–8.
32. Dayton S, Pearce ML, Hashimoto S *et al.* A controlled clinical trial of a diet high in unsaturated fat preventing complications in atherosclerosis. *Circulation* 1969; **39/40**(Suppl II):63–88.
33. Furberg CD. Natural statins and stroke risk. *Circulation* 1999; **99:**185–8.

7

Antiaggregants, old and new: which ones? In what cases? Mode of action

Natan M Bornstein

INTRODUCTION

Stroke remains a major cause of worldwide morbidity and mortality, imposing an enormous economic burden that knows no borders. In most industrialized countries, it is the third leading cause of death and the most important cause of physical disability in people over 60 years of age. Stroke has been predicted to become an even greater burden within the next 25 years, given the aging of the population and the increase in other risk factors.[1] Recurrent stroke is also a major cause of mortality and morbidity among stroke survivors.[2] The high incidence and serious consequences of stroke make it one of the most important challenges faced by contemporary medicine. The limited effectiveness of current therapeutic approaches for acute stroke dictates that the emphasis be placed on strategies for prevention and, thanks to large clinical trials conducted worldwide, we have been privileged to see great progress in this area over the past decade. In this chapter, we will review the current knowledge of antiaggregant strategies in stroke prevention and how the results of recently published studies have impacted upon our conceptual approach to preventing stroke. We will review the current information on aspirin, ticlopidine, clopidogrel and dipyridamole in order to choose the appropriate drug for the stroke patient in daily clinical practice.

ASPIRIN

Aspirin (acetylsalicylic acid), originally obtained from the bark of the white willow (*Salix alba*), is the most widely used preventive medical therapy in patients with ischemic cerebral events.

Mechanism of action

Aspirin completely and irreversibly inhibits the action of the enzyme cyclo-oxygenase, thereby suppressing the production of thromboxane A_2 (TXA_2) in platelets, which induces platelet aggregation and vasoconstriction. On the other hand, aspirin reduces the production of prostacyclin (PGI_2) in the vessel wall which inhibits platelet aggregation and induces vasodilation and, therefore, might have some antithrombogenic effect.[3] In addition to its antiaggregate effect, aspirin has other actions which may potentially play a role in stroke prevention, namely, anti-inflammatory and antioxidant activities. Aspirin is rapidly absorbed in the stomach and upper intestine: the peak plasma concentration occurs 15–20 min after ingestion and the antiaggregate activity within 1 h after administration. Thus, the inhibitory effect is rapid and lasts for the life-span of the platelet.

Primary prevention

Two trials aimed at investigating the use of aspirin for primary prevention of stroke have been performed with inconclusive results. The US Physician Health Study[4] and the British Doctors' Trial,[5] both of which included only men and had small numbers of stroke end-points, reached the conclusion of there being a possible but statistically non-significant 21% (±13%) increase of stroke among all low-risk patients (i.e., primary prevention).[6]

Recently Kronmal *et al.*[7] reported the intriguing results that, in a cohort of 5011 elderly people from the Cardiovascular Health Study (CHS) followed for a mean of 4.2 years, aspirin-use was associated with increased risk for ischemic stroke in women and hemorrhagic stroke in both men and women. They found that frequent aspirin-use was associated with an increased risk of ischemic stroke compared with non-users (relative risk = 1.6; 95% CI, 1.2–2.2; $P = 0.001$). After adjusting for other risk factors, only women but no men had a 1.8-fold (95% CI, 1.2–2.8) increased risk of ischemic stroke. The authors mentioned the possibility of there having been some confounding of results stemming from aspirin-use itself as opposed to cause and effect.

In another randomized study, the Hypertension Optimal Treatment (HOT),[8] in which 9391 hypersensitive patients were assigned to receive 75 mg/day aspirin and 9391 patients received placebo, a significant beneficial effect of aspirin on myocardial infarction (36%) was reported, but there was no effect on stroke. In these studies, there was a small but definite chance of adverse events (i.e., bleeding) with about 1 per 1000 excess of bleeding due to aspirin.

In the light of these findings, it emerges that there are presently no approved prescription indications for aspirin in the primary prevention of cerebrovascular disease, and that formal policy recommendations need to await the results of the randomized trials. In the meantime, the American Heart Association suggests that aspirin may outweigh the harm in men with high risk for coronary disease but no guidelines have been issued for women.

Secondary prevention

Since the late 1970s, many clinical trials have been conducted to determine the value of aspirin in the prevention of ischemic stroke. The first placebo-controlled randomized trial which was done in Canada[9] involved almost 600 patients (290 patients assigned to the two groups that included aspirin treatment were compared with 295 patients assigned to one of the two groups that did not take the drug) and showed that 1300 mg/day aspirin reduced the incidence of stroke and death by 31%.

Another randomized controlled study conducted in France on 604 patients with previous transient ischemic attacks (TIA) (18%) or completed stroke (84%) showed that 1000 mg/day of aspirin significantly reduced the risk of stroke (40%) in both sexes but the mortality rate was not reduced.[10] In this study, co-treatment with dipyridamole did not offer additional benefits. Since then, several other trials have been conducted with different doses of aspirin, ranging from 30 to 1000 mg/day.

The results of three trials were published in 1991. One was the final report of the UK-TIA aspirin trial,[11] in which 2435 patients with TIA or minor stroke were randomly allocated to receive 'blind' treatment with aspirin 1200 mg/day, 300 mg/day aspirin or placebo, with the patients being followed for a mean of about 4 years. The outcome, i.e., death, myocardial infarction (MI) and stroke, was similar in the two groups allocated aspirin—neither dose of aspirin was significantly better than placebo. It is noteworthy that the number of patients in each aspirin group was 815 and 806, which might be too small to rule out a type II error. In the final analysis, when both aspirin dose groups were combined, the investigators found a significant 15% reduction in the risk of death, MI and stroke, but only a 7% reduction in disabling stroke and death and 3% in disabling stroke and vascular death. It is important to mention that the population of the UK-TIA study was somewhat different from other stroke studies in that there was a relative low annual rate of stroke (3.2%) in the placebo group compared to 5.9–7.3% reported in other studies.[9,12]

A randomized double-blind Dutch TIA trial[12] compared the effectiveness of 30 mg/day aspirin to 283 mg/day aspirin on the occurrence of non-fatal stroke, MI and vascular death in patients after TIA or minor stroke (there was no placebo group). A total of 3131 patients were included and followed for an average of 2.6 years. No significant difference was found in vascular events between the 30 mg/day group (14.7%) compared with the 283 mg/day group (15.2%).

The Swedish Aspirin Low-Dose Trial (SALT)[13] was a double-blind randomized trial which compared 75 mg/day aspirin with placebo for the prevention of stroke and death following TIA or minor stroke. The 1360 study patients were followed for a mean of 32 months. There was a significant 18% reduction in the primary outcome events (stroke or death).

In 1994, the antiplatelet Trialists' Collaboration published the results of a meta-analysis[6] in which they analyzed 18 placebo-controlled clinical trials in 10 000 patients with TIAs or minor stroke: allocation to a mean duration of 33 months antiplatelet therapy produced a highly significant ($2P > 0.00001$) reduction of 37 per 1000 in risk of suffering another vascular event (i.e., MI, stroke or vascular death) with a standard deviation (SD) of 8. The proportional reduction in important vascular events in these trials was 22% (SD 5%).

Acute ischemic stroke

Evidence for the effectiveness of early intervention with antiaggregants was lacking until the result of the International Stroke Trial (IST)[14] and the Chinese Acute Stroke Trial (CAST)[15] were published in 1997.

The IST was a large (19 435 patients) randomized open study of antithrombotic therapy started within 48 h of stroke onset. For the aspirin part of this factorial design study, the IST suggests that aspirin given in a dose of 300 mg/day will reduce the recurrent stroke and death risk within 14 days by 10 per 1000 patients treated. Similar results were obtained by the CAST study where 10 000 patients were treated with 160 mg/day aspirin for 4 weeks and 10 000 patients received placebo. Together, the IST and CAST included almost 40 000 patients and, when analyzed together, they showed that 160–300 mg/day aspirin started within 48 h of stroke onset reduces early recurrent ischemic stroke by about one-quarter (2.5 vs. 3.2%; $P = 0.00002$) and increases the risk of hemorrhagic stroke. This means that treating 1000 stroke patients with aspirin prevents five recurrent strokes (seven fewer recurrent ischemic strokes but two more hemorrhagic strokes) and nine non-fatal stroke and deaths in the first few weeks ($2P < 0.001$).

In summary, although immediate administration of 300 mg aspirin has no effect on the course of the initial stroke, fewer recurrences and deaths could be achieved.

Dose of aspirin

The issue of what is the optimal dose of aspirin is still controversial[16–21] and will remain unresolved until a proper trial comparing low doses (~100 mg/day) to a high dose (1000 mg/day) will be conducted. In any event, a medium dose of aspirin (75–325 mg/day) is now the most widely used regimen as antiplatelet therapy for secondary stroke prevention.[22,23]

Adverse effects

Regular use of aspirin increases the risk of gastrointestinal side-effects, such as epigastric pain, peptic ulcer, gastritis and gastrointestinal bleeding. Administration of enteric-coated aspirin, but not the buffered type, may lessen the damage to the gastric mucosa.[24–26] In both the UK-TIA and the Dutch TIA trials, the bleeding complications were more frequent in the higher aspirin dose group. In the UK-TIA trial, gastrointestinal bleeding occurred in 1.6% of patients on placebo, 2.6% on 300 mg aspirin and 4.7% on 1200 mg aspirin, and approximately one-half of the patients in each group required hospitalization. It is a widely held view that all-site bleeding with aspirin is not dose-related.[16] In the Dutch TIA, although major bleeding occurred only slightly less in the 30 mg group, minor bleeds were significantly less in the 30 mg group.

Regarding aspirin and hemorrhagic stroke, in a recent[27] meta-analysis of 16 randomized controlled trials with 55 462 participants, aspirin-use was associated with an absolute risk increase in hemorrhagic stroke of 12 events per 10 000 persons (95% CI, 5–20; $P < 0.001$). In the CHS,[7] there was a four-fold (95% CI, 1.6–10.0) increase in risk of hemorrhagic stroke for both frequent and infrequent users of aspirin ($P = 0.003$).

TICLOPIDINE

Mechanism of action

Ticlopidine hydrochloride is a potent inhibitor of platelet aggregation with a different mechanism of action than that of aspirin, although its mechanism of action is uncertain.[28] It appears that ticlopidine selectively inhibits adenosine diphosphate (ADP)-induced fibrinogen binding to platelets, but the exact molecular mechanism by which this is accomplished is unknown. Since ticlopidine is not a cyclo-oxygenase inhibitor, it has no effect on prostacyclin production. Ticlopidine is extensively metabolized by the liver, and steady-state plasma concentrations are obtained only after a few days (unlike aspirin) of repeated administration of 250 mg twice daily.

Secondary stroke prevention

Two major trials were conducted to determine the efficacy of ticlopidine in secondary stroke prevention. The Ticlopidine Aspirin Stroke Study (TASS)[29] was a 'triple'-blind study comparing the effect of 1300 mg/day aspirin vs. 250 mg ticlopidine twice daily in 3069 patients with TIA (1300) and minor stroke who were followed for up to 5.8 years. The primary analysis was an 'intention-to-treat' assessment of death from all causes of non-fatal stroke. Ticlopidine produced a 13% greater reduction than aspirin in the primary endpoints and a reduction of 21% in the 3-year event rate for fatal or non-fatal stroke. It was interesting to note that there was a 42% relative risk reduction (RRR) for stroke and death in the first year and a 47% RRR for stroke and stroke death. This was largely maintained over the next 2 years, but the RRR declined to 21% after 3 years. The superiority of ticlopidine over aspirin in the reduction of stroke was seen in both males and females.

The Canadian–American Ticlopidine Study (CATS)[30] was a randomized double-blind placebo-controlled trial which involved 1072 patients with a substantial completed stroke, rather than a TIA or minor stroke as in TASS. Patients were randomly allocated to receive 250 mg ticlopidine twice daily or a matching placebo. The primary outcome events were a combination of recurrent non-fatal stroke, non-fatal MI and vascular death. The follow-up lasted for an average of 2 years. This appears to be the biggest trial which assessed stroke recurrence in patients who experienced a major stroke. Using the efficacy approach, the cumulative events rate for the primary endpoints per year was 15.3% in the placebo group and 10.8% in the ticlopidine group (RRR 30.2%, $P = 0.006$). Intention-to-treat analysis gave a RRR of 23.3% ($P = 0.02$). Efficacy was found in both sexes.

To complete the picture, there was also a Japanese TIA study[31] wherein 170 patients received 200 mg/day ticlopidine and 170 received 500 mg aspirin. The outcome events included TIA stroke and MI. Ticlopidine was found to be superior to aspirin, but the difference in this small study was not statistically significant.

Adverse effects

Of the side-effects enumerated in both the CATS and TASS trials, the commonly described adverse effects of ticlopidine were mild gastrointestinal complaints, mainly diarrhea (20.4%), and skin rash (12%). The most important and threatening hematological side-effect, which occurred within 3 months of treatment onset, was severe neutropenia (less than 450 mL) with a frequency of 0.8–0.9%. All adverse side-effects were reversed with cessation of the study drug. Another major severe side-effect of ticlopidine was recently reported: thrombotic thrombocytopenic purpura (TTP) with a mortality rate possibly as high as 33%.[32] Due to above-mentioned side-effects, complete blood count and white cell differentials monitoring is required. In summary, TASS showed ticlopidine to be superior to aspirin in the prevention of all strokes and stroke plus death. CATS data provided strong evidence that ticlopidine conveys a clinically important reduction in the risk of stroke in patients with completed ischemic stroke. In general, we can assume that it reduces the risk of vascular events by another 10–20% over the 15–20% effect of aspirin, with only a small (0.86%) risk of reversible severe neutropenia.

CLOPIDOGREL

Clopidogrel is a new thienopyridine derivative which is chemically related to ticlopidine.

Mechanism of action

Clopidogrel blocks activation of platelets by adenosine diphosphate (ADP). This is achieved by selectively and irreversibly inhibiting the binding of this agonist to its receptor on platelets, thereby affecting ADP-dependent activation of the GpIIb–IIIa complex platelet surface.[33]

Secondary prevention

A large (19 185 patients) randomized blinded, international trial of clopidogrel vs. aspirin in patients at risk of ischemic events (CAPRIE) was conducted and reported in 1996.[34] CAPRIE was the largest clinical trial of a secondary prevention strategy to prevent various vascular endpoints in a high-risk population. The trial was designed to assess the relative efficacy of 75 mg/day clopidogrel and 325 mg/day aspirin reducing the risk of a composite outcome cluster of ischemic stroke, MI, or vascular death. Three groups of patients at significant risk of vascular events, those with recent ischemic stroke (6431), recent MI (6302), or symptomatic peripheral arterial disease (PAD) (6452), were followed for 1–3 years. The result of the outcome cluster showed a significant RRR of 8.7% in favor of clopidogrel (95% CI, 0.3–16.5; $P = 0.043$) and an absolute risk reduction of 0.51%. There were no significant differences in adverse events between the two regimens: specifically, there was no increased risk of neutropenia in the clopidogrel group. In a post-hoc analysis, there were significant differences in the RRR for each of the three entry groups (stroke, MI and PAD), with the most striking effect appearing to be in patients with PAD (RRR 23.8%; 95% CI, 8.9–36.2). For stroke patients, there was non-significant benefit for clopidogrel over aspirin (RRR 7.3%; 95% CI, 5.7–18.7). However, the trial was not able to detect a realistic treatment effect in each of the three clinical subgroups. Moreover, an additional analysis of these patients in the ischemic stroke and PAD subgroups with a previous history of MI demonstrated clear benefit for clopidogrel over aspirin. Hence, the conclusion of this study appears to confirm strongly, and be consistent with, the previous ticlopidine studies. When the absolute risk reduction of 0.5% is taken in consideration, it is calculated that 200 patients per year would need to be treated with clopidogrel rather than aspirin to save one endpoint. Thus, it seems probable that clopidogrel will replace ticlopidine but that it is less likely to replace aspirin as the first-line therapy for secondary stroke prevention, given its only modest superiority and presumed higher cost.

DIPYRIDAMOLE

Mechanism of action

There are three principal mechanisms by which dipyridamole (DP) has been assumed to inhibit platelet function.[35]

1. Inhibition of phosphodiesterase in platelets, resulting in an increase in intraplatelet cAMP levels and a consequent potentiation of the platelet-inhibiting action of PGI_2.
2. Direct stimulation of the release of PGI_2 by the vascular endothelium.
3. Inhibition of the cellular uptake and metabolism of adenosine, thereby increasing its level at the platelet–vascular interface.

The absorption of DP from conventional formulations is quite variable and may result in low systemic bioavailability of the drug. A new modified-release formulation of DP with low-dose aspirin was developed with improved bioavailability and with a half-life of 10 h (DP is eliminated by biliary excretion).

Secondary prevention

The recently completed second European Stroke Prevention Study (ESPS-2) was a randomized, placebo-controlled, double-blind trial comparing the effect of low-dose aspirin (50 mg/day) and modified-release DP (400 mg/day), and the combination of both drugs with the effects of placebo in 6602 patients with prior ischemic stroke or TIA.[36] The investigators reported that the combined therapy was more effective in preventing stroke (37% reduction) than aspirin alone (18.1% reduction) or DP alone (16.3 reduction). For the combination endpoint of stroke death, the combination regimen was associated with a 24.4% risk reduction. The combination of aspirin and DP compared with aspirin alone was associated with 12.9% (95% CI, 0–25; $P = 0.056$) relative risk reduction in primary outcome event of stroke and death, and 22% (95% CI, 9–33) relative event vascular death, non-fatal stroke or non-fatal MI.[37,38] None of the treatments significantly reduced the risk of death alone or of fatal stroke.

Before ESPS-2, the four studies that had compared the combination of aspirin and DP with aspirin alone in TIA/stroke patients had collectively shown that the combination of the two drugs was associated with only a 3% (95% CI, −22 to 22) reduction in vascular events compared with aspirin alone.[3,9] These results are somewhat different from the result obtained by EPSP-2. A meta-analysis of all trials, including ESPS-2, indicated that among the 2473 patients with prior stroke or TIA who were assigned to the combination of aspirin and DP, 356 (14.6%) experienced a vascular event compared with 419 (17.2%) of 2436 patients assigned to receive aspirin—a relative risk reduction of 15% ($P = 0.012$).[38] If the results of this meta-analysis are correct, the combination of aspirin and DP prevents twice as many vascular events as does aspirin alone. However, it is known that large randomized trials may contradict previous meta-analyses.

The results of ESPS-2 were criticized on several issues.

1. There were ethical concerns regarding the use of a placebo arm when the efficacy of aspirin was proven.
2. There were concerns that one of the participating centers was excluded from analysis after 438 fictitious patients were enrolled.
3. Among the 25% of patients who withdrew from the study, most were in the DP and the combination groups and compliance was higher among DP patients (97%) than in the aspirin groups (84%).
4. The low dose of aspirin (50 mg/day) was regarded by many as a placebo.
5. The predominant effect of the combination regimen was in reducing non-fatal stroke with little effect on MI and fatal stroke, which is different from the effect of other antiplatelet agents.

Adverse effects

Headache is the most common adverse effect. Bleeding was reported in 4.7% of the patients assigned to receive DP and it occurred in 8.8% of the combination regimen patients in the ESPS-2 trial. Gastrointestinal bleeding occurred in 1.6% of DP alone patients and 1.7% of those on placebo.

In summary, given the questions that remain, especially the difference between the ESPS-2 results and those of previous studies, the superiority of the combination regimen over aspirin alone awaits confirmation by another large, randomized clinical trial.

GPIIB/IIIA ANTAGONISTS

Although they are effective in preventing thromboembolic complications, the efficacy of currently used antiplatelet drugs is limited, and a significant number of serious thromboembolic events still occur. Recently, GPIIb/IIIa antagonists were identified as the final common pathway for all platelet antagonists.[39] The binding of adhesive proteins, such as fibrinogen, to GPIIb/IIIa causes platelets to aggregate. Thus, many research groups have concentrated on developing small-molecule GPIIb/IIIa antagonists in order to find an agent that inhibits platelet activations in response to all agonists of platelet activators.[40] In cardiology, the combination of aspirin and a parenteral GPIIb/IIIa blocker was proven to be significantly more effective than aspirin alone in reducing the 30-day rate of death or non-fatal MI for patients with unstable angina or non-Q-wave MI, or undergoing percutaneous coronary intervention.[41] These agents are now in the early stages of clinical trials and, in the future, we may have at our disposal a potent and more efficacious antiplatelet drug for preventing ischemic thromboembolic events.

SUMMARY

Primary prevention

There is no substantial evidence to recommend aspirin for primary stroke prevention in high-risk groups. Aspirin could be even harmful considering its adverse side-effects. However, in certain patients with non-vascular atrial fibrillation who are considered as low in risk (i.e., less than 65 years old, no high-risk features) for embolic stroke (~1% per year) or when warfarin is contraindicated 325 mg/day aspirin is recommended.

Secondary prevention

Antiplatelets are the pivotal drugs in preventing recurrent stroke or other major vascular events in patients who have undergone TIA or stroke.

Aspirin
Aspirin is the most widely used although its effect is very modest (RRR, 20%), and in spite of the fact that the optimal dose has not been determined, most physicians use between 100 and 325 mg/day as a maintenance dose. For patients who develop stroke on aspirin treatment, the options are either to increase the dose of aspirin or to administer another antiaggregate. No study has yet been performed to support these approaches.

Clopidogrel and dipyridamole
In patients who cannot tolerate aspirin, the options are 75 mg/day clopidogrel, or 400 mg dipyridamole combined with 50 mg aspirin.

Combined aspirin/clopidogrel
An approach which is very appealing but not yet proven is to combine different antiplatelet drugs with different modes of action, such as aspirin and clopidogrel, in order to achieve a better and more effective antithrombotic effect. Further controlled trials are needed to justify this approach.

REFERENCES

1. Kaste M, Fogelholm R, Rissanen A. Economic burden of stroke and the evaluation of new therapies. *Pub Hlth* 1998; **112:**103–12.
2. Bornstein NM, Korczyn AD. Prevention of recurrent stroke. In: *Prevention of Stroke* (Norris JW, Hachinski V, eds), pp. 261–8. New York; Springer-Verlag: 1985.
3. Patrono C. Aspirin as an antiplatelet drug. Review article. *N Engl J Med* 1994; **330:**1287–94.
4. Steering Committee of the Physicians' Health Study Research Group. Final report on the aspirin component of the ongoing physicians health study. *N Engl J Med* 1989; **321:**129–35.
5. Peto R, Gray R, Collins R *et al.* Randomised trial of prophylactic daily aspirin in British male doctors. *Br Med J* 1988; **296:**313–6.
6. Antiplatelet Trialists' Collaboration. The aspirin papers. Aspiring benefits patients with vascular disease and those undergoing revascularisation. Collaborative overview of randomised trials of antiplatelet therapy. I: Prevention of death, myocardial infarction, and stroke by prolonged antiplatelet therapy in various categories of patients. *Br Med J* 1994; **308:**71–106.
7. Kronmal RA, Hart RG, Manolio TA *et al.* Aspirin use and incident stroke in cardiovascular health study. *Stroke* 1998; **29:**887–94.
8. Hansson L, Zanchetti A, George S. Effects of intensive blood-pressure lowering and low-dose aspirin in patients with hypertension: principal results of the Hypertension Optimal Treatment (HOT) randomised trial. *Lancet* 1998; **351:**1755–62.
9. Canadian Cooperative Study Group. A randomized trial of aspirin and sulfinpyrazone in threatened stroke. *N Engl J Med* 1978; **299:** 53–9.
10. Bousser MG, Eschwege E, Haguemau M *et al.* 'AICLA' Controlled trial of ASA and dipyridamole in the secondary prevention of atherothrombotic cerebral ischemia. *Stroke* 1983; **15:**5–14.
11. UK-TIA Study Group. The United Kingdom Transient Ischemic Attack (UK-TIA) Aspirin Trial, Final results. *J Neurol Neurosurg Psychiatry* 1991; **54:**1044–54.
12. The Dutch TIA Study Group. A comparison of two doses of aspirin (30 mg vs. 283 mg a day) in patients after a transient ischemic attack of minor ischemic stroke. *N Engl J Med* 1991; **325:**1261–6.
13. The SALT Collaborative Group. Swedish Aspirin Low-Dose Trial (SALT) of 75 mg aspirin as secondary prophylaxis after cerebrovascular ischemic events. *Lancet* 1991; **338:** 1345–9.
14. International Stroke Trial Collaborative Group. The International Stroke Trial (IST): a randomised trial of aspirin, subcutaneous heparin, both, or neither among 19 435 patients with acute ischaemic stroke. *Lancet* 1997; **349:**1569–81.
15. CAST (Chinese Acute Stroke Trial) Collaborative Group. CAST: randomised placebo-controlled trial of early aspirin use in 20 000 patients with acute ischaemic stroke. *Lancet* 1997; **349:**1641–9.
16. Adams HP, Bendixen BH. Low versus high dose aspirin in prevention of ischemic stroke. *Clin Neuropharmacol* 1993; **16:**485–500.
17. Algra A, Van Gijn J. Aspirin at any dose above 30 mg offers only modest protection after cerebral ischaemia. *J Neurol Neurosurg Psychiatry* 1996; **60:**197–9.
18. Dyken ML, Barnet HJM, Easton DJ *et al.* Low-dose aspirin and stroke 'It Ain't Necessarily So'. *Stroke* 1992; **23:**1395–9.
19. Hart RG, Harrison MJG. Aspirin Wars. The optimal dose of aspirin to prevent stroke. *Stroke* 1996; **27:**585–7.
20. Barnett HJM, Kaste M, Meldrum H *et al.* Aspirin dose in stroke prevention. Beautiful hypotheses slain by ugly facts. *Stroke* 1996; **27:**588–92.
21. Patrono C, Roth GJ. Aspirin in ischemic cerebrovascular disease. How strong is the case for a different dosing regimen? *Stroke* 1996; **27:**756–60.
22. Hennerici MG. Aspirin dosage—a never-ending story? *Cerebrovasc Dis* 1995; **5:**308–9.
23. Goldstein LB, Farmer A, Matchar DB. Primary care physician-reported secondary and tertiary stroke prevention practices. A comparison between the United States and the United Kingdom. *Stroke* 1997; **28:**746–51.
24. Robbins DC, Schwartz RS, Kutny K *et al.* Comparative effects of aspirin and enteric-coated aspirin on loss of chromium. *Clin Ther* 1984; **6:**461–6.
25. Lanza FL, Rover GL, Nelson RS. Endoscopic evaluation of the effects of aspirin, buffered aspirin, and enteric-coated aspirin on gastric and duodenal mucosa. *N Engl J Med* 1990; **303:**136–8.
26. Kelly JP, Kaufman DW, Jurgelson JM *et al.* Risk of aspirin-associated major upper-gastrointestinal bleeding with enteric-coated or buffered product. *Lancet* 1996; **348:**1413–6.
27. Jiang H, Whelton PK, Vu B *et al.* Aspirin and risk of hemorrhagic stroke. A meta-analysis of

randomized controlled trials. *J Am Med Assoc* 1998; **280:**1930–5.
28. Kent RA. Ticlopidine. *Lancet* 1991; **337:** 459–60.
29. Hass WK, Easton JD, Adams HP *et al.* A randomized trial comparing ticlopidine hydrochloride with aspirin for the prevention of stroke in high-risk patients. *N Engl J Med* 1989; **321:** 501–7.
30. Gent M, Blakely JA, Easton JD *et al.* The Canadian American Ticlopidine Study (CATS) in thromboembolic stroke. *Lancet* 1989; **i:** 1215–20.
31. Toghi H, Murakami M. The effect of ticlopidine on TIA compared with aspirin: a double-blind, twelve-month follow-up study and open 24-month follow-up study. *Jpn J Med* 1987; **26:**117–9.
32. Bennett CL, Weinberg PD, Rozenberg-Ben-Dror K *et al.* Thrombotic thrombocytopenic purpura associated with ticlopidine. *Ann Intern Med* 1998; **128:**541–4.
33. Herber JM, Frehel D, Valleee E *et al.* Clopidogrel, a novel antiplatelet and antithrombotic agent. *Cardiovasc Drug Rev* 1993; **11:**180–98.
34. CAPRIE Steering Committee. A randomised, blinded trial of clopidogrel versus aspirin in patients at risk of ischemic events (CAPRIE). *Lancet* 1996; **348:**1329–39.
35. Kappelle LJ, Adams HP, Bendixen BH. Antiaggregant therapy for stroke prevention. In: *Cerebrovascular Disease: Pathophysiology, Diagnosis and Management* (Ginsberg MD, Bogousslavsky J, eds), pp. 1826–38. Oxford; Blackwell Science: 1998.
36. Diener H, Cunha L, Forbes C *et al.* European Stroke Prevention Study. Dipyridamole and acetylsalicylic acid in the secondary prevention of stroke. *J Neurol Sci* 1996; **143:**1–13.
37. Van Gijn J, Algra A. Secondary stroke prevention with antithrombotic drugs: what to do next? *Cerebrovasc Dis* 1997; **7**(Suppl 6):30–2.
38. Hankey GJ. One year after CAPRIE, IST and ESPS-2. Any changes in concepts? *Cerebrovasc Dis* 1998; **8**(Suppl 5):1–7.
39. Philips DR, Charo IF, Scharborough RM. GPIIb/IIIa: the responsive integrin. *Cell* 1991; **65:**359–62.
40. Mousa SA, DeGrado WF, Mu D-X *et al.* Oral antiplatelet, antithrombotic efficacy of DMP 728, a novel platelet GPIIb/IIIa antagonist. *Circulation* 1996; **93:**537–43.
41. Topol EJ. Toward a new frontier in myocardial reperfusion therapy. Emerging platelet prominence. *Circulation* 1998; **97:**211–8.

8

When to anticoagulate? At what dosage?

Richard Kay

CONTENTS • **Theory and practice** • **Primary prevention** • **Secondary prevention** • **Acute treatment** • **Conclusion**

THEORY AND PRACTICE

Anticoagulants have the theoretical value of preventing the formation, propagation, and embolization of thrombus. A thrombus, commonly called a blood clot, is a mixture of fibrin and blood cells. Some authorities differentiate clots into white clots and red clots. White clots, or arterial thrombi, are formed under conditions of high flow, and are composed mainly of platelet aggregates linked together by strands of fibrin. Red clots, or venous thrombi, are formed in areas of low flow, and are composed mainly of red cells trapped in a large network of fibrin. In the arterial system, white clots are usually formed at sites where atherosclerotic plaques rupture and expose the thrombogenic components of the endothelium to platelets and coagulation proteins. When these platelet-rich thrombi become occlusive, secondary stasis develops and a red clot is superimposed. Blood coagulation and platelet aggregation augment each other: thrombin is a potent activator of platelets and platelet phospholipid is required for several of the steps in the coagulation cascade, including the conversion of prothrombin to thrombin. Arterial thrombosis is therefore a product of two inseparable systems, to which a third system, the fibrinolytic system, also contributes. Antiaggregants, anticoagulants, and fibrinolytic drugs are all potentially effective in the prevention or treatment of ischemic stroke.[1,2]

Most ischemic strokes begin with the occlusion of a cerebral vessel by an in situ thrombus or a distant embolus. This is followed by the deterioration of the local circulation in which initially ischemic, but functional, brain tissues progress to a non-functional state and ultimately to infarction. This process may take place over 24 h or longer, depending on factors such as the adequacy of collateral flow and the metabolic status of the patient.[3] During this time, anticoagulents may have a beneficial effect by altering the balance between ongoing thrombosis and thrombolysis, and thus potentially affecting the flow of blood to the ischemic penumbra.[4–10]

It is, however, in the area of stroke prevention that anticoagulants (and antiaggregants) have found most support from clinical trials. The evidence is strongest with regard to the primary and secondary prevention of stroke in patients with non-valvular atrial fibrillation (NVAF). Nine randomized controlled trials (RCTs) have not only proven the value of long-term warfarin for primary prevention, but have fine-tuned the dosage and solved the question of whether the addition of aspirin would help to decrease the intensity of anticoagulation required (unfortunately it did not help).[11–19] The European Atrial Fibrillation Trial also confirmed that warfarin has an equal value for secondary prevention.[20]

In practice, therefore, anticoagulants may be considered for:

- primary prevention (against occurrence),
- secondary prevention (against recurrence), and
- acute treatment (against progression).

PRIMARY PREVENTION

For primary prevention, the patient is asymptomatic but has one or more risk factors that predispose to a future stroke. Stroke risk factors, for which subsequent stroke occurrence may be modified by anticoagulation, include atrial fibrillation (see Chapter 9) and other heart diseases (see Chapter 3), and hematological conditions including the prothrombotic states (see Chapter 4).

Oral anticoagulants, particularly warfarin, are usually used for primary prevention and the timing of starting therapy is not critical. After ensuring that the platelet count, liver function, and prothrombin time (expressed as an international normalized ratio, INR) are normal, most physicians would start with a loading dose of 10 mg/day for 2 days, followed by smaller daily doses adjusted according to the patient's INR and the range of INR being targeted.

Concerns have been expressed that the traditional 10-mg loading dose might produce excessive anticoagulation while potentially causing a transient hypercoagulable state through the precipitous fall of protein C during the first 36 h of warfarin therapy. Compared with the 10-mg regimen, regimens employing a 5-mg loading dose resulted in a four-fold reduction in the incidence of excessive anticoagulation, while the time to reach stable anticoagulation remained unchanged.[21,22] Since for primary prevention the full effects of anticoagulation are not needed urgently, warfarin should in general be started on a 5-mg induction regime.

The optimal range of INR for patients with NVAF is 2.0–3.0,[23–25] except for elderly patients in whom a range of 1.6–2.5 may be safer and yet retain 90% of the protection afforded by the standard ranges.[26,27] Higher ranges are recommended for patients with mechanical heart valves (2.5–3.5),[28] and for patients with prothrombotic states such as the antiphospolipid–antibody syndrome (≥3).[29] For many other cardiac, vascular, or hematological conditions, the optimal ranges of INR have not been established, but the general recommendation is 2.0–3.0 if stroke prevention is the goal.[30]

Apart from the target intensity of anticoagulation and the age of the patient, major factors that will affect the maintenance dose of warfarin include vitamin K intake and race.[31] Unexpected fluctuations in dose requirement could be due to changes in diet, undisclosed drug use, poor patient compliance or intermittent alcohol consumption.[32]

SECONDARY PREVENTION

For secondary prevention, the patient will have already suffered a stroke or transient ischemic attack (TIA) at some time before the anticoagulants are considered. The goal of therapy is to prevent a recurrence of the stroke, or the occurrence of some other vascular event such as myocardial infarction, systemic embolism, or vascular death (see Chapter 10). The European Atrial Fibrillation Trial, which enrolled patients up to 3 months after a TIA or minor ischemic stroke, found that oral warfarin (target INR 3.0) was significantly more effective than aspirin (300 mg/day) in reducing the composite outcome of vascular death, any stroke, myocardial infarction, or systemic embolism.[20] The study was not designed to address the timing of anticoagulation for acute cardioembolic strokes.

Opinion is divided on whether there is a particular need to start anticoagulating patients with cardioembolic strokes early, or even immediately, with intravenous heparin. Conversely, there is the perception that early recurrences are common if there is a cardiac source of emboli, and there is the risk of caus-

Table 8.1 Frequency of early cerebral recurrence after cardioembolic stroke

In retrospective studies					
	Days observed	*Number observed*	*Number anticoagulated*	*Overall recurrence (%)*	*Recurrence in untreated patients (%)*
Furlan (1982)[35]	7	54	25	13	22
Koller (1982)[36]	28	44	15	9	14
Hart (1983)[37]	10	35	12	3	4
Sage (1983)[38]	90	59	0	2	2
In prospective studies					
	Days observed	*Number observed*	*Number anticoagulated*	*Overall recurrence (%)*	*Cardiac condition*
Rothrock (1989)[55]	14	90	49	2	mixed
Sacco (1989)[41]	30	246	?	4	mixed
Bogousslavsky (1990)[43]	30	159	?	3	NVAF
Sandercock (1992)[42]	30	97	?	1	AF
Broderick (1992)[40]	30	318	?	2	mixed
Hornig (1993)[46]	21	566	?	3	mixed
In randomized studies					
	Days observed	*Number randomized*	*Number anticoagulated*	*Recurrence in treated patients (%)*	*Recurrence in control patients (%)*
CESG (1983)[39]	14	45	24	0	10
IST (AF subgroup)[80]	14	3169	1557	2.8	4.9
TOAST (CE subgroup)[81]	7	266	143	0	1.6
FISS (CE subgroup)[84]	10	43	27	3.7	6.3

AF, atrial fibrillation; NVAF, non-valvular AF; CE, cardioembolic.

ing hemorrhagic transformation in the process of giving heparin to patients with acute cerebral infarcts.

Early recurrence after ischemic stroke (Table 8.1)

The frequency of early cerebral recurrence after cardioembolic stroke in untreated patients is generally quoted as 1% per day, or about 12% (2–22%), in the first 2 weeks.[33,34] This impression was formed in the early 1980s based on retrospective studies of patients who were not systematically anticoagulated.[35–38] Results of a randomized study published in 1983,[39] in which none of 24 heparinized patients and two of 21 untreated patients had early recurrence, gave support to a practice that has remained largely unchanged today. This practice recommends that for acute cardioembolic stroke, heparin followed by warfarin should be given to non-hypertensive patients with small to moderately-sized infarcts, provided that a period of at least 48 h has lapsed since the onset of stroke and a CT scan done at the end of that period has ruled out any hemorrhagic transformation.[30] Patients with large infarcts or uncontrolled hypertension will have to have anticoagulant therapy further postponed or curtailed.

In more recent prospective studies, the frequencies of early cerebral recurrence after cardioembolic stroke were found to be considerably less than previously reported, ranging from 2% in the Rochester Epidemiology Project[40] to 4% in the NINDS Stroke Data Bank.[41] Patients with atrial fibrillation had even lower recurrence rates, from 1% in the Oxfordshire Community Stroke Project[42] to 3% in the Lausanne Stroke Registry.[43] Furthermore, the rate of early recurrence after cardioembolic stroke is not always higher than the rate after non-cardioembolic strokes. In the NINDS Stroke Data Bank, in which 40 (3.3%) of 1273 patients with cerebral infarction had a recurrence within 30 days, the risk for recurrence was greatest for large-artery atherothrombotic infarction (7.9%), followed by cardioembolic infarction (4.3%), infarction of undetermined cause (3.0), and lacunar infarction (2.2%). In the Rochester Epidemiology Project, the 30-day stroke recurrence rate (2%) was similar among patients with or without a cardiac source of emboli.

Thus, for patients with NVAF as the presumed embolic source, intravenous heparin may not be necessary. Oral warfarin may be initiated once the CT scan (≥48 h after onset) has ruled out hemorrhagic transformation or a large infarct.[30] Since warfarinization will take 2 days, it would be reasonable to start warfarin immediately provided the initial CT scan shows no hemorrhage and the patient's stroke is not major. In order to make a case for giving intravenous heparin, one has to look for other risk factors that predict a substantial risk of early re-embolization.

Among the many risk factors that have been suggested to predict early recurrence of cardioembolic stroke (e.g. history of hypertension, diabetes mellitus or alcohol abuse; diastolic hypertension or elevated blood glucose on admission; increased weakness, dehydration or nausea and vomiting; presence of atrial fibrillation, congestive heart failure, valvular heart disease, mechanical heart valves or intracardiac thrombi),[40,41,43–46] only valvular heart disease has been shown consistently to carry a clear risk of early re-embolization.[34,40,44–46] In practical terms, since the prevalence of rheumatic heart disease has declined sharply in the developed world, the absolute need for giving intravenous heparin for acute embolic stroke is now rarely encountered. However, it is likely that patients with mechanical heart valves or intracardiac thrombi (e.g. after acute myocardial infarction) will also have a risk of early recurrence high enough to justify intravenous heparin.

Patients who develop a stroke after acute myocardial infarction may have the stroke from causes other than embolism from the heart (e.g. hemodynamic causes, air or particulate embolism from cardiac catheterization, cerebral hemorrhage associated with thrombolytic treatment), and it is essential that these causes are excluded before heparin is considered. Transesophageal echocardiography and transcranial Doppler ultrasonography (for the detection of microemboli), in addition to the CT brain scan, will be useful in deciding which patient with acute cardioembolic stroke needs early heparinization.[47–49]

For patients with thrombi demonstrated in the aorta or in a large extracranial or intracranial artery, no RCTs supporting anticoagulation, whether early or late, have been reported. Results of the WARSS (Warfarin-Antiplatelet Recurrent Stroke Study) and the WASID (Warfarin–Aspirin Symptomatic Intracranial Disease) trials,[50,51] when they are available, will provide useful information on the effects of anticoagulants on these arterial lesions.

Hemorrhagic transformation of the infarct (Table 8.2)

The frequency of hemorrhagic transformation of the infarct (HTI) in patients receiving heparin for ischemic stroke ranged from 4% to 16% in studies conducted in the 1980s.[35–37,39,52–58]

Table 8.2 Frequency of hemorrhagic transformation of the infarct in patients receiving early anticoagulation

In comparative studies (all presumed embolic strokes)

	Number of patients anticoagulated	*Overall HTI in anticoagulated patients*	*Symptomatic HTI in anticoagulated patients*	*Overall HTI in untreated patients*
Furlan (1982)[35]	25	1 (4%)	0	0/29
Koller (1982)[36]	15	?	0	0/29
Hart (1983)[37]	12	?	0	?/23
Lodder (1983)[52]	21	2 (10%)	0	0/10
Calandre (1984)[53]	25	4 (16%)	3 (12%)	3/17 (18%)
Kelley (1984)[54]	14	2 (14%)	1 (7%)	2/19 (11%)
Rothrock (1989)[55]	49	4 (8%)	1 (2%)	3/41 (7%)

In non-comparative studies

	Number of patients anticoagulated	*Overall HTI in anticoagulated patients*	*Symptomatic HTI in anticoagulated patients*	*Indication for anticoagulation*
R-Lassepas (1986)[56]	132	?	2 (2%)	ischemic stroke
Haley (1988)[57]	36	?	1 (3%)	progressive stroke
Slivka (1990)[58]	69	?	2 (3%)	progressive stroke
Dahl (1994)[62]	52	?	1 (2%)	progressive stroke
Camerlingo (1994)[63]	45	6 (13%)	2 (4%)	ischemic stroke
Chamorro (1995)[64]	83	20 (24%)	7 (8%)	embolic stroke
Total	417	–	3.6%	

In randomized controlled trials

	Number of patients anticoagulated	*Overall HTI in anticoagulated patients (%)*	*Symptomatic HTI in anticoagulated patients (%)*	*Overall HTI in untreated patients (%)*	*Symptomatic HTI in untreated patients (%)*
CESG (1983)[39]	24	0	0	10	0
Duke (1986)[79]	112	0	0	0	0
IST (all patients)[80]	9717	?	1.2	?	0.4
IST (AF subgroup)[80]	1557	?	2.1	?	0.4
TOAST[81]	638	9.6	2.2	8.6	0.6
FISS[84]	203	7.4	0	12	1.0
FISS bis (high-dose)[85]	228	45	6.1	47	2.8
FISS bis (low-dose)[85]	255	44	3.7	47	2.8

Cardiac sources of emboli were not more prevalent in patients with HTI than in those with other causes of cerebral infarction.[40] Large infarcts with midline shift, acute hypertension, and early heparinization (less than 48 h after stroke onset) were believed to contribute to HTI.[59–61] In the last decade, the detection rate of HTI by CT scanning has increased to nearly a quarter of patients given intravenous heparin for acute ischemic stroke.[62–64]

Of more relevance is the frequency of HTI with symptomatic deterioration. This was documented in approximately 4% of patients given intravenous heparin, and it was clear that the occurrence of HTI more often than not resulted in no clinical worsening. Indeed, anticoagulation may have no serious consequences even when continued in the presence of HTI.[65] Very early (less than 5 h from onset) administration of heparin did not appear in one study to have caused an excessive number of symptomatic HTI,[63] and five out of seven symptomatic

HTIs in another study occurred 5 days or more after stroke onset.[64] The target range of activated partial thromboplastin time (aPTT) in the latter study was 1.5–2 times the control, but in four out of seven patients with symptomatic HTI, the last aPTT was greater than 3.0 times the control. With intravenous heparin therapy, what is targeted may not be what is always achieved, and both under-dosing and over-dosing regularly occur.

In summary, the risk of symptomatic HTI associated with intravenous heparin therapy is substantial, and administration 5 days or more after stroke onset may not be protective. In the presence of valvular heart disease, mechanical heart valve or intracardiac thrombi, immediate anticoagulation using heparin (but without a bolus dose) may be justified. Large infarcts should probably not be anticoagulated at all since anticoagulation will not affect what has already occurred (namely a major disabling stroke).[66] Compounds safer than standard heparin (e.g. low molecular weight heparin or heparinoid) can be considered (see below). For NVAF, oral warfarin may be used without loss of protection. For large artery thrombi, neither the risk of early recurrence nor the benefit of anticoagulation is known.

ACUTE TREATMENT

Another goal of giving anticoagulants during the acute phase of ischemic stroke is to limit the progression of the stroke, so that the eventual infarct volume might be smaller than it would have been otherwise. Traditionally, strokes that are clearly progressing are targeted for immediate heparinization. This practice of treating stroke by time course has been much criticized.[67] In the past few years, results of a number of RCTs of anticoagulation for the treatment of acute ischemic stroke have been published. These trials have in common the same pragmatic hypothesis that early anticoagulation, irrespective of the underlying mechanism, affects the long-term functional outcomes of stroke.

Progressing stroke

The concept of progressing or progressive stroke, or stroke-in-evolution, first proposed in the 1950s, has always been controversial.[68,69] It has been described as a clinical entity with no accepted name, no accepted definition, no accepted underlying mechanism and no accepted treatment.[70] Some degree of progression can be expected in 12–42% of patients hospitalized for stroke.[71] It is often assumed that the increasing deficits are due to propagation or embolization of the arterial thrombus, in which case heparin may be of some benefit. On the other hand, had the progression been due to brain edema, hemorrhagic transformation, fever, changes in blood glucose or blood pressure, or cellular mechanisms such as leukocycte accumulation or glutamate release,[72] anticoagulants would not be expected to be of any value.

The tradition of using heparin in patients who progress, began with clinical trials that were reported between 1958 and 1962.[73–75] These pre-CT era trials, which generally showed that heparin had a positive effect, were heavily criticized a decade ago,[76–78] and are now of historical interest only. In 1986 Duke *et al.* published a RCT of intravenous heparin for the prevention of stroke progression in 'acute partial stable stroke'.[79] This trial, which enrolled 225 patients, had the distinction of being the first trial of stroke therapy in which the power of the study (80% change of detecting a 30% difference with an alpha error of 5%) was predetermined and accomplished. But it did not answer the question whether heparin was beneficial to patients with progressive stroke, since those who were actually progressing or had atrial fibrillation had been specifically excluded. Nevertheless, 17% of the heparin-treated patients did progress further during treatment, compared with 19.5% of placebo-treated patients. The difference of 2.5% between the two groups was not statistically significant ($P = 0.62$, 95% CI −8.7 to 13.7%).

In a prospective study, Haley *et al.* administered intravenous heparin to 36 patients who had documented worsening or fluctuation after admission to hospital.[57] Overall, 50% of the patients showed continued progression despite receiving heparin. In a retrospective study of 69 patients treated with heparin for progressive stroke, 36% continued to deteriorate without regard to the intensity of anticoagulation.[58] However, in another retrospective study of 52 heparinized patients, only 21% continued to deteriorate.[62] The rates of serious HTI were under 3% in all three studies, although total bleeding complications were nearly 15% in the former two studies.[57,58]

With the currently available data, some authorities regard heparin anticoagulation for 3–5 days as reasonable in the setting of progressing ischemic stroke, especially those involving the vertebrobasilar circulation.[30] Others prefer aspirin.

Recent clinical trials of anticoagulation for acute ischemic stroke (Table 8.3)

The International Stroke Trial (IST)

IST was conceived in the late 1980s, inspired by the 'mega-trials' for myocardial infarction that were prevailing in Oxford, England. The aim of IST was to provide, by means of a large sample size, a 'reasonable estimate' of the effects of

Table 8.3 Trials of heparin, low molecular weight heparin and low molecular weight heparinoid for the treatment of acute ischemic stroke

	IST	*FISS*	*FISS bis*	*TOAST*
Patients randomized	19435	308	767	1281
Time window (h)	48	48	24	24
Mean time to treatment (h)	19	27	14	16
Main outcome measure	death or dependency	death or dependency	death or Barthel <85	'favorable outcome'*
Interim follow-up	none	3 months	3 months	7 days
High-dose group (%)	–	53	65	59
Low-dose group (%)	–	60	62	–
Control group (%)	–	64	61	54
P value	–	0.12	0.41	0.07
Final follow-up	6 months	6 months	6 months	3 months
High-dose group (%)	62.6	45	59	75
Low-dose group (%)	63.1	52	57	–
Placebo group (%)	62.9	65	57	74
P value	NS	0.005	0.62	0.49
Main safety measure	any death	any HTI	symptomatic ICH	serious ICH
Measured at	14 days	10 days	6 months	10 days
High-dose group (%)	9.3	6.2	6.1	2.4
Low-dose group (%)	8.7	8.6	3.7	–
Placebo group (%)	9.3	12.0	2.8	0.8
P value	NS	0.19	NS	0.05

* Combination of Glasgow Outcome Scale of I or II and modified Barthel Index of 12 or greater. HTI, hemorrhagic transformation of the infarct; ICH, intracranial hemorrhage.

subcutaneous heparin (in twice daily doses of 5000 IU or 12 500 IU) or oral aspirin (300 mg/day) on death and other major clinical events during the first 14 days after acute ischemic stroke, and on death and dependency in activities of daily living at 6 months after stroke. The fundamental criterion of inclusion was that the participating physician was uncertain whether or not to administer either or both of the trial treatments to a particular patient.[80]

Nearly 20 000 patients from 36 countries were randomized, and the outcome data were over 99% complete. CT scanning was obtained in 67% of patients before randomization, and in a further 29% after randomization. Treatment was given without blinding, but the 6-month outcome was assessed largely by blinded means (letter or telephone).

The main results of IST are shown in Table 8.3. The IST collaborative group concluded that neither heparin regimen offered any clinical advantage at 6 months after stroke, but for aspirin there was a suggestion of worthwhile improvement (approximately 1% in absolute terms). In the secondary analyses, patients allocated to heparin vs. no heparin had fewer recurrent ischemic strokes (2.9% vs. 3.8%) but more hemorrhagic strokes (1.2% vs. 0.4%) at 14 days. In the subgroup of patients with atrial fibrillation, heparin was associated with a larger than average reduction of recurrent ischemic stroke (Table 8.1), but there was also a larger than average increase in hemorrhagic stroke (Table 8.2). Patients with a posterior circulation syndrome derived no definite benefit from heparin therapy when observed at 6 months, although the confidence interval was wide.

The Trial of ORG 10172 in Acute Stroke Treatment (TOAST)

TOAST was a double-blind, placebo-controlled trial which was also conceived in the late 1980s,[81] when low molecular weight heparin and heparinoids were showing promise as safer alternatives to standard heparin. ORG 10172 (danaparoid) is a mixture of heparinoids, namely dermatan sulfate, heparan sulfate, and chondroitin sulfate, with a mean molecular weight of 5500 daltons. The antithrombotic action of danaparoid is derived chiefly from heparan sulfate, which, like the low molecular weight heparins, has greater antifactor Xa activity than antifactor IIa activity, and has only a modest effect in prolonging global tests of coagulation. Compared with heparin, these low molecular weight compounds have almost no effect on platelets, so that in patients treated with them bleeding is less likely and heparin-induced thrombocytopenia rarely occurs. They are potentially more useful than heparin clinically because of their better bioavailability, longer half-life, and having a dose-dependent clearance, resulting in a more predictable anticoagulant response even when given subcutaneously without monitoring in fixed or weight-adjusted dosages.[82,83]

TOAST enrolled 1281 patients with acute ischemic stroke within 24 h of onset. Patients assigned to danaparoid received it initially as a bolus, followed by continuous infusion for 7 days, with rates adjusted to maintain an antifactor Xa activity at 0.6–0.8 antifactor Xa U/ml. The main outcome measure of efficacy was a 'favorable outcome', defined as the combination of a Glasgow Outcome Scale score of I or II and a modified Barthel Index of 12 (on a scale of 0 to 20) or greater, at 7 days and at 3 months after stroke.

The main results of TOAST are shown in Table 8.3. At 7 days, 59.2% of 635 patients given danaparoid and 54.3% of 633 receiving placebo had favorable outcomes ($P = 0.07$). At 3 months, 75.2% of patients given danaparoid and 73.7% of patients receiving placebo had favorable outcomes ($P = 0.49$). Serious intracranial bleeding occurred in 2.4% of danaparoid-treated patients and in 0.8% of placebo-treated patients ($P = 0.05$). Among patients with large-artery atherosclerosis, 68.1% of 113 who received danaparoid, and 54.7% of 117 who received placebo had favorable outcomes at 3 months, a difference that was significant (odds ratio 1.77, 95% CI, 1.04–3.03).

The TOAST investigators concluded that despite an apparent positive response to treatment at 7 days, emergent administration of danaparoid was not associated with an improvement in favorable outcome at 3 months. However, they found the positive response at both 7 days and 3 months among patients who had stroke secondary to large-artery atherosclerosis intriguing, and recommended a further prospective study for this group of patients.

The Fraxiparine in Ischemic Stroke Study (FISS)

FISS was a small trial of the low molecular weight heparin, Fraxiparine (nadroparin), performed entirely on Chinese patients.[84] It used the IST method of outcome assessment, and also had two dosage regimens, which were nadroparin 3800 anti-Xa IU,* once daily for the low-dose group and twice daily for the high-dose group. Treatment was given subcutaneously within 48 h of onset of CT-proven ischemic stroke, for a total of 10 days.

The main results of FISS are show in Table 8.3. At 3 months, 53% of 100 patients in the high-dose group, 60% of 101 patients in the low-dose group, and 64% of 105 patients in the placebo group were dead or dependent on others for activities of daily living ($P = 0.12$). At 6 months, 45% of patients in the high-dose group, 52% of patients in the low-dose group, and 65% of patients in the placebo group were dead or dependent ($P = 0.005$). There was no significant difference in the rates of any HTI among the three groups at 10 days; symptomatic HTI occurred in only one patient in the placebo group. There were too few patients to allow for any subgroup analysis.

The FISS investigators concluded that nadroparin, given at a dosage of 3800 anti-Xa IU twice daily for 10 days, was superior to placebo in treating patients with acute ischemic stroke. However, they were not sure if their results could be generalized to other populations.

*The dosage of Fraxiparine quoted in previous publications was 4100 anti-Xa IU, but this should be changed to 3800 anti-Xa IU, in accordance with the current definition of anti-Xa international units (European Pharmacopoeia).

The FISS bis study

FISS bis was a bigger trial that took place mainly in Europe.[85] Compared with FISS, it had a shorter time window (24 h), a weight adjusted dosage of nadroparin, and a requirement that patients must have significant weakness (Unified Neurological Stroke Scale motor score ≥10/15) before participation. The weight-adjusted dosage meant that for persons weighing 60–69 kg, 5700 anti-Xa IU of nadroparin would be administered, once daily for those assigned to the low-dose group and twice daily for those assigned to the high-dose group. Treatment was given for a total of 10 ± 2 days.

The main results of FISS bis are shown in Table 8.3. At 3 months, 65% of patients in the high-dose group, 62% of patients in the low-dose group, and 61% of patients in the placebo group were dead or had a Barthel Index of <85 ($P = 0.41$). At 6 months, 59% of patients in the high-dose group, 57% of patients in the low-dose group, and 57% of patients in the placebo group were dead or had a Barthel Index of <85 ($P = 0.62$). Unlike the TOAST patients, patients in FISS bis with large-artery atherosclerosis showed no better outcomes after treatment with nadroparin than with placebo. There was a non-significant trend towards more symptomatic HTI with higher dosages of nadroparin.

The FISS bis group concluded that there was no overall benefit in the primary endpoint (death or Barthel Index <85 at 6 months) at either dose. There was only a significantly lower rate of pulmonary embolism with both doses.

Relationship between anticoagulation and symptomatic HTI in clinical trials

Commentators stress the risk of symptomatic HTI if stroke patients are treated acutely with anticoagulants, but how large is the risk? The baseline risk of symptomatic HTI in untreated patients is less than 1% in IST, FISS and TOAST (FISS bis 2.8%—see below). In all but the FISS study, there is an excess of symptomatic HTI in patients receiving anticoagulation. The absolute difference is small, from 0.8% in IST, 1.6% in TOAST, to 2.0% in FISS bis.

In IST, the excess of symptomatic HTI comes almost entirely from the 12 500 IU twice daily heparin group. Anticoagulant response to heparin given subcutaneously is highly variable; in most patients there is hardly any effect on anticoagulation, while in others the clotting times are much prolonged. This variability may paradoxically make heparin seem ineffective, for most patients will have insufficient drug in the circulation, while an increase in side-effects may be observed in the small number of patients with very high concentrations, which appears to be what is observed in IST.[86]

In TOAST, danaparoid was given initially as a bolus, then by infusion at a rate adjusted to produce an antifactor Xa activity of 0.6–0.8 U/ml. This method of delivery and the dose range were tested in pilot studies,[87,88] but small increases in risks might have been overlooked. In the main study, patients who weighed less than 56.2 kg had a higher antifactor Xa activity and a greater risk of serious bleeding when given danaparoid.

In FISS, antifactor Xa activity was not measured. Based on the pilot study,[89] it was unlikely to be more than 0.6 U/ml on average in the high-dose group. Compared with TOAST, the dose given in FISS was not only smaller but also given later (mean interval to treatment 27 vs. 16 h), and subcutaneously rather than intravenously. The overall (symptomatic and asymptomatic) rates of HTI in treated patients were slightly less in FISS (7.4%) than in TOAST (9.6%), and symptomatic HTI occurred only in TOAST (2.2%), suggesting that the FISS regimen was safer.

In FISS bis, the dose of nadroparin was higher and given earlier than in FISS. An average patient in FISS bis would receive 50% more drug and 13 h earlier than he would in FISS. The overall rates of HTI, in the order of 45% irrespective of treatment, were very high in FISS bis, suggesting that a different standard of reading CT scans had been used. For symptomatic HTI, the baseline rate of 2.8% was already higher than in other studies. The excess

Table 8.4 Suggested timing and dosage for using anticoagulants in ischemic stroke

	Timing	*Dosage*
For primary prevention		
NVAF	Start warfarin anytime	Aim for INR 2.0–3.0
Mechanical heart valves	Start warfarin anytime	Aim for INR 3.0–4.0
Other conditions*	Start warfarin anytime	Aim for INR 2.0–3.0
For secondary prevention (after acute stroke)		
Valvular heart disease	Start heparin after 48 h†	Aim for aPTT 1.5–2 × control
Mechanical heart valves	Start heparin after 48 h†	Aim for aPTT 1.5–2 × control
Intracardiac thrombi	Start heparin after 48 h†	Aim for aPTT 1.5–2 × control
NVAF	Start warfarin after 48 h‡	Aim for INR 3.0
Other conditions*	Start warfarin after 48 h‡	Aim for INR 3.0
For acute treatment		
Progressive stroke	No evidence that anticoagulation is effective in stopping progression	
All ischemic stroke	No evidence that anticoagulation is beneficial for long-term outcomes	
Stroke with specific etiology	No evidence available from randomized controlled trials	

* For which anticoagulation is indicated.
† Or immediately without a bolus dose if the stroke is not major (after CT to exclude cerebral hemorrhage).
‡ Or immediately on 5-mg induction if the stroke is not major (after CT to exclude cerebral hemorrhage).

of 3.3% in the high-dose group represented an increase of 1.2 times over the baseline rate, which is less than the proportions seen in IST and TOAST.

In summary, while there is a definite risk of symptomatic HTI in patients anticoagulated for ischemic stroke, under clinical trial conditions the increase in absolute risk is no more than 2%. Large doses of heparin, even when given subcutaneously, should be avoided. Low molecular weight heparin or heparinoid can cause significant increases in symptomatic HTI, which appears to occur in a dose-dependent manner. There should be no need to give this group of drugs intravenously, which only increases the risk of bleeding. Lastly, anticoagulation after the first 24 h of stroke may cause fewer hemorrhagic transformations that are symptomatic.

CONCLUSION

A suggested approach to the administration of anticoagulants for the prevention and treatment of ischemic stroke is shown in Table 8.4. The list is not exhaustive and many conditions have been left out, mainly because there is no clear consensus for their management. For the acute treatment of stroke, future research should be in the direction of testing therapies, anticoagulants included, for specific causes of brain ischemia.[90,91]

REFERENCES

1. Caplan LR (ed.). *Brain Ischemia*. London; Springer-Verlag: 1995.
2. Moulin T, Bogousslavsky J. Anticoagulation in stroke. In: *Cerebrovascular Disease: Pathophysiology, Diagnosis, and Management* (Ginsberg MD, Bogousslavsky J, eds), pp. 1839–53. Oxford; Blackwell Science: 1998.
3. Fisher M, Garcia JH. Evolving stroke and the ischemic penumbra. *Neurology* 1996; **47:** 884–8.
4. del Zoppo GJ. Microvascular changes during cerebral ischemia and reperfusion. *Cerebrovasc Brain Metabolic Rev* 1994; **6:**47–96.
5. Thomas WS, Mori E, Copeland BR, Yu JQ, Morrissey JH, del Zoppo GJ. Tissue factor contributes to microvascular defects after focal cerebral ischemia. *Stroke* 1993; **24:**847–53.
6. Uchiyama S, Yamazaki M, Hara Y, Iwata M. Alterations of platelet, coagulation, and fibrinolysis markers in patients with acute ischemic stroke. *Semin Thromb Hemost* 1997; 23: 535–41.
7. Takano K, Yamaguchi T, Kato H, Omae T. Activation of coagulation in acute cardioembolic stroke. *Stroke* 1991; **22:**12–6.
8. Toghi H, Kawashima M, Tamura K, Suzuki H. Coagulation-fibrinolysis abnormalities in acute and chronic phases of cerebral thrombosis and embolism. *Stroke* 1990; **21:**1663–7.
9. Fisher M, Francis R. Altered coagulation in cerebral ischemia: platelet, thrombin, and plasmin activity. *Arch Neurol* 1990; **47:**1075–9.
10. Landi G, D'Angelo A, Boccardi E *et al.* Hypercoagulability in acute stroke: prognostic significance. *Neurology* 1987; **37:**1667–71.
11. Petersen P, Boysen G, Godtfredsen J, Andersen ED, Andersen B. Placebo-controlled, randomised trial of warfarin and aspirin for prevention of thromboembolic complications in chronic atrial fibrillation: The Copenhagen AFASAK study. *Lancet* 1989; **i:**175–9.
12. Stroke Prevention in Atrial Fibrillation Study Group Investigators. Stroke Prevention in Atrial Fibrillation Study: Final results. *Circulation* 1991; **84:**527–9.
13. The Boston Area Anticoagulation Trial for Atrial Fibrillation Investigators. The effect of low-dose warfarin on the risk of stroke in patients with nonrheumatic atrial fibrillation. *N Engl J Med* 1990; **323:**1505–11.
14. Connolly SJ, Laupacis A, Gent M, Roberts RS, Cairns JA, Joyner C. Canadian Atrial Fibrillation Anticoagulation (CAFA) Study. *J Am Coll Cardiol* 1991; **18:**349–55.
15. Ezekowitz MD, Bridgers SL, James KE *et al.* Warfarin in the prevention of stroke associated with nonrheumatic atrial fibrillation. *N Engl J Med* 1992; **327:**1406–12.
16. Stroke Prevention in Atrial Fibrillation Investigators. Warfarin versus aspirin for prevention of atrial fibrillation: Stroke Prevention in Atrial Fibrillation II Study. *Lancet* 1994; **343:**687–91.
17. Stroke Prevention in Atrial Fibrillation Investigators. Adjusted-dose warfarin versus low-intensity, fixed-dose warfarin plus aspirin for high-risk patients with atrial fibrillation:

Stroke Prevention in Atrial Fibrillation III randomised clinical trial. *Lancet* 1996; **348:**633–8.

18. Gullov AL, Koefoed BG, Petersen P *et al.* Fixed minidose warfarin and aspirin alone and in combination vs adjusted-dose warfarin for stroke prevention in atrial fibrillation: Second Copenhagen Atrial Fibrillation, Aspirin, and Anticoagulation Study. *Arch Int Med* 1998; **158:**1513–21.
19. Pengo V, Zasso A, Barbero F *et al.* Effectiveness of fixed minidose warfarin in the prevention of thromboembolism and vascular death in nonrheumatic atrial fibrillation *Am J Cardiol* 1998; **82:**433–7.
20. EAFT (European Atrial Fibrillation Trial) Study Group. Secondary prevention in non-rheumatic atrial fibrillation after transient ischaemic attack or minor stroke. *Lancet* 1993; **342:**1255–62.
21. Harrison L, Johnston M, Massicotte MP, Crowther M, Moffat K, Hirsh J. Comparison of 5-mg and 10-mg loading doses an initiation of warfarin therapy. *Ann Int Med* 1997; **126:** 133–6.
22. Tait RC, Sefcick A. A warfarin induction regimen for out-patient anticoagulation in patients with atrial fibrillation. *Br J Haematol* 1998; **101:**450–4.
23. Lancaster T, Mant J, Singer DE. Stroke prevention in atrial fibrillation: warfarin is most effective when the INR lies between 2.0 and 4.0 [Editorial]. *Br Med J* 1997; **314:**1563–4.
24. Hylek EM, Skates SJ, Sheehan MA, Singer DE. An analysis of the lowest effective intensity of prophylactic anticoagulation for patients with nonrheumatic atrial fibrillation. *N Engl J Med* 1996; **335:**540–6.
25. The European Atrial Fibrillation Trial Study Group. Optimal oral anticoagulant therapy in patients with nonrheumatic atrial fibrillation and recent cerebral ischaemia. *N Engl J Med* 1995; **333:**5–10.
26. Hart RG. Intensity of anticoagulation to prevent stroke patients with atrial fibrillation [Letter]. *Ann Int Med* 1998; **128:**408.
27. Booth F, Mehta A. Stroke prevention in atrial fibrillation: suggested range of international normalised ratio may lead to overanticoagulation [Letter]. *Br Med J* 1997; **315:**1019.
28. Cannegieter SC, Rosendaal FR, Wintzen AR, van der Meer FJ, Vandenbroucke JP, Briet E. Optimal oral anticoagulant therapy in patients with mechanical heart valves. *N Engl J Med* 1995; **333:**11–17.
29. Khamashta MA, Cuadrado MJ, Mujic F, Taub NA, Hunt BJ, Hughes GRV. The management of thrombosis in the antiphospholipid–antibody syndrome. *N Engl J Med* 1995; **332:** 993–7.
30. Sherman DG, Dyken ML Jr, Gent M, Harrison MJG, Hart RG, Mohr JP. Antithrombotic therapy for cerebrovascular disorders: an update. *Chest* 1995; **108**(Suppl):444–56.
31. Yu HCM, Chan TYK, Critchley JAJH, Woo KS. Factors determining the maintenance dose of warfarin in Chinese patients. *Q J Med* 1996; **89:**127–35.
32. Hirsh J, Dalen JE, Deykin D, Poller L, Bussey H. Oral anticoagulants: mechanism of action, clinical effectiveness, and optimal therapeutic range. *Chest* 1995; **108**(Suppl):231–46.
33. Cerebral Embolism Task Force. Cardiogenic brain embolism. *Arch Neurol* 1986; **43:**71–84.
34. Cerebral Embolism Task Force. Cardiogenic brain embolism: the second report of the Cerebral Embolism Task Force. *Arch Neurol* 1989; **46:**727–43.
35. Furlan AJ, Cavalier SJ, Hobbs RE, Weinstein MA, Modic MT. Hemorrhage and anticoagulation after nonseptic embolic brain infarction. *Neurology* 1982; **32:**280–2.
36. Koller RL. Recurrent embolic cerebral infarction and anticoagulation. *Neurology* 1982; **32:**283–5.
37. Hart RG, Coull BM, Hart D. Early recurrent embolism associated with nonvalvular atrial fibrillation: a retrospective study. *Stroke* 1983; **14:**688–93.
38. Sage JI, Van Uitert RL. Risk of recurrent stroke in patients with atrial fibrillation and non-valvular heart disease. *Stroke* 1983; **14:**537–40.
39. Cerebral Embolism Study Group. Immediate anticoagulation of embolic stroke: a randomized trial. *Stroke* 1983; **14:**668–76.
40. Broderick JP, Phillips SJ, O'Fallon M, Frye RL, Whisnant JP. Relationship of cardiac disease to stroke occurrence, recurrence and mortality. *Stroke* 1992; **23:**1250–6.
41. Sacco RL, Foulkes MA, Mohr JP, Wolf PA, Hier DB, Price TR. Determinants of early recurrence of cerebral infarction. *Stroke* 1989; **20:**983–9.
42. Sandercock P, Bamford J, Dennis M *et al.* Atrial fibrillation and stroke: prevalence in different types of stroke and influence on early and long term prognosis (Oxfordshire community stroke project). *Br Med J* 1992; **305:**1460–5.
43. Bogousslavsky J, Van Melle G, Regli F, Kappenberger L. Pathogenesis of anterior circulation stroke in patients with nonvalvular atrial fibrillation: The Lausanne Stroke Registry. *Neurology* 1990; **40:**1046–50.

44. Yasaka M, Yamaguchi T, Oita J, Sawada T, Shichiri M, Omae T. Clinical features of recurrent embolization in acute cardioembolic stroke. *Stroke* 1993; **24:**1681–5.
45. Arboix A, Garcia-Eroles L, Oliveres M, Massons JB, Targa C. Clinical predictors of early embolic recurrence in presumed cardioembolic stroke. *Cerebrovasc Dis* 1998; **8:**345–53.
46. Hornig CR, Dorndorf W. Early outcome and recurrence after cardiogenic brain embolism. *Acta Neurol Scand* 1993; **88:**26–31.
47. Di Pasquale G, Urbinati S, Pinelli G. New echocardiographic markers of embolic risk in atrial fibrillation. *Cerebrovasc Dis* 1995; **5:**315–22.
48. Infeld B, Bowser DN, Gerraty RP. Cerebral microemboli in atrial fibrillation detected by transcranial Doppler ultrasonography. *Cerebrovasc Dis* 1996; **6:**339–45.
49. Valton L, Larrue V, Pavy Le Traon A, Géraud A. Cerebral microembolism in patients with stroke or transient ischaemic attack as a risk factor for early recurrence. *J Neurol Neurosurg Psychiatry* 1997; **63:**784–7.
50. Mohr JP and the WARSS Group. Design considerations for the Warfarin–Antiplatelet Recurrent Stroke Study. *Cerebrovasc Dis* 1995; **5:**156–7.
51. Chimowitz MI, Kokkinos J, Strong J *et al.* The Warfarin–Aspirin Symptomatic Intracranial Disease Study. *Neurology* 1995; **45:**1488–93.
52. Lodder J, van der Lugt PJ. Evaluation of the risk of immediate anticoagulant treatment in patients with embolic stroke of cardiac origin. *Stroke* 1983; **14:**42–6.
53. Calandre L, Ortega JF, Bermejo F. Anticoagulation and hemorrhagic infarction in cerebral embolism secondary to rheumatic heart disease. *Arch Neurol* 1984; **41:**1152–4.
54. Kelley RE, Berger JR, Alter M, Kovacs AG. Cerebral ischemia and atrial fibrillation: Prospective study. *Neurology* 1984; **34:**1285–91.
55. Rothrock JF, Dittrich HC, McAllen S, Taft BJ, Lyden PD. Acute anticoagulation following cardioembolic stroke. *Stroke* 1989; **20:**730–4.
56. Ramirez-Lassepas M, Quinones MR, Nino HH. Treatment of acute ischemic stroke: open trial with continuous intravenous heparinization. *Arch Neurol* 1986; **43:**386–90.
57. Haley EC Jr, Kassell NF, Torner JC. Failure of heparin to prevent progression in progressing ischemic infarction. *Stroke* 1988; **19:**10–14.
58. Slivka A, Levy D. Natural history of progressive ischemic stroke in a population treated with heparin. *Stroke* 1990; **21:**1657–62.
59. Lodder J. CT-detected hemorrhagic infarction; relation with the size of the infarct, and the presence of midline shift. *Acta Neurol Scand* 1984; **70:**329–35.
60. Cerebral Embolism Study Group. Immediate anticoagulation of embolic stroke: brain hemorrhage and management options. *Stroke* 1984; **15:**779–89.
61. Cerebral Embolism Study Group. Cardioembolic stroke, early anticoagulation, and brain hemorrhage. *Arch Int Med* 1987; **147:**636–40.
62. Dahl T, Sandset PM, Abildgaard U. Heparin treatment in 52 patients with progressive ischemic stroke. *Cerebrovasc Dis* 1994; **4:**101–5.
63. Camerlingo M, Casto L, Censori B *et al.* Immediate anticoagulation with heparin for first-ever ischemic stroke in the carotid artery territories observed within 5 hours of onset. *Arch Neurol* 1994; **51:**462–7.
64. Chamorro A, Vila N, Saiz A, Alday M, Tolosa E. Early anticoagulation after large cerebral embolic infarction: a safety study. *Neurology* 1995; **45:**861–5.
65. Pessin MS, Estol CJ, Lafranchise F, Caplan LR. Safety of anticoagulation after hemorrhagic infarction. *Neurology* 1994; **43:**1298–303.
66. Lodder J. Safety of heparin in acute ischemic stroke [Letter]. *Neurology* 1996; **47:**589.
67. Caplan LR. To heparinize or not: an unsettled issue [Letter]. *Stroke* 1989; **20:**968.
68. Gautier JC. Stroke-in-progression. *Stroke* 1985; **16:**729–33.
69. Caplan LR. Treatment of 'progressive' stroke [Letter]. *Stroke* 1991; **22:**694–5.
70. Asplund K. Any progress on progressing stroke? [Editorial] *Cerebrovasc Dis* 1992; **2:**317–9.
71. Rödén-Jüllig Å. Progressing stroke: epidemiology. *Cerebrovasc Dis* 1997; **7**(Suppl 5):2–5.
72. Dávalos A, Castillo J. Potential mechanisms of worsening. *Cerebrovasc Dis* 1997; **7**(Suppl 5): 19–24.
73. Fisher CM. Use of anticoagulants in cerebral thrombosis. *Neurology* 1958; **8:**311–32.
74. Carter AB. Anticoagulant treatment in progressing stroke. *Br Med J* 1961; **2:**70–3.
75. Baker RN, Broward JA, Fang HC *et al.* Anticoagulant therapy in cerebral infarction: report on co-operative study. *Neurology* 1962; **12:**823–35.
76. Sage JI. The use and overuse of heparin in therapeutic trials [Editorial]. *Arch Neurol* 1985; **42:**315–7.
77. Miller VT, Hart RG. Heparin anticoagulation in acute brain ischemia. *Stroke* 1988; **19:**403–6.

78. Estol CJ, Pessin MS. Anticoagulation: Is there still a role in atherothrombotic stroke? *Stroke* 1990; **21:**820–4.
79. Duke RJ, Bloch RF, Turpie AGG, Trebilcock R, Bayer N. Intravenous heparin for the prevention of stroke progression in acute partial stable stroke: a randomized controlled trial. *Ann Intern Med* 1986; **105:**825–8.
80. International Stroke Trial Collaboration Group. The International Stroke Trial (IST): a randomised trial of aspirin, subcutaneous heparin, both or neither among 19435 patients with acute ischaemic stroke. *Lancet* 1997; **349:**1569–81.
81. TOAST investigators. Low molecular weight heparinoid, ORG 10172 (danaparoid), and outcome after acute ischemic stroke. *J Am Med Assoc* 1998; **279:**1265–72.
82. Gordon DL, Linhardt R, Adams HP Jr. Low-molecular-weight heparins and heparinoids and their use in acute or progressing ischemic stroke. *Clin Neuropharmacol* 1990; **13:**522–43.
83. Weitz JI. Low-molecular-weight heparins. *N Engl J Med* 1997; **337:**688–98.
84. Kay R, Wong KS, Yu YL *et al.* Low-molecular-weight heparin for the treatment of acute ischemic stroke. *N Engl J Med* 1995; **333:**1588–93.
85. Hommel M. Fraxiparine in Ischaemic Stroke Study (FISS bis) [Abstract]. *Cerebrovasc Dis* 1998; **8**(Suppl 4):19.
86. Cohen A. Interpretation of IST and CAST stroke trials [Letter]. *Lancet* 1997; **350:**440.
87. Biller J, Massy EW, Marler JR *et al.* A dose escalation study of ORG 10172 (low molecular weight heparinoid) in stroke. *Neurology* 1989; **39:**262–5.
88. Massey EW, Biller J, Davis JN *et al.* Large-dose infusions of heparinoid ORG 10172 in ischemic stroke. *Stroke* 1990; **21:**1289–92.
89. Kay R, Wong KS, Woo J. Pilot study of low-molecular-weight heparin in the treatment of acute ischemic stroke. *Stroke* 94; **25:**684–5.
90. Hankey GJ. Heparin in acute ischaemic stroke: The T wave is negative and it's time to stop. *Med J Aust* 1998; **169:**534–6.
91. Caplan LR. Stroke treatment: promising but still struggling [Editorial]. *J Am Med Assoc* 1998; **279:**1304–6.

9

Atrial fibrillation

David G Sherman

CONTENTS • **Introduction** • **Diagnosis** • **Clinical trials** • **Summary**

INTRODUCTION

Atrial fibrillation (AF) is a common cardiac arrhythmia, especially in older individuals. The prevalence of AF increases progressively after the age of 60. The median age of individuals with AF is 75 years old. Thus AF is a disease affecting the elderly. AF is present in over one-third of individuals aged 80–89 with acute ischemic stroke.[1] The causes of AF are multiple. Mitral stenosis often leads to AF as pressures increase within the left atrium. Thyrotoxicosis may cause AF in which case reversion to sinus rhythm occurs with successful treatment of the hyperthyroidism. In patients without mitral stenosis, 'non-valvular' AF, there is often coexistent hypertension, diabetes mellitus or coronary artery disease. These largest groups of patients with AF are thought to have 'degenerative' changes in the cardiac conduction system that is responsible for their AF although these changes may be adversely influenced by coexistent cardiovascular disorders. Estimates are that there are over 3 million individuals in the United States with AF with the number of cases increasing. Atrial fibrillation has been described as one of the 'epidemics' in cardiovascular disease with the number of hospital discharges with this diagnosis more than doubling over a decade.[2] Efforts to maintain sinus rhythm in patients with AF have not been widely successful suggesting that for the foreseeable future, management strategies will still be largely directed towards preventing the adverse consequences of AF rather than eliminating the rhythm disturbance.

Atrial fibrillation is a well-established risk factor for stroke. Epidemiological studies have shown that AF conveys about a five-fold increased risk for stroke.[3] This risk is even greater in those patients with mitral stenosis and AF where there is a 17-fold increase in risk. The importance of AF as a risk factor for stroke increases with age. The attributable risk in the 80–89-year-old age group of AF patients is 23% in the Framingham study.[4] In this very elderly population AF emerges as the most powerful risk factor for stroke while the other recognized risk factors, i.e., hypertension, diabetes, hyperlipidemia, become less dominant as predictors of stroke. The randomized clinical trials of AF have confirmed an overall annual stroke incidence of about 5% in the general population of patients with AF.[5–8] An important principal that has emerged from these trials is that of variable risk depending on the presence or absence of coexisting conditions in patients with AF. The details of this risk stratification will be presented later.

About 15% of patients with ischemic stroke have associated AF. This proportion more than doubles in patients with ischemic stroke over the age of 80.[1] These patients often have other risk factors as a potential cause for their stroke. They commonly have hypertension and evidence of atherosclerotic cerebrovascular disease. They may have cardiac abnormalities other than AF that could be a potential source of embolus. At the conclusion of a diagnostic evaluation, about two-thirds of patients with ischemic stroke and AF are found to have their stroke due to an embolus originating from a thrombus in the left atrium. This observation underscores the need for consideration of alternative stroke mechanisms and a diagnostic evaluation for other potential causes of stroke in these patients.

DIAGNOSIS

There are no clinical features that are highly specific in establishing AF as the mechanism for stroke in a given patient. Stroke symptoms tend to be sudden and maximal at onset. Preceding transient ischemic attacks (TIAs) are uncommon but may be part of the history. Unconsciousness or seizures at onset are symptoms that are suggestive of a cardiogenic stroke mechanism.[9] Any vascular territory may be affected but the middle cerebral artery (MCA) territory is most common. Posterior cerebral artery territory strokes have a somewhat higher likelihood of being of cardiogenic embolic mechanism, as do strokes involving the 'top of the basilar'.[10] The assumption is that emboli entering a vertebral artery are prone to occlude the distal basilar artery or enter one or both posterior cerebral arteries. Compared to other causes, AF-related strokes tend to be larger, more disabling and more often fatal.[11,12] The Oxfordshire community stroke project found the 30-day case fatality rate to be significantly higher (23%) than that in patients with sinus rhythm (8%).[13] Similar findings of increased mortality at 30 days and handicap at 6 months associated with AF were found by Censori *et al.* in a study of prognostic factors in ischemic stroke.[14]

The diagnostic evaluation of a patient with acute stroke and AF is directed at establishing that an embolus arising from a left atrial thrombus and not an alternative stroke mechanism was the probable cause for an individual's stroke. As with most acute stroke patients the initial screening neuroimaging study is a non-contrasted computerized tomographic (CT) scan. The CT scan may be normal, or it may show signs of early ischemia in the region of ischemia. One may be able to visualize the embolus by demonstrating the 'dense middle cerebral artery' sign. A cortical abnormality is more common with cardiogenic embolus than a lacunar location. Large lacunes, more than 1.5 cm in diameter, should raise the possibility of a mechanism other than small artery occlusive disease, and increase suspicions of an embolic stroke mechanism. Visualization of previous brain infarcts in arterial territories remote from the current stroke raises suspicion of an embolic mechanism that may have already caused brain infarcts with or without obvious symptoms.

The diagnosis of AF, when present, is not difficult. An electrocardiogram (ECG) confirms the abnormal rhythm in a patient with an irregularly irregular heart rate or pulse. The diagnostic difficulty lies with those patients with intermittent AF who on presentation for medical evaluation are in sinus rhythm. Patients with bouts of AF may experience palpitations, dyspnea or lightheadedness related to the rapid ventricular response and drop in cardiac output. Other patients with AF may be asymptomatic. Long-term monitoring of cardiac rhythm in patients with intermittent AF suggests that many episodes of symptoms thought by the patient to be due to AF are not accompanied by this arrhythmia and conversely patients with intermittent AF fail to recognize over 80% of the documented episodes of AF. More than half of the patients with AF and stroke had not been diagnosed with AF prior to onset of stroke.[15] It is also not uncommon for a patient with an acute ischemic stroke and no clinical or ECG evidence of a cardiac abnormality to develop an episode of AF during their acute hospitalization exposing the possibility of an embolic stroke arising from a left atrial thrombus. Thus it seems probable that many individuals with intermittent AF are unaware of this dysrhythmia that may come to light only after a disabling stroke.

Once AF is recognized studies are generally undertaken to uncover potential causes and associated abnormalities. Hyperthyroidism is considered with appropriate diagnostic studies. Transthoracic echocardiography may suggest or confirm mitral stenosis or rarely an atrial myxoma. Left atrial size may be increased especially in patients with chronic AF. Left ventricular dysfunction may be noted and has been shown to be a predictor of increased stroke risk. Other findings predictive of heightened stroke risk are left ventricular mass, and mitral annular calcification. Many patients with AF have associated cardiovascular risk factors, especially hypertension and coronary ischemic disease. Transthoracic echocardiography may reveal other potential cardiac causes of embolus such as a left ventricular thrombus or abnormalities of the aortic or mitral valve.

Transesophageal echocardiography (TEE) is particularly sensitive in detecting abnormalities in the left atrium, interatrial septum and mitral valve. The decision to proceed with TEE in addition to, or instead of, transthoracic echocardiography varies depending on the clinical situation. In the patient with AF and stroke, presumably due to an embolus from the left atrium, long-term anticoagulation is indicated and it is unlikely that information from TEE will alter management. In this setting many clinicians would elect not to proceed with TEE. Some clinicians advocate TEE in patients with AF to guide management decisions. TEE is consistently superior to transthoracic echocardiography in identifying left atrial thrombi and other features considered potentially important as predictors of thromboembolic risk in patients with AF.

Spontaneous echo contrast (SEC) is the smoke-like signal detected in the atria of some patients with AF. This phenomenon is thought to indicate stasis and erythrocyte or platelet microaggregates. SEC is associated with an increased prevalence of atrial thrombus and considered to possibly be an important marker for thromboembolic risk. In one study SEC was more common in patients with rheumatic valve disease (67%) than non-valvular AF (33%), more common in patients with chronic (40%) than paroxysmal (5.6%) AF, and more often associated with enlarged left atrium. Thrombi were observed in 23% of the 26 patients with SEC and in only 1.9% of the 54 patients without SEC.[16] TEE studies in the Stroke Prevention in Atrial Fibrillation (SPAF) III trial showed that SEC was more likely in AF patients with higher blood fibrinogen concentrations and that dense SEC was predictive of thrombi within the left atrium.[17] TEE has the additional advantage over transthoracic echocardiography of visualizing the aortic arch. This potential source of emboli has become an important stroke mechanism that was difficult to document prior to the use of TEE.[18]

CLINICAL TRIALS

Prior to the first randomized clinical treatment trial in AF there was considerable debate as to whether, and how, to manage patients with AF for the prevention of stroke. There was even debate as to the relevance of AF as a cause of stroke. Because of this uncertainty a series of randomized clinical treatment trials were undertaken. These trials yielded remarkably similar results confirming the importance of AF as a risk factor for stroke, establishing the value of long-term anticoagulation for stroke prevention, and suggesting that stroke risk varies depending on the coexistence of other cardiovascular factors.

The first study reported was the Copenhagen Atrial Fibrillation, Aspirin, Anticoagulation Study (AFASAK) that began in November 1985, and by June 1988 had enrolled 1007 out-patients with chronic non-rheumatic AF. Patients were randomized with 335 receiving anticoagulation with warfarin openly, and in a double-blind study 336 received 75 mg aspirin once daily and 336 placebo. Each patient was followed up for 2 years or until termination of the trial. The primary endpoint was a thromboembolic complication (stroke, transient cerebral ischemic attack, or embolic complications to the viscera and extremities). The secondary endpoint was death. The incidence of thromboembolic complications and vascular mortality were significantly lower in the warfarin group than in the aspirin and placebo groups, which did not differ significantly. Five patients on warfarin had thromboembolic complications compared with 20 patients on aspirin and 21 on placebo. Twenty-one patients on warfarin were withdrawn because of non-fatal bleeding complications compared with two patients on aspirin and none on placebo. Thus, anticoagulation therapy with warfarin was recommended to prevent thromboembolic complications in patients with chronic non-rheumatic AF.[5]

The Stroke Prevention in Atrial Fibrillation (SPAF) Study began in June 1987. It was a 15-center randomized clinical trial examining the risks and benefits of warfarin (prothrombin time of 1.3–1.8 times control) and aspirin (325 mg/day) in patients with constant or intermittent atrial fibrillation. Candidates for anticoagulation (group I) were randomized to receive warfarin (in an open-label fashion), aspirin, or placebo; the last two treatments were given in a double-blind fashion. Warfarin-ineligible patients (group II) were randomized to receive aspirin or placebo in a double-blind fashion. The primary end-points were ischemic stroke and systemic embolism. Secondary end-points were death, transient ischemic attack, myocardial infarction, and unstable angina pectoris. Analysis was based on the intention-to-treat principle. High-risk subgroups identified by clinical and echocardiographic criteria were sought prospectively. By November 1989, 1244 patients had been followed for a mean of 1.13 years. The event rates were 1.6% per year in the 393 patients who made up the two active treatment arms (warfarin and aspirin) of group 1, and 8.3% per year in the 195 patients who made up the placebo arm ($P < 0.00005$) (risk reduction, 81%; 95% CI, 56–91). In all 517 patients given aspirin, the rate of primary events (3.2% per year) was lower than that in the 528 patients given placebo (6.3% per year; $P = 0.014$) (risk reduction, 49%; 95% CI, 15–69). However, the study was unable to show a benefit of aspirin in patients over 75 years of age.[6]

In 1991 the Canadian Atrial Fibrillation Anticoagulation Study was reported. This was a randomized double-blind placebo-controlled trial to assess the potential of warfarin to reduce systemic thromboembolism and its inherent risk of hemorrhage. This study was stopped early before completion of its planned recruitment of 630 patients. There were 187 patients randomized to warfarin and 191 to placebo. Permanent discontinuation of study medication occurred in 26% of warfarin-treated patients and 23% of placebo-treated patients. The target range of the international normalized ratio was 2–3. For the warfarin-treated patients, the international normalized ratio was within the target range during 43.7% of the study days, above the target range on 16.6% of the study days and below the target range on 39.6% of the study days. Fatal or major bleeding occurred at annual rates of 2.5% in warfarin-treated and 0.5% in placebo-treated patients. Minor bleeding occurred in 16% of patients receiving warfarin and 9% receiving placebo. The primary outcome event cluster was non-lacunar stroke, non-central nervous systemic embolism, and fatal or intracranial hemorrhage. Events were included in the primary analysis of efficacy if they occurred within 28 days of permanent discontinuation of the study medication. The annual rates of the primary outcome event cluster were 3.5% in warfarin-treated and 5.2% in placebo-treated patients, with a relative risk reduction of 37% (95% CI, −63.5 to 75.5% $P = 0.17$).[8]

The Veterans Affairs Administration organized a double-blind randomized placebo-controlled study to evaluate low-intensity anticoagulation with warfarin (prothrombin-time ratio, 1.2–1.5) in 571 men with chronic non-rheumatic atrial fibrillation, 46 of these patients had previously had a stroke, the remainder had not. The primary endpoint was cerebral infarction; secondary endpoints were cerebral hemorrhage and death. Among the patients with no history of stroke, cerebral infarction occurred in 19 of the 265 patients in the placebo group during an average follow-up of 1.7 years (4.3% per year) and in the four of the 260 patients in the warfarin group during an average follow-up of 1.8 years (0.9% per year). The reduction in risk with warfarin therapy was 0.79 (95% CI, 0.52–0.90; $P = 0.001$). The annual event rate among the 228 patients over 70 years of age was

4.8% in the placebo group and 0.9% in the warfarin group (risk reduction, 0.79; $P = 0.02$). The only cerebral hemorrhage occurred in a 73-year-old patient in the warfarin group. Other major hemorrhages, all gastrointestinal, occurred in 10 patients: four in the placebo group, at a rate of 0.9% per year, and six in the warfarin group, at a rate of 1.3% per year. There were 37 deaths that were not preceded by a cerebral endpoint, 22 in the placebo group and 15 in the warfarin group (risk reduction, 0.31; $P = 0.19$). Cerebral infarction was more common among patients with a history of cerebral infarction (9.3% per year in the placebo group and 6.1% per year in the warfarin group) than among those without such a history.[19]

The SPAF-II study aimed to compare aspirin and warfarin and to assess the differential effects of the two treatments according to age. SPAF-II compared warfarin (prothrombin time ratio, 1.3–1.8; international normalized ratio, INR 2.0–4.5) with 325 mg/day aspirin for the prevention of ischemic stroke and systemic embolism (primary events) in two parallel randomized trials involving 715 patients aged 75 years or less and 385 patients older than 75. In the younger patients, warfarin decreased the absolute rate of primary events by 0.7% per year (95% CI, −0.4 to 1.7). The primary event rate per year was 1.3% with warfarin and 1.9% with aspirin (relative risk, RR, 0.67; $P = 0.24$). The absolute rate of primary events in low-risk younger patients (without hypertension, recent heart failure, or previous thromboembolism) on aspirin was 0.5% per year (95% CI, 0.1–1.9). Among older patients, warfarin decreased the absolute rate of primary events by 1.2% per year (95% CI, −1.7 to 4.1). The primary event rate per year was 3.6% with warfarin and 4.8% with aspirin (RR 0.73; $P = 0.39$). In this older group, the rate of all strokes with residual deficit (ischemic or hemorrhagic) was 4.3% per year with aspirin and 4.6% per year with warfarin (RR 1.1). Younger patients without risk factors had a low rate of stroke when treated with aspirin. In older patients the rate of stroke (ischemic and hemorrhagic) was substantial, irrespective of which agent was given. SPAF-II concluded that patient age and the inherent risk of thromboembolism should be considered in the choice of antithrombotic prophylaxis for patients with atrial fibrillation.[20]

The European Atrial Fibrillation Trial (EAFT) was exclusively a secondary prevention trial. A total of 1007 non-rheumatic AF patients with a recent TIA or minor ischemic stroke were randomized to open anticoagulation or double-blind treatment with either 300 mg/day aspirin or placebo (group 1, 669 patients). Patients with contraindications to anticoagulation were randomized to receive aspirin or placebo (group 2, 338 patients). The measure of outcome was death from vascular disease, any stroke, myocardial infarction, or systemic embolism. During a mean follow-up of 2.3 years, the annual rate of outcome events was 8% in patients assigned to anticoagulants vs. 17% in placebo-treated patients in group 1 (hazard radio, HR, 0.53; 95% CI, 0.36–0.79). The risk of stroke alone was reduced from 12% to 4% per year (HR 0.34; 95% CI, 0.20–0.57). Among all patients assigned to aspirin (groups 1 and 2), the annual incidence of outcome events was 15%, against 19% for those on placebo (HR 0.83; 95% CI, 0.65–1.05). Anticoagulation was significantly more effective than aspirin (HR 0.60; 95% CI, 0.41–0.87). The incidence of major bleeding events was low, both on anticoagulation (2.8% per year) and on aspirin (0.9% per year).[7]

Another secondary prevention randomized trial was reported from Italy. In the Studio Italiano Fibrillazione Atriale (SIFA) trial a total of 916 patients with non-rheumatic AF and a recent (≤15 days) cerebral ischemic episode were randomized to either indobufen (100 or 200 mg b.i.d.) or warfarin (to obtain an international normalized ratio of 2.0–3.5) for 12 months. The two groups (462 on indobufen and 454 on warfarin) were well balanced in terms of their main baseline characteristics. The primary outcome of the study was the combined incidence of non-fatal stroke) including intracerebral bleeding), pulmonary or systemic embolism, non-fatal myocardial infarction, and vascular death. At the end of follow-up, the incidence of primary outcome events was 10.6% in the indobufen group (95% CI, 7.7–13.5) and 9.0% in the warfarin group (95% CI, 6.3–11.8), with no statistically significant difference between treatments. The frequency of non-cerebral major bleeding complications was low: only four cases (0.9%) of gastrointestinal bleeding were observed, all of them in the warfarin group.[21]

Data on individual patients with atrial fibrillation were pooled from the first five randomized trials comparing warfarin (all studies) or aspirin (the AFASAK and the SPAF studies) with control. The purpose of the analysis was: (1) to identify patient features predictive of a high or low risk or stroke; (2) to assess the efficacy of antithrombotic therapy in major patient subgroups (e.g., women); and (3) to obtain the most precise estimate of the efficacy and risks of antithrombotic therapy in atrial fibrillation. For the warfarin–control comparison there were 1889 patient-years receiving warfarin and 1802 in the control group. For the aspirin–placebo comparison there were 1132 patient-years receiving aspirin and 1133 receiving placebo. The daily dose of aspirin was 75 mg in the AFASAK study and 325 mg in the SPAF study. At the time of randomization the mean age was 69 years and the mean blood pressure was 142/82 mmHg. Forty-six per cent of the patients had a history of hypertension, 6% had a previous transient ischemic attack or stroke, and 14% had diabetes. Risk factors that predicted stroke on multivariate analyses in control patients were increasing age, history of hypertension, previous transient ischemic attack or stroke, and diabetes. Patients younger than 65 years who had none of the other predictive factors (15% of all patients) had an annual rate of stroke of 1.0%, 95% CI, 0.3–3.0. The annual rate of stroke was 4.5% for the control group and 1.4% for the warfarin group (RR 68%; 95% CI, 50–79). The efficacy of warfarin was consistent across all studies and subgroups of patients. In women, warfarin decreased the risk of stroke by 84% (95% CI, 55–95) compared with 60% (95% CI, 35–76) in men. The efficacy of aspirin was not as consistent. The risk reduction with 75 mg aspirin in the AFASAK study was 18% (95% CI, 60–58), and with 325 mg aspirin in the SPAF study the risk reduction was 44% (95% CI, 7–66). When both studies were combined the risk reduction was 36% (95% CI, 4–57). The annual rate of major hemorrhage (intracranial bleeding or a bleed requiring hospitalization or 2 units of blood) was 1.0% for the control group, 1.0% for the aspirin group, and 1.3% for the warfarin group. This combined analysis of these five randomized trials showed that warfarin consistently decreased the risk of stroke in patients with atrial fibrillation (a 68% reduction in risk) with virtually no increase in the frequency of major bleeding. Patients with atrial fibrillation younger than 65 years without a history of hypertension, previous stroke or transient ischemic attack, or diabetes were at very low risk of stroke even when not treated. The efficacy of aspirin was less consistent.[22]

The SPAF III study was designed to compare the accepted standard for warfarin therapy (INR 2.0–3.0), to low fixed-dose warfarin plus aspirin in high-risk AF patients. A total of 1044 patients with AF and with at least one thromboembolic risk factor (i.e., congestive heart failure or left ventricular fractional shortening ≤25%, previous thromboembolism, systolic blood pressure of more than 160 mmHg at study enrolment, or being a woman aged over 75 years), were randomly assigned either a combination of low-intensity, fixed-dose warfarin (INR 1.2–1.5 for initial dose adjustment) and aspirin (325 mg/day) or adjusted-dose warfarin (INR 2.0–3.0). Drugs were given open-labeled. The mean INR during follow-up of patients taking combination therapy ($N = 521$) was 1.3, compared with 2.4 for those taking adjusted-dose warfarin ($N = 523$). During follow-up, 54% of INRs in patients taking combination therapy were 1.2–1.5 and 34% were less than 1.2. The trial was stopped after a mean follow-up of 1.1 years when the rate of ischemic stroke and systemic embolism (primary events) in patients given combination therapy (7.9% per year) was significantly higher than in those given adjusted-dose warfarin (1.9% per year) at an interim analysis ($P < 0.0001$). This difference represented an absolute reduction of 6.0% per year (95% CI, 3.4–8.6) by adjusted-dose warfarin. The annual rates of disabling stroke (5.6% vs. 1.7%; $P = 0.0007$) and of primary event or vascular death (11.8% vs. 6.4%; $P = 0.002$), were also higher with combination therapy. The rates of major bleeding were similar in both treatment groups.[23]

SPAF III also incorporated a prospective cohort study with a mean duration of follow-up of 2.0 years, conducted between 1993 and 1997. Patients with AF categorized as 'low risk' based on the absence of the four thromboembolic risk factors used in the 'high-risk' portion of SPAF III were given 325 mg/day aspirin. The primary outcome events were ischemic stroke and systemic embolism. Among 892 participants, the mean age was 67 years, 78% were men, and histories of hypertension, diabetes, and ischemic heart disease were present in 46%, 13%, and 16%, respectively. The rate of primary events was 2.2% per year (95% CI, 1.6–3.0), of ischemic stroke was 2.0% per year (95% CI, 1.5–2.8), and of disabling ischemic strokes was 0.8% per year (95% CI, 0.5–1.3). Those with a history of hypertension had a higher rate of primary events (3.6% per year) than those with no history of hypertension (1.1% per year) ($P < 0.001$). The rate of disabling ischemic stroke was low in those with and without a history of hypertension (1.4% per year and 0.5% per year, respectively). The rate of major bleeding during aspirin therapy was 0.5% per year.[24]

SPAF III demonstrated that low doses of warfarin, even with aspirin, were ineffective in preventing thromboembolism in high-risk patients with AF. Other investigators have addressed the optimal range of the international normalized ratio (INR) to prevent stroke and minimize the risk for major bleeding, especially intracerebral bleed. An analysis of the 214 patients who received anticoagulant therapy in the European Atrial Fibrillation Trial calculated incidence rates for both ischemic and major hemorrhagic events as they related to the patient's INR. The optimal intensity of anticoagulation was found to lie between an INR of 2.0 and an INR of 3.9. No treatment effect was apparent with anticoagulation below an INR of 2.0. The rate of thromboembolic events was lowest at INRs from 2.0 to 3.9 and most major bleeding complications occurred with treatment at intensities with INRs of 5.0 or above.[25]

Another case–control study concluded that the optimal INR range was 2.0–3.0 although some effect in prevention of thromboembolism was noted with INRs below 2.0.[26] Given the difficulties in maintaining a consistent INR level

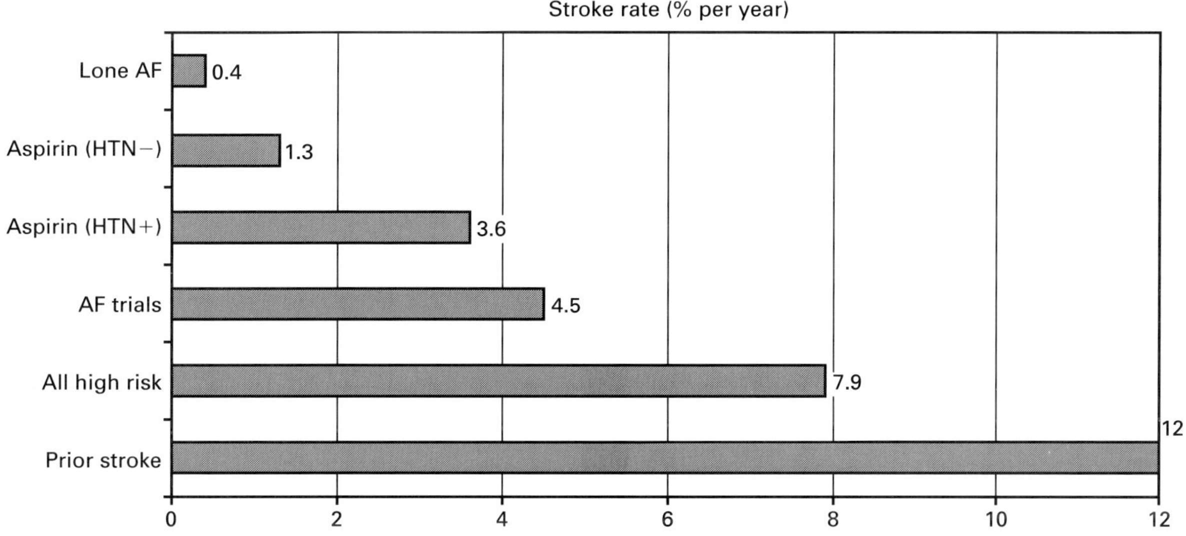

Figure 9.1 Spectrum of stroke risk in atrial fibrillation. Aspirin (HTN−) = AF patients without a history of hypertension treated with aspirin only. Aspirin (HTN+) = AF patients with a history of hypertension as their only risk predictor and treated with aspirin only.

over time it seems most prudent to target an INR of 2.5 (range 2.0–3.0). The randomized trials have observed that about 20% of INR levels over an extended period of time will fall below the target range, thus the practice of targeting a low INR in an attempt to avoid bleeding complications risks periods of inadequate anticoagulation, placing the patient at risk for stroke. The major predictor of intracerebral hemorrhage seems to be advanced age. Poorly controlled hypertension is also considered to increase the risk of intracerebral bleed.

SUMMARY

The past decade has witnessed the consistent and powerful demonstration of the importance of AF as a risk factor for stroke and the value of warfarin for the prevention of stroke. The value of warfarin is compelling in those patients with 'high-risk' predictors of stroke accompanying their AF. One of the clear messages arising from the randomized treatment trials is that treatment decisions must be based on the estimated risk for stroke, and the risk of bleeding with warfarin, in a given patient (Fig. 9.1). The patient with lone AF or the patient without high-risk predictors has a low risk of stroke on aspirin alone or perhaps on no therapy. Conversely the patient with prior stroke and AF has a stroke risk of alarming proportion that demands anticoagulation therapy in the absence of clear contraindications. A suggested approach to the management of AF patients is outlined in Fig. 9.2.

Atrial fibrillation is a major cause of stroke with a growing population of at risk individuals. While strategies to reverse and prevent AF are being investigated, the mainstay of management for the vast majority of the affected population is appropriate antithrombotic therapy to prevent stroke. In high-risk patients, warfarin anticoagulation is highly effective in preventing stroke. The goal is to identify patients with AF and begin treatment before the unheralded occurrence of a disabling stroke.

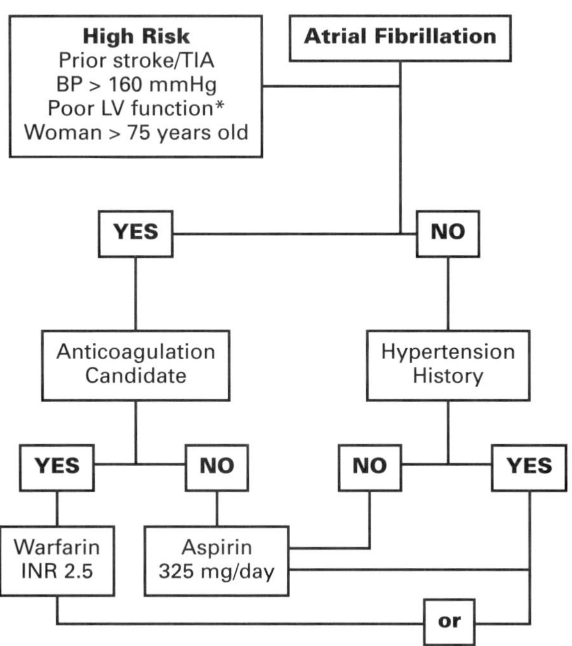

Figure 9.2 Management of atrial fibrillation patients.

* Poor LV function = A history of congestive heart failure within the past 3 months or fractional shorting of less than 25% on a transthoracic echocardiogram.

REFERENCES

1. Wolf PA, Abbott RD, Kannel WB. Atrial fibrillation: a major contributor to stroke in the elderly. The Framingham Study. *Arch Intern Med* 1987; **147:**1561–4.
2. Braunwald E. Shattuck lecture—cardiovascular medicine at the turn of the millennium: triumphs, concerns, and opportunities [see comments]. *N Engl J Med* 1997; **337:**1360–9.
3. Wolf PA, Dawber TR, Thomas HE Jr, Kannel WB. Epidemiologic assessment of chronic atrial fibrillation and risk of stroke: the Framingham study. *Neurology* 1978; **28:**973–7.
4. Wolf PA, Abbott RD, Kannel WB. Atrial fibrillation as an independent risk factor for stroke: the Framingham Study. *Stroke* 1991; **22:**983–8.
5. Petersen P, Boysen G, Godtfredsen J, Andersen ED, Andersen B. Placebo-controlled, randomised trial of warfarin and aspirin for prevention of thromboembolic complications in chronic atrial fibrillation. The Copenhagen AFASAK study. *Lancet* 1989; **i:**175–9.

6. Stroke Prevention in Atrial Fibrillation Investigators. Preliminary report of the Stroke Prevention in Atrial Fibrillation Study [see comments]. *N Engl J Med* 1990; **322:**863–8.
7. European Atrial Fibrillation Trial Study Group. Secondary prevention in non-rheumatic atrial fibrillation after transient ischaemic attack or minor stroke. EAFT (European Atrial Fibrillation Trial) Study Group [see comments]. *Lancet* 1993; **342:**1255–62.
8. Connolly SJ, Laupacis A, Gent M, Roberts RS, Cairns JA, Joyner C. Canadian Atrial Fibrillation Anticoagulation (CAFA) Study. *J Am Coll Cardiol* 1991; **18:**349–55.
9. Bogousslavsky J, Cachin C, Regli F, Despland PA, Van Melle G, Kappenberger L. Cardiac sources of embolism and cerebral infarction—clinical consequences and vascular concomitants: the Lausanne Stroke Registry. *Neurology* 1991; **41:**855–9.
10. Caplan LR. 'Top of the basilar' syndrome. *Neurology* 1980; **30:**72–9.
11. Jorgensen HS, Nakayama H, Reith J, Raaschou HO, Olsen TS. Acute stroke with atrial fibrillation. The Copenhagen Stroke Study. *Stroke* 1996; **27:**1765–9.
12. Wolf PA, Mitchell JB, Baker CS, Kannel WB, D'Agostino RB. Impact of atrial fibrillation on mortality, stroke, and medical costs. *Arch Intern Med* 1998; **158:**229–34.
13. Sandercock P, Bamford J, Dennis M *et al.* Atrial fibrillation and stroke: prevalence in different types of stroke and influence on early and long term prognosis (Oxfordshire community stroke project). *Br Med J* 1992; **305:**1460–5.
14. Censori B, Camerlingo M, Casto L *et al.* Prognostic factors in first-ever stroke in the carotid artery territory seen within 6 hours after onset. *Stroke* 1993; **24:**532–5.
15. Sherman DG, Goldman L, Whiting RB, Jurgensen K, Kaste M, Easton JD. Thromboembolism in patients with atrial fibrillation. *Arch Neurol* 1984; **41:**708–10.
16. De Belder MA, Lovat LB, Tourikis L *et al.* Left atrial spontaneous contrast echoes–markers of thromboembolic risk in patients with atrial fibrillation. *Eur Heart J* 1993; **14:**326–35.
17. Zabalgoitia M, Halperin JL, Pearce LA *et al.* Transesophageal echocardiographic correlates of clinical risk of thromboembolism in nonvalvular atrial fibrillation. Stroke prevention in atrial fibrillation III investigators. *J Am Coll Cardiol* 1998; **31**(7):1622–6.
18. Amarenco P, Duyckaerts C, Tzourio C, Henin D, Bousser MG, Hauw JJ. The prevalence of ulcerated plaques in the aortic arch in patients with stroke. *N Engl J Med* 1992; **326:**221–5.
19. Ezekowitz MD, Bridgerws SL, James KE *et al.* Warfarin in the prevention of stroke associated with nonrheumatic atrial fibrillation. *N Engl J Med* 1992; **327:**1406–12.
20. Stroke Prevention in Atrial Fibrillation Investigators. Warfarin versus aspirin for prevention of thromboembolism in atrial fibrillation: Stroke Prevention in Atrial Fibrillation II Study. *Lancet* 1994; **343:**687–91.
21. Morocutti C, Amabile G, Fattapposta F *et al.* Indobufen versus warfarin in the secondary prevention of major vascular events in nonrheumatic atrial fibrillation. SIFA (Studio Italiano Fibrillazione Atriale) Investigators. *Stroke* 1997; **28:**1015–21.
22. Atrial Fibrillation Investigators. Risk factors for stroke and efficacy of antithrombotic therapy in atrial fibrillation. Analysis of pooled data from five randomized controlled trials [published erratum appears in *Arch Intern Med* 1994; **154:**2254]. *Arch Intern Med* 1994; **154:**1449–57.
23. Stroke Prevention in Atrial Fibrillation Investigators. Adjusted-dose warfarin versus low-intensity, fixed-dose warfarin plus aspirin for high-risk patients with atrial fibrillation: Stroke Prevention in Atrial Fibrillation III randomised clinical trial [see comments]. *Lancet* 1996; **348:**633–8.
24. Stroke Prevention in Atrial Fibrillation Investigators. Patients with nonvalvular atrial fibrillation at low risk of stroke during treatment with aspirin: Stroke Prevention in Atrial Fibrillation III Study. The SPAF III Writing Committee for the Stroke Prevention in Atrial Fibrillation Investigators [see comments]. *J Am Med Assoc* 1998; **279:**1273–7.
25. European Atrial Fibrillation Trial Study Group. Optimal oral anticoagulant therapy in patients with nonrheumatic atrial fibrillation and recent cerebral ischemia. *N Engl J Med* 1995; **333:**5–10.
26. Hylek EM, Skates SJ, Sheehan MA, Singer DE. An analysis of the lowest effective intensity of prophylactic anticoagulation for patients with nonrheumatic atrial fibrillation. *N Engl J Med* 1996; **335:**540–6.

10

Prevention of recurrent stroke: risk of hemorrhage

Gudrun Boysen

CONTENTS • **Introduction** • **Rates of recurrent stroke** • **Antiplatelet therapy** • **Discussion**

INTRODUCTION

Secondary stroke prevention is the responsibility of the medical profession, i.e., doctors and nurses, primary-care physicians, neurologists, internists, vascular surgeons and many more, whereas primary prevention should start early in life by the incorporation of healthy life-styles. Primary prevention, therefore, is the responsibility of the family, the school, the politicians and the government in collaboration with the medical profession. As in primary prevention, modification of life-style factors also plays a role in secondary stroke prevention; however, there is much less scientific evidence to support this. Table 10.1 gives a list of factors to be considered in a patient for whom secondary stroke prevention is planned.

The background factors are either predestined or, as in the case of education, not subject to modification once people have reached 'stroke age'. Life-style factors may always be modified—at least in theory. Our knowledge about the effect of changing life-style after a stroke is, however, almost nil and we have to rely on evidence from epidemiological, observational, and intervention studies in primary prevention.[1]

Among the life-style variables, smoking is the most important, and this is a risk factor which ought to be easily eliminated. A reasonable level of physical activity should be encour-

Table 10.1 Risk factors for stroke

Background:	Age
	Sex
	Family history
	Education
Life-style:	Smoking
	Physical activity
	Diet
	Alcohol
	Drugs
Disease markers:	Hypertension
	Cardiac disease
	Atrial fibrillation
	Myocardial infarction
	Valvular heart disease
	Cardiomyopathy
	Persistent foramen ovale
	Mitral valve prolapse
	Carotid artery disease
	Peripheral arterial disease
	Cholesterol
	Diabetes
	Homocysteinemia
	Polycythemia
	Sickle cell anemia
	Antiphospholipid antibodies
	Coagulation defects
	Thyroid function

aged, and a diet rich in fish, fruit and vegetables may be advisable. Among the alcoholic beverages, an observational study[2] found that wine in small quantities reduced the risk of stroke, while intake of beer and strong liquor in small amounts did not influence stroke risk. Stroke recurrence was significantly increased among patients with prior heavy alcohol use.[3] Whether reduction of alcohol intake in heavy drinkers will reduce stroke risk has not been determined.

Among the disease markers, hypertension suffers from a paucity of studies in secondary stroke prevention. Hypertension is such an important risk factor for first stroke, and it seems likely that the same is true for recurrent stroke. In primary prevention antihypertensive treatment reduces the risk of stroke by about 40%.[4] In secondary prevention, two older trials of antihypertensive treatment gave conflicting results: the American Study[5] found no significant reduction in stroke recurrence, while the British Trial[6] did. Further studies are needed to determine the optimal intensity of blood pressure lowering after a stroke. However, due to the lack of clear scientific evidence, our policy is to start antihypertensive treatment if blood pressure remains elevated above 160/90 mmHg a couple of weeks after stroke.

Plasma cholesterol level is another controversial issue. Few studies have demonstrated a relationship between increasing plasma cholesterol level and risk of stroke,[7] while a meta-analysis showed no such relationship.[8] After myocardial infarction (MI),[9] however, treatment with cholesterol-lowering drugs has demonstrated reduced risk not only of acute AMI but also of stroke. It is possible that future studies will show an effect of cholesterol-lowering even in transient ischemic attack (TIA) and ischemic stroke patients. However, there is no clear evidence to recommend such treatment at the present.

Whether diabetes increases the risk of stroke recurrence is uncertain, but it seems likely, and an optimal regulation of blood glucose should be attempted.

In this chapter the focus will be on the prevention of non-cardioembolic stroke by antiplatelet therapy with emphasis on the risk of hemorrhage. Carotid endarterectomy and cardiac diseases including atrial fibrillation and hematological risk factors will be discussed in separate chapters.

RATES OF RECURRENT STROKE

The annual risk of having a stroke in patients with TIA or ischemic stroke was estimated by Wilterdink and Easton[10,11] (Tables 10.2 and 10.3).

Table 10.2 Estimates of vascular event rates for individuals with various features of atherothrombotic cerebrovascular disease (Reproduced with permission from Wilterdink and Easton[10])

Cerebrovascular features	*Annual probability (%) of:*	
	Stroke	*Vascular death*
General elderly male population	0.6	
Asymptomatic carotid disease	1.3	3.4
Transient monocular blindness	2.2	3.5
Transient ischemic attack	3.7	2.3
Minor stroke	6.1	3.2
Major stroke	9.0	3.5
>70% CS with symptoms	15	2

Table 10.3 Incidence of stroke recurrence. (Reproduced with permission from Easton[11])

Ischemic stroke	*Annual probability (%)*
Year 1	6–12
Years 2–5	5–8
By 5 years	30–40
Myocardial infarction	15
Vascular death	15

There was a gradual increase in the annual risk from 2.2% in amaurosis fugax to 9% in major stroke. After lacunar infarction the annual risk of stroke recurrence was found to be 7% per year during the first 2 years, and during the following years it was reduced to 3% per year.[12] The risk of recurrent stroke after lacunar infarction was not different from the risk after territorial infarctions.[13]

ANTIPLATELET THERAPY

In patients with TIA or ischemic stroke of non-cardioembolic origin, antiplatelet therapy is the best documented preventive intervention. Many trials have studied the effect of aspirin in these patients. Some studies have shown reduction in the risk of stroke, acute MI and vascular death[14–16] while other studies have failed to do so.[17–19] The Antiplatelet Trialists' Collaboration[20] collected all available trials in a systematic overview from which 13 trials of aspirin were analyzed separately by Algra and van Gijn,[21] who found a risk reduction of the combined endpoint: stroke, acute MI and vascular death of 13% (95% CI, 4–21). This risk reduction is clearly much lower than 20–25% that is usually quoted. The latter applies to the complete overview which included other drugs than aspirin and mainly consisted of patients with prior acute MI.

Bleeding complications have been given little attention in aspirin treatment in general. The first hint of the problem was given by the Physicians' Health Study,[22] where more hemorrhagic strokes occurred in the aspirin-treated group than in the placebo group. Although this was not statistically significant, it was a contributing factor to not recommending aspirin as a primary preventive measure. Because the risk of hemorrhagic complication is small, it takes large studies to detect it. Bleeding complications do, however, become important when large scale use of aspirin or other antithrombotic drugs is contemplated.

In the systematic overviews the rate of hemorrhagic stroke was slightly higher in the antiplatelet group than in the control group,[20] but the difference was not statistically significant. There were no data on systemic hemorrhages and the meta-analysis did not give a clear impression of the magnitude of bleeding complication. Therefore, in this chapter, focus will be placed on newer antiplatelet trials with description of bleeding events, such as the Swedish Aspirin Low-dose Trial,[14] the Dutch TIA Trial,[23] the European Stroke Prevention Study 2 (ESPS 2),[16] the Canadian American Ticlopidine Study (CATS),[24] the Ticlopidine Aspirin Stroke Study (TASS),[25] the Clopidogrel vs. Aspirin in Patients at Risk of Ischemic Events (CAPRIE),[26] the International Stroke Trial (IST), [27] and the Chinese Acute Stroke Trial (CAST).[28] The data on hemorrhagic complications as well as on recurrent strokes in these studies are of variable quality. However, they provide the best sources of information available on these important questions. In general, for intracerebral hemorrhage to be diagnosed a CT scan was required, and such bleedings were rated as severe. Asymptomatic hemorrhagic transformation of cerebral infarcts was not likely to be counted as a hemorrhagic complication, since the event analyzed was a recurrent stroke, and hemorrhagic transformation often occurs without clinical deterioration. For each trial the definitions used will be quoted. Severe systemic hemorrhagic complications usually mean a bleed requiring either a transfusion or an operation, or a fatal bleed.

Table 10.4 Antiplatelet randomized placebo-controlled trials in patients with TIA and ischemic stroke

Trials	*Drugs*	N	*Patient-years at risk*	*Outcome events per 100 treatment years* N	*Vascular events per 100 treatment years*	*Vascular events avoided* N	*Severe or fatal bleeds* N	*Bleeds per 100 treatment years*	*Excess bleeds per 100 treatment years*	*95% CI*
					Strokes, MI, v.d.					
SALT	Aspirin 75 mg/day	676	1802	137	7.60	2.05	20	1.11	0.62	0.04–1.20
	Placebo	684	1824	176*	9.65		9	0.49		
					Strokes					
ESPS 2	Aspirin 50 mg	1649	3298	206*	6.25	1.33	20	0.61	0.40	0.09–0.71
	Dipyridamole retard 200 mg twice daily	1654	3308	211*	6.38	1.20	6	0.18	0.61	0.27–0.95
	Aspirin + dipyridamole	1650	3300	157*	4.74	2.82*	27	0.82		
	Placebo	1649	3298	250	7.58		7	0.21		
					Strokes, MI, v.d.					
CATS	Ticlopidine 500 mg/day	525	683	74	10.8	4.5	2	0.29	0.16	−0.29–0.61
	Placebo	528	773	118	15.3		1	0.13		

* Statistically significant difference, $P < 0.05$; v.d., vascular death.

The Swedish Aspirin Low-dose Trial[14] compared 75 mg/day aspirin with placebo in patients with TIA or minor stroke. In that study CT scan or necropsy was carried out in 98% of patients, who had a fatal or non-fatal stroke. There were six fatal intracranial bleeds in the aspirin group vs. nil in the placebo group. Gastrointestinal bleeding was not clearly defined; nine instances were listed as severe in the aspirin group vs. four in the placebo group. Table 10.4 shows that two vascular events were avoided per 100 treatment-years at the expense of an excess of 0.6 (95% CI, 0.04–1.20) severe or fatal bleeds. The Dutch TIA Trial[23] compared 30 mg/day aspirin with 283 mg/day aspirin in 3131 patients (Table 10.5). Fatal bleeding had to be documented by convincing clinical evidence or autopsy. Non-fatal bleeds were considered major if a hospital visit and treatment were necessary. An incidence of major bleeding events of 2.6% in the 30 mg group and 3.2% in the 283 mg group was reported. Calculated as events per 100 treatment-years, given a mean duration of follow-up of 31 months, the risk of major bleeds was 0.99 and 1.3 per 100 treatment-years, respectively. Without a placebo group the excess risk is unknown, as well as the number of vascular events avoided. However, this study shows that a dose of aspirin as low as 30 mg/day is associated with an appreciable risk of bleeding complications.

ESPS 2[16] evaluated the effect of dipyridamole, aspirin, and dipyridamole plus aspirin, vs. placebo in patients with TIA or ischemic stroke. Bleeding episodes were recorded as mild, moderate, severe, or fatal, but were not otherwise defined. As shown in Table 10.4, aspirin prevented 1.3 strokes per 100 treatment-years at the expense of an excess risk of 0.4 (95% CI, 0.09–0.71) severe or fatal bleeds. Dipyridamole alone prevented 1.2 strokes without any excess bleeds. The combination of dipyridamole and aspirin prevented 2.8 strokes at the expense of an excess of 0.6 (95% CI, 0.27–0.95) severe or fatal bleeds. The risk of bleeding complications was maintained over the 2 years of treatment, in contrast to the side-effects to dipyridamole, headache and diarrhea, which mainly occurred in the early phase of treatment.

Antithrombotic therapy is no longer tested against placebo since it is unethical to withhold antithrombotic therapy from patients at risk of ischemic stroke. However, the IST[27] and CAST[28] studies of acute stroke did contain large groups of placebo-treated patients providing ample evidence of the bleeding risk associated with aspirin in the acute phase of stroke. In IST (Table 10.6), symptomatic intracranial hemorrhage within 14 days was a secondary outcome as well as major extracranial hemorrhage including any bleed that required transfusion or caused death within 14 days. Fourteen days of 300 mg/day aspirin following acute stroke prevented 1.2 ischemic strokes or strokes of unknown etiology per 100 patients treated at the expense of an excess of 0.41 (95% CI, 0.05–0.77) intracerebral hemorrhages, transfused, or fatal bleeds. In CAST,[28] 160 mg aspirin for 4 weeks after acute stroke (Table 10.6) prevented 0.89 deaths or non-fatal ischemic strokes per 100 patients treated at the expense of 0.48 (95% CI, 0.13–0.83) severe or fatal intracranial or extracranial bleeds.

Ticlopidine,[24] another antiplatelet drug, significantly reduced stroke risk in patients with ischemic strokes when compared with placebo (Table 10.4). The risk of bleeding seemed to be twice as high as in the placebo group, 34 events vs. 16, but severe bleeds were rare in both groups. However, there was no clear definition of severe bleeds, and it may have differed from other studies. In TASS, 500 mg/day ticlopidine was compared with 1300 mg/day aspirin (Table 10.5).[25] In this study peptic ulcer and gastrointestinal hemorrhage were listed among adverse experiences without precise definitions and the severity of intracerebral hemorrhage was not described. The ticlopidine group had a significantly lower rate of vascular events, and a lower gastrointestinal bleeding risk, than that of the aspirin group, while the number of intracerebral bleeds was equal. A rare but severe adverse event, granulocytopenia, is associated with ticlopidine and in many countries the drug is not registered. Clopidogrel,[26] a drug with similar biochemical properties to ticlopidine but with fewer side-effects, was compared with

Table 10.5 Antiplatelet randomized aspirin-controlled trials in patients with TIA and ischemic stroke

Trials	*Drugs*	N	*Patient years at risk*	*Outcome-events* N	*Vascular events per 100 treatment years*	*Severe or fatal bleeds* N	*Bleeds per 100 treatment years*
			Strokes, MI, v.d.				
Dutch TIA trial	Aspirin 30 mg/day	1555	4017	228	5.67	40	1.00
	Aspirin 283 mg/day	1576	4071	240	5.89	53	1.30
TASS	Ticlopidine 500 mg/day	1529	5014	306	6.10	14	0.28
	Aspirin 1300 mg/day	1540	5008	349	6.97*	28	0.56
CAPRIE	Clopidogrel 75 mg/day	9599	17 636	939	5.32	77	0.44
	Aspirin 325 mg/day	9586	17 519	1021	5.83*	109	0.62

* Statistically significant difference, $P < 0.05$; v.d., vascular death.

Table 10.6 Antiplatelet randomized placebo-controlled trials in acute ischemic stroke during 2–4 weeks

Trials	*Drugs*	N	*Strokes of ischemic or unknown etiology* N	*Events per 100 treated patients*	*Events avoided per 100 patients*	*Severe or fatal bleeds* N	*Bleeds per 100 treated patients*	*Excess bleeds per 100 treated patients*	*95% CI*
IST	Aspirin 300 mg/day	4858	156	3.2	1.2	49	1.01	0.41	0.05–0.77
	Placebo	4859	214	4.4*		29	0.60		
			Death or non-fatal ischemic stroke						
CAST	Aspirin 160 mg/day	10 335	430	4.16	0.89	201	1.94	0.48	0.13–0.83
	Placebo	10 320	521	5.04*		151	1.46		

* Statistically significant difference, $P < 0.05$.

325 mg/day aspirin in a large study in which the study population was composed of one-third with TIA and ischemic stroke, one-third with AMI, and one-third with peripheral vascular disease. The risk of vascular events was slightly but significantly lower in the clopidogrel group than in the aspirin group. However, when the group which entered the study with TIA and ischemic stroke was analyzed separately, the risk reduction by clopidogrel was not statistically significant, nor was the occurrence of ischemic stroke in all patients significantly lower in the clopidogrel arm. The gastrointestinal and intracerebral hemorrhages were reported as 'any ever occurring' or 'severe' without any further definition of severity. Clopidogrel was accompanied by a lower risk of gastrointestinal bleeding than aspirin (Table 10.5), whereas the risk of intracerebral hemorrhage was not significantly different. Clopidogrel may be considered an alternative to aspirin, but can hardly be said, on the basis of the present evidence, to be superior to aspirin in patients with TIA and ischemic stroke.

The association of gastrointestinal bleeding and aspirin intake has been analyzed in several studies. The UK-TIA trial[17] reported that the risk of gastrointestinal bleeding was significantly higher with aspirin 1200 mg/day than with 300 mg, which again had a higher risk than placebo. A review of the gastrointestinal toxicity of aspirin[29] including all vascular disease prevention trials from the Antiplatelet Trialists' Collaboration in which direct aspirin to placebo comparison was possible, found an odds ratio of 2.0 (99% CI, 1.5–2.8) for gastrointestinal bleeding. The odds ratio for developing peptic ulcer was 1.3 (99% CI, 1.0–1.6). From that analysis, however, it was not possible to extract the number of severe and fatal bleeds for any given period of treatment. The risk of hospitalization for bleeding peptic ulcers was analyzed in 1121 patients,[30] who were matched with hospital and community controls. In the peptic ulcer group 12.8% had been regular users of aspirin compared with 9.0% of the hospital controls and 7.8% of the community controls. Odds ratios for gastrointestinal bleeding were significantly raised for all doses of aspirin between 75 mg/day and 300 mg/day. Addition of non-steroidal anti-inflammatory drugs (NSAIDs) increased the risk of gastric bleeding.

DISCUSSION

In secondary stroke prevention modification of risk factors should be discussed with each patient. If at all possible a healthier life-style should be adopted.

Hypertension should be treated properly. If cardioembolism is suspected anticoagulation therapy should be considered. In non-cardioembolic ischemic cerebrovascular events antithrombotic therapy is universally accepted. Aspirin remains the most widely used drug. Low-dose regimens are to be preferred as they cause less dyspepsia. In any dose, aspirin causes bleeding complications and for the severe bleeds there seems to be little difference between high and low dose. In this survey, the number of vascular events avoided per 100 treatment-years is confronted with the number of excess severe bleeds. In the patient group with TIA and/or ischemic stroke aspirin may prevent one to two strokes or vascular events per 100 treatment-years at the expense of 0.4–0.6 severe excess bleeds.

Although the benefit/risk ratio is clearly in favor of aspirin, the analyses show the necessity of inquiring about peptic ulcer and dyspepsia before starting antithrombotic therapy. It may be necessary to institute proper therapy for peptic ulcer before embarking on antiplatelet therapy. Other NSAIDs should be avoided, or in cases where this is not possible, aspirin should be stopped.

The newer antiplatelet drugs ticlopidine and clopidogrel cause less severe bleeds than aspirin. Ticlopidine is slightly more effective in stroke prevention, but may have serious side-effects. Clopidogrel may be an alternative to aspirin, if the price is of no concern.

Dipyridamole did not in itself increase bleeding risk. Furthermore the ESPS 2, with the combination of dipyridamole and aspirin, had a favorable benefit/risk ratio with 2.8 strokes avoided at the expense of an excess risk of bleeds of 0.6.

Future antithrombotic agents in secondary stroke prevention will have to be tested against aspirin or another known drug. It is therefore of great importance to know as precisely as possible the risk reduction as well as the risk of side-effects of the drug to which new therapies are compared.

It is likely that the higher the thromboembolic event rate is in a given population, the more favorable will the benefit/risk ratio be. If the event rate is low, the number of events that can be prevented will be low and the risk/benefit ratio may approach unity. It is therefore unlikely that aspirin will ever be beneficial as a primary preventive measure for stroke.

In the acute phase of stroke, the risk of hemorrhagic complications is much increased compared to that in the stable phase weeks or months after a stroke. In IST and CAST the 2- and 4-week rate of excess severe bleeds was about 0.4 per 100 patients treated, which is similar to the risk during a whole year of aspirin treatment in the stable phase. Thus, prevention of stroke and other vascular events by aspirin, although economically very favorable, has a cost in the way of severe or fatal bleeds. An ideal alternative antithrombotic therapy should be more effective than aspirin with fewer side-effects at an affordable price.

REFERENCES

1. Boysen G. Medical intervention: Clinical trials and population-based observational studies. In: *Stroke: Populations, Cohorts, and Clinical Trials*. (Whisnant JP, ed.) pp. 187–207. Butterworth Heinemann: 1993.
2. Truelsen T, Grønbæk M, Schnohr P, Boysen G. Intake of beer, wine, and spirits and risk of stroke. The Copenhagen City Heart Study. *Stroke* 1998; **29:**2467–72.
3. Sacco RL, Shi T, Zamanillo MC, Kargman DE. Predictors of mortality and recurrence after hospitalized cerebral infarction in an urban community: The Northern Manhattan Stroke Study. *Neurology* 1994; **44:**626–34.
4. Collins R, Peto R, MacMahon S *et al.* Blood pressure. Stroke, and coronary heart disease: part 2. Short-term reductions in blood pressure: overview of randomised drug trials in their epidemiological context. *Lancet* 1990; **335:**827–38.
5. Hypertension-Stroke Cooperative Study Group. Effect of antihypertensive treatment on stroke recurrence. *J Am Med Assoc* 1974; **229:** 409–18.
6. Beevers DG, Fairman MJ, Hamilton M, Harpur JE. Antihypertensive treatment and the course of established cerebral vascular disease. *Lancet* 1973; **i:**1407–9.
7. Lindenstrøm E, Boysen G, Nyboe J. Influence of total cholesterol, high density lipoprotein cholesterol, and triglycerides on risk of cerebrovascular disease: The Copenhagen City Heart Study. *Br Med J* 1994; **309:**11–15.
8. Prospective Studies Collaboration. Cholesterol, diastolic blood pressure, and stroke, 13000 strokes in 450000 people in 45 prospective cohorts. *Lancet* 1995; **346:**1647–53.
9. Sacks FM, Pfeffer MA, Moye LA *et al.* The effect of pravastatin on coronary events after myocardial infarction in patients with average cholesterol levels. *N Engl J Med* 1996; **335:**1001–9.
10. Wilterdink JL, Easton JD. Vascular event rates in patients with atherosclerotic cerebrovascular disease. *Arch Neurol* 1992; **49:**857–63.
11. Easton JD. Epidemiology of stroke recurrence. *Cerebrovasc Dis* 1997; **7**(Suppl 1):2–4.
12. Salgado AV, Ferro JM, Gouveia-Oliveira A. Long-term prognosis of first-ever lacunar strokes. A hospital-based study. *Stroke* 1996; **27:**661–6.
13. Boiten J, Lodder J. Prognosis for survival, handicap and recurrence of stroke in lacunar and superficial infarction. *Cerebrovasc Dis* 1993; **3:**221–6.
14. SALT Collaborative Group. Swedish aspirin low-dose trial (SALT) of 75 mg aspirin as secondary prophylaxis after cerebrovascular events. *Lancet* 1991; **338:**1345–9.
15. Bousser MG, Eschwege E, Haguenau M *et al.* AICLA Controlled trial of aspirin and dipyridamole in the secondary prevention of atherothrombotic cerebral ischema. *Stroke* 1983; **14:**5–14.
16. Diener HC, Cunha L, Forbes C, Sivenius J, Smets P, Löwenthal A. European Stroke Prevention Study 2. Dipyridamole and acetylsalicylic acid in the secondary prevention of stroke. *J Neurol Sci* 1996; **143:**1–13.
17. UK-TIA Study Group. United Kingdom

transient ischaemic attack (UK-TIA) aspirin trial: interim results. *Br Med J* 1988; **296:**316–20.

18. Britton M, Helmers C, Samuelsson K. High-dose acetylsalicylic acid after cerebral infarction: a Swedish cooperative study. *Stroke* 1987; **18:**325–34.
19. Boysen G, Soelberg PS, Juhler M *et al.* Danish very-low-dose aspirin after carotid endarterectomy trial. *Stroke* 1988; **19:**1211–5.
20. Antiplatelet Trialists' Collaboration. Collaborative overview of randomised trial of antiplatelet therapy—I: Prevention of death, myocardial infarction, and stroke by prolonged antiplatelet therapy in various categories of patients. *Br Med J* 1994; **301:**81–106.
21. Algra A, van Gijn J. Aspirin at any dose above 30 mg offers only modest protection after cerebral ischaemia. *J Neurol Neurosurg Psychiat* 1996; **60:**197–9.
22. Physicians' Health Study Research Group. Final report on the aspirin component of the ongoing physicians' health study. *N Engl J Med* 1989; **321:**129–35.
23. Dutch TIA Trial Study Group. A comparison of two doses of aspirin (30 mg vs. 283 mg a day) in patients after a transient ischaemic attack or minor ischaemic stroke. *N Engl J Med* 1991; **325:**1261–6.
24. Gent M, Easton JD, Hachinski VC *et al.* The Canadian American ticlopidine study (CATS) in thromboembolic stroke. *Lancet* 1989; **i:** 1215–20.
25. Hass WK, Easton JD, Adams HP *et al.* For the Ticlopidine Aspirin Stroke Study Group. A randomised trial comparing ticlopidine hydrochloride with aspirin for the prevention of stroke in high-risk patients. *N Engl J Med* 1989; **321:**501–7.
26. Caprie Steering Committee. A randomised, blinded, trial of clopidogrel versus aspirin in patients at risk of ischaemic events (CAPRIE). *Lancet* 1996; **348:**1329–39.
27. International Stroke Trial Collaborative Group. The International Stroke Trial (IST): a randomised trial of aspirin, subcutaneous heparin, both, or neither among 19.435 patients with acute ischaemic stroke. *Lancet* 1997; **349:**1569–81.
28. CAST (Chinese Acute Stroke Trial) Collaborative Group. CAST: randomised placebo-controlled trial of early aspirin use in 20 000 patients with acute ischaemic stroke. *Lancet* 1997; **349:**1641–9.
29. Roderick PJ, Wilkes HC, Meade TW. The gastrointestinal toxicity of aspirin: an overview of randomised controlled trials. *Br J Clin Pharmacol* 1993; **35:**219–26.
30. Weil J, Colin-Jones D, Langman M *et al.* Prophylactic aspirin and risk of peptic ulcer bleeding. *Br Med J* 1995; **310:**827–30.

11

Prevention after lacunar infarction: what changes?

Danilo Toni and Anne Falcou

CONTENTS • **Introduction** • **Risk factors for lacunar infarcts** • **Stroke recurrence in patients with index lacunar infarct** • **Conclusion: what kind of preventive treatment?**

INTRODUCTION

Adequate prevention of stroke recurrence should theoretically be targeted to the pathogenetic mechanisms causing the first stroke, assuming that subsequent recurrent strokes are likely to be the same type as the first one. However, in case this assumption were not true in all cases, and the pattern of stroke recurrence was more heterogeneous, knowledge of the incidence of the possible types of new events and of the underlying pathogenetic mechanisms would more effectively guide the choice of preventive treatments.

As regards lacunar infarction, such knowledge cannot as yet be considered unequivocal. The 'lacunar hypothesis', on the one hand, and doubts on the appropriateness of considering lacunes as a nosological entity, on the other, are but the two extremes of a long-lasting debate which has already produced numerous publications worldwide.[1]

It is well known that in a series of first-ever stroke patients, lacunes represent approximately 20% of the total.[1] Following the initial observations by Fisher,[2,3] lacunes appeared to be a specific type of stroke characterized by a peculiar arterial lesion called lipohyalinosis[3] and by the high frequency, and likely pathogenetic role, of hypertension.[2] It is of some interest that, more recently, Fisher himself reviewed this topic suggesting that lipohyalinosis is the pathological process underlying smaller infarcts with a diameter of 2–5 mm, whereas those over 5 mm which become symptomatic are consequences of microatheroma or embolism.[4] As to signs and symptoms, it was again Fisher who first suggested that lacunes have specific clinical pictures subsequently called the classic lacunar syndromes (pure motor hemiplegia,[5] pure sensory stroke,[6] ataxic hemiparesis,[7] dysarthria-clumsy hand[8] and sensorimotor stroke[9]).

The above observations initiated the 'lacunar hypothesis', which states that a lacunar syndrome is a synonym for lacunar infarct which is a stroke subtype due to small-vessel disease.[10] As we will see, most of the studies aimed at investigating risk factors and potential pathogenetic mechanisms of lacunes begin with this assumption, with the eventual corollary view that CT must either show a lacune or be completely negative.

But in how many cases can deep infarcts of the size of lacunes underlie signs and symptoms not classifiable as one of the classic lacunar syndromes and, conversely, how frequently may non-lacunar infarcts give rise to a clinical picture resembling a lacunar syndrome? Not many studies have addressed these two questions. As to the former, in a study of 350 patients hospitalized more than 24 h after stroke onset, 9% of those presenting a non-lacunar syndrome had a lacunar infarct,[11] whereas in a study of a larger series of 517 consecutive patients first seen within 12 h of stroke onset, 4% of those with a non-lacunar syndrome had a lacune and an additional 12% had a permanently normal CT. Half these patients with a normal CT improved over the subsequent days and their 'cortical' signs and symptoms cleared, but the remaining half kept showing a non-lacunar syndrome. All these patients were considered as having lacunes.[12] This assumption was based on the comment made by Fisher that 'the number of clinical patterns or syndromes linked to penetrator occlusion has grown to at least 70', to include aphasia, homonymous hemianopia, and neglect,[4] i.e., the signs and symptoms whose presence, according to the 'lacunar hypothesis', would exclude a lacune.[13] Hence, it is hardly tenable that, irrespective of the clinical picture, patients with a permanent neurological deficit and an infarct not visible at CT some days after stroke onset, might have anything but a very small lacune. In different studies, normal CT scans were found in 20–49% of patients with a non-lacunar syndrome.[14–16] Bearing in mind that CT examinations were not systematically performed in the whole series of patients, and considering differences in CT devices and in the timing of the CT examination after stroke onset with possible 'fogging effect', 10–20% of patients with a non-lacunar syndrome may mistakenly be diagnosed as having a non-lacunar infarct. This is in keeping with the results of an autoptic study which demonstrated that 20% of symptomatic lacunes had presented with aphasia in addition to right hemiparesis.[17]

The question of non-lacunar infarcts diagnosed as lacunar ones on the basis of the clinical picture is even more controversial. Some studies have, in fact, suggested a positive predictive value of lacunar syndromes as high as 80–94%,[11,13,18–21] whereas others observed that only 42–70% of patients with lacunar syndrome had a lacunar stroke.[12,22–24] Again, taking account of a series of variables that may lead to the false clinical diagnosis of small deep infarcts, such as inadequate testing of speech disorders and, above all, of non-dominant higher function,[10,11,25] we may conclude that 20–40% of non-lacunar infarcts may be misdiagnosed as lacunar on the basis of the clinical picture alone.

The aim of this long preamble was to introduce the issues of the search for risk factors and of stroke recurrence in patients with lacunar infarcts. In fact, according to the definition of lacunar infarcts adopted, we can distinguish three main groups of studies.

1. Clinical diagnosis: based on the description of a lacunar syndrome, which implies both false-positive and false-negative clinical diagnoses; included in this group are the studies which for the diagnosis relied exclusively or predominantly (i.e., not submitting all patients to CT) on the clinical picture.
2. Clinical and radiological diagnosis: patients presenting a lacunar syndrome and CT which shows a lacune or is completely normal, which excludes false-positive but includes false-negative clinical diagnoses.
3. Radiological diagnosis: based on CT data, irrespective of the clinical picture, which excludes both false-positive and false-negative clinical diagnoses, provided that the classification as lacunes of the few cases of non-lacunar syndrome with negative CT does not represent a false-positive radiological diagnosis.

RISK FACTORS FOR LACUNAR INFARCTS

Table 11.1 summarizes the prevalence of risk factors for stroke in lacunar and non-lacunar infarcts in the studies we have reviewed.

Hypertension

The association between lacunes and hypertension (HT) was first suggested by Fisher who reported that 97% of subjects with

Table 11.1 Prevalence of risk factors for stroke in lacunar and non-lacunar infarct patients

Definition of lacunar infarct	*No. of lacunar patients (%)*	*HT (%)*	*DM (%)*	*IHD (%)*	*PCES (%)*	*ICS (%)*	*pTIA (%)*	*Smoke (%)*
Clinical								
Sacco[27]	159 (12)	81/70	14/16	NE	12/28	21/27	NE	NE
Lodder[15]	102 (33)	44/47	13/9	39/50	*10/22	14/13	18/18	68/68
Landi[16]	88 (46)	65/52	19/16	24/50	12/32	18/27	23/15	41/45
[a]Toni[25]	219 (42)	49/50	17/17	41/51	*18/25	NE	19/13	34/26
Clinical and radiological								
[b]Gandolfo[26]	108 (100)	65	21	37	*8	NE	34	55
[c]Norrving[14]	61 (50)	52/44	8/10	8/25	NE	3.3/66	NE	51/52
[d]Arboix[21]	227 (100)	72	28	26	NE	NE	18	NE
[e]Chamorro[28]	316 (47)	75/64	26/21	24/65	NE	NE	13/21	NE
[c]Tegeler[29]	55 (51)	60/56	35/30	NE	NE	13/41	31/37	38/70
[f]Horowitz[30]	108 (100)	68	37	NE	18	23	27	NE
[f]Miyao[31]	215 (100)	59	12	19	*4	NE	NE	NE
Boiten[32]	103 (52)	50/37	27/27	26/36	*10/30	13/37	NE	NE
[fg]Clavier[33]	178 (100)	76	40	16	†19	NE	47	46
[f]Salgado[34]	145 (100)	72	25	NE	†10	2	18	NE
[h]Yamamoto[35]	19 (22)	63/78	42/18	16/33	47/54	NE	NE	37/58
[c]Schmal[36]	242 (61)	59/58	23/33	26/30	NE	20/50	NE	18/19
Radiological								
[i]Ghika[23]	42 (42)	71/50	31/41	NE	21/13	28/27	28/27	31/34
[a]Toni[25]	170 (33)	56/46	16/17	37/52	*15/26	NE	23/12	32/28

Pairs of values separated by slash indicate prevalence of risk factors in lacunar/non-lacunar infarcts.
NE = not evaluated.
HT = hypertension; DM = diabetes mellitus; pTIA = previous transient ischemic attack.
IHD = ischemic heart diseases (see text for definition).
PCES = potential cardioembolic sources (see text for definition).
ICS = ipsilateral internal carotid stenosis.
[a]Lacunar infarcts diagnosed first on clinical grounds alone and then on the basis of CT data alone assuming that all normal control CT were lacunes irrespective of clinical presentation.
[b]Compared with non-stroke controls whose data are hence not reported.
[c]Cardioembolic strokes excluded.
[d]Compared with 56 lacunar syndrome patients with non-lacunar infarcts ($N = 26$) or parenchymal hemorrhage ($N = 30$) whose data are hence not reported.
[e]Lacunar infarct defined also by absence of cardiac and/or arterial embolic sources on non-invasive testing.
[f]Studies only on lacunar infarcts, without comparison with non-lacunar ones.
[g]Previous stroke considered together with previous TIA.
[h]Study only on patients who had a recurrence.
[i]Study only on subcortical infarcts.
*Only atrial fibrillation.

lacunes detected by autopsy had been hypertensive during life. Obviously, the point of view of necropsy might have been biased towards the observation of patients with more severe cardiovascular diseases, including hypertension. Moreover, the threshold for HT set by Fisher at blood pressure (BP) values >140/90 mmHg may have influenced the results of that study, which were not confirmed by a more recent autoptic study on lacunar infarcts which found a 64% prevalence of HT, defined as BP values >160/95 mmHg.[17]

The prevalence of HT in clinical studies varies widely from 44 to 81%,[14–16,21,23,25–36] indicating substantial differences in the populations studied and in the definitions of HT adopted. The studies reporting data on lacunar infarcts alone show the highest prevalence of HT but, as a comparison with non-lacunar infarcts is lacking, we do not know what the global prevalence of HT was in the populations from which lacunar patients were drawn.[21,26,30,31,33,34]

By examining the studies comparing lacunar to non-lacunar infarcts, we find that HT is 1–13% more frequent in the former than in the latter,[14,16,25,27–29,32,36] and this figure rises to 21% when only subcortical infarcts of different size are considered.[23] Two studies are apparently at variance with this contention. In one study which relied on the clinical picture alone to classify stroke subtypes,[15] the slightly higher prevalence of HT in non-lacunar infarct patients may be explained by the aforementioned possible misdiagnosis. This is also suggested by the change in the prevalence of all risk factors for stroke observed when lacunar infarcts are diagnosed on the basis of CT data rather than on clinical grounds.[25] Another study reporting a 63% prevalence of HT in lacunar infarcts and a 78% prevalence in non-lacunar infarcts was retrospective and focused exclusively on a small group of patients with different subtypes of first stroke who had had a recurrent event.[35] In the same study, the prevalence of diabetes mellitus was far higher in lacunar than in non-lacunar infarcts and the authors emphasize this association, omitting to comment on the apparent paradox of a possible protective effect of HT against stroke recurrence in lacunar infarcts.[35] On the other hand, in the population of patients from which this subgroup was extracted, HT was, as is the general rule, more prevalent among lacunar infarcts.[37]

Considering all these caveats and the non-immediate comparability of the studies, it emerges that, although HT is, as generally believed, more frequent in lacunar than in non-lacunar infarcts, this difference may not be so significant[38] and above all, that approximately 20–50% of patients with lacunar infarcts may not be hypertensive.

Diabetes mellitus

Except for the aforementioned study reporting a high prevalence of diabetes mellitus (DM) in lacunar infarct patients who experienced stroke recurrence,[35] in general DM prevalence is comparable in lacunar and non-lacunar infarcts, whatever the diagnostic procedure.[14–16,25,28,29,32] However, the wide variability of data among studies is confirmed, DM prevalence ranging from 8 to 40%, as is the higher prevalence of DM observed in studies that focused on lacunar infarcts alone.[21,30,33,34] Finally, two studies report a 10% higher prevalence of DM in non-lacunar infarcts,[23,36] and in one of these, a history of DM was found to be significantly associated with risk of cortical infarct.[36]

Cardiopathies and potential cardioembolic sources

In lacunar infarcts the prevalence of ischemic heart disease (IHD), which include angina pectoris, congestive heart failure, coronary by-pass or non-recent myocardial infarction, varies from 8 to 37%, as compared to 25 to 52% in non-lacunar infarcts.[14–16,25,32,35,36]

In one study, which also included the absence of carotid and cardiac embolic sources at non-invasive testing in its definition of lacunar infarcts, the prevalence of IHD in lacunar infarcts was nevertheless 29%, though this was offset by an expectedly overwhelming 65% in non-lacunar infarcts,[28] and is similar to the 26% reported in another study in which the same diagnostic criteria were adopted.[21] Moreover, in both these studies cardiac dysrythmias were considered together with IHD and their relative prevalence was not specified. When atrial fibrillation is considered separately, however, its prevalence in lacunar infarcts varies from 4 to 15%[15,25,26,31,32] as compared to 22 to 30% in non-lacunar infarcts.[15,25,32] Finally, when in addition to atrial fibrillation other potentially high risk cardioembolic sources (PCES) were considered, such as sick sinus syndrome, mitral/aortic valve diseases, prosthetic valves, recent myocardial infarction, left ventricular aneurysm or thrombus, left ventricular dyskinesia, endocarditis and cardiomyopathy,[39] the overall prevalence of PCES was 12–18% in lacunar infarcts[16,27,30] as compared to 28–32% in non-lacunar ones.[16,27]

Two studies are apparently at variance with this finding and are worthy of a short comment. In one study, focused on subcortical lacunar and non-lacunar infarcts, the prevalence of PCES was 21% in the former and 13% in the latter, thus indicating a higher prevalence of PCES in lacunar infarcts compared not only to lacunar infarcts in other studies but also, contrary to what is generally believed,[1] to subcortical large infarcts.[23] An even more interesting, and apparently surprising result is that, in the study on patients who experienced stroke recurrence, prevalence of PCES was 47% in those with an initial lacunar infarct and 54% in non-lacunar ones.[35] Hence in that study, prevalence of PCES, both in the whole series and particularly in lacunar infarct patients, was definitely higher than in other studies, a result which may at least in part be explained by the use of more refined diagnostic tools such as transesophageal echocardiography.[40,41]

Concomitant ipsilateral internal carotid stenosis

Internal carotid stenosis ipsilateral to the lacunar infarct was quantified in different ways in the studies reviewed. In two studies, 'cervical bruits' were found in 14% and 21% of lacunar infarcts as opposed, respectively, to 13% and 27% of non-lacunar infarcts.[15,27] Significant carotid stenosis, defined as a reduction of the carotid lumen ≥50%, was found, respectively, in 3.3% and 13% of lacunar infarcts and in 66% and 37% of non-lacunar ones,[14,32] whereas a stenosis >50% was detected in 2–20% of lacunar infarcts[16,34,36] as compared to 27–50% of non-lacunar ones,[16,36] and finally a stenosis ≥75% was found in 28% lacunar and 27% non-lacunar subcortical infarcts.[23] Thus, it is evident that there is a wide variability between studies as regards the prevalence of concomitant large artery disease, which makes it difficult to draw general conclusions; furthermore, there is no agreement on how to interpret this observation. In fact, it might either indicate a potential arterial source of embolism[38,42,43] or be a finding determined merely by chance. Whatever the underlying reasons, however, it should be considered at least as an index that small and large vessels may concomitantly be harmed by the same noxious conditions.

Other risk factors

In comparative studies, the prevalence of previous transient ischemic attacks in lacunar infarcts ranged from 13 to 32% and is similar to,[15,23] higher[16,25] or lower[28,36] than that in non-lacunar infarcts, whereas in non-comparative studies it ranged from 18 to 47%.[21,26,30,33,34]

Finally, cigarette smoking is largely comparable in the two groups in all[14–16,23,25,26,36] but two studies,[29,35] with a wide variability between studies which probably reflects different attitudes toward tobacco use in different populations.[14–16,23,25,26,29,33,35,36]

This short review highlights, on the one hand, a less exclusive pathogenetic role of HT in lacunar infarcts than previously believed, and, on the other, the fact that in a considerable proportion of cases lacunar infarcts share similar stroke risk factors with non-lacunar infarcts. One might object that the possible concomitance of HT with ICS or with PCES may mask the actual pathogenetic role of HT,[16] but in this regard it is noteworthy that the concomitance does not affect more than one-third of cases[23,30,35] and above all, that its prevalence is similar to that of ICS and PCES without HT.[30] Finally, as mentioned above, the wider use of more refined and sensitive diagnostic techniques, such as transesophageal echocardiography will probably improve the definition of the pathogenetic mechanisms underlying each stroke subtype, including lacunes.[44]

STROKE RECURRENCE IN PATIENTS WITH INDEX LACUNAR INFARCT

Rates of stoke recurrence and types of recurrent events in patients with index lacunar infarct are summarized in Table 11.2

First of all, let us consider the dimensions of the problem. The rate of early stroke recurrence within 1 month of an index lacunar infarct varies from 0.75 to 4%,[10,16,18,27,46,48] and is 2.5–5 times lower than in non-lacunar infarct patients in all[10,16,18,46,48] but one study in which early recurrence in the former was two-fold that in the latter.[27] The rate of stroke recurrence 1 year after a lacunar infarct varies from 3.6 to 11.8%,[10,16,18,27,31,33,44,46,48–50] and is similar to,[49] higher[27,46] or lower,[16,48] than that of non-lacunar infarcts which ranges from 2 to 12%.[16,27,46,48,49] However, in two studies which further separated lacunar from non-lacunar atherothrombotic (AHT), cardioembolic (CE) and cryptogenic (CRY) infarcts,[46,48] the rate of 1-year recurrence in patients with non-lacunar ATH infarcts is 1.5[46] to 2.5[48] times higher than that in patients with lacunar infarcts, whereas the recurrence rate in patients with non-lacunar CE and CRY infarcts is comparable to that in lacunar infarct patients. The highest 1-month and 1-year rate of recurrence in both patients with lacunar and non-lacunar infarcts is reported in a study[47] in which the definition of stroke recurrence adopted may, however, have led to patients with stroke recurrence being mixed up with patients experiencing late progression of the initial stroke.[51] Also this study performed a separate analysis of different stroke subtypes, from which we learn that the 1-year recurrence rate in patients with an index ATH non-lacunar infarct was approximately 1.5 times higher than that in patients with lacunar infarcts, whereas the recurrence rate in patients with CE infarcts was less than half that in lacunar infarct patients.[47] The total recurrence rate obviously varies according to the duration of follow-up in the different studies. However, it is noteworthy that in the studies with the longest follow-up the risk of recurrent stroke in patients with an index lacunar infarct changes little over time, the annual risk of recurrence varying from 5 to 10%.[27,34,45,48,50]

The question of the type of second and further strokes in patients with an index lacunar infarct, however, is the one that yields the most interesting and surprising data. In some series, in fact, recurrent stroke was a lacunar infarct in 50–86%[31,34,47,50] or in a non-specified 'majority' of cases,[46,48] although never in all cases. In other series, by contrast, recurrent stroke was more frequently a non-lacunar infarct[27,33,35,45,49] which represented up to 69% of recurrences.[27] In one study that further separated recurrent atherothrombotic from cardioembolic non-lacunar infarcts in patients with an index lacunar infarct, the former accounted for 31% and the latter for 17% of recurrent events as compared to 48% of recurrences due to a new lacunar infarct.[35] Finally, recurrent stroke was a parenchymal hemorrhage in 3.5–15% of cases.[27,31,33–35,49,50]

These data allow us to speculate on the pathophysiology not only of recurrent events but also of the index lacunar infarct. The point of view of those who found that recurrent stroke was generally of the same type as index stroke is best represented by the statement that 'lacunar infarcts occur as a result of occlusion of a single perforating artery, and thus any recurrent event would require the occlusion of another artery'.[13] This would also account for the lower rate of early recurrence in lacunar than in non-lacunar infarct patients[10,16,18,46,48] since 'an active source of embolism that might give rise to a series of events close together is a less likely mechanism'.[13] The observation that recurrent infarcts were more frequently lacunar also in patients with PCES and/or carotid stenosis[34] would additionally support this contention. Finally, the observation of a far higher frequency of lacunar infarct recurrence in patients with index lacunar infarct and leukoaraiosis than in those without leukoaraiosis[31] would further support the aforementioned statement. The diffuse arteriosclerosis[52,53] and the impaired cerebral circulation[54,55] frequently associated with leukoaraiosis, are postulated to play a role in the higher recurrent rate. However, other studies have not confirmed the association between leukoaraiosis and lacunar infarct recurrence.[33,34]

Table 11.2 Early and late recurrence rates and types of recurrent events in patients with index lacunar and non-lacunar infarct

Definition of lacunar infarct	*No. of patients*	*Longest follow-up (months)*	*Recurrence rate during follow-up (%): 1 month*	*1 year*	*total*	*Type of recurrent stroke (%): LI*	*NLI*	*PH*	*UK*
Clinical									
Bamford[10]	102	12	1	11.8	11.8	NE			
Bamford[18]	137	12	0.75/5.5	9/15.7	9/15.7	NE			
Landi[16]	88	48	1.1/2	7.9/11.4	13.6/30.7	NE			
Clinical and radiological									
Gandolfo[45]	107	70	NE	4.7	33.6	30	38	8	*25
Sacco[27]	78	60	4/2	10/8	26/27	17	69	14	/
[a]Hier[46]	337	24	2.2/7.9	10.6/8.8	14.6/13.8	NE			
Miyao[31]	190	36	NE	9	17.8	76	12	12	/
Boiten[33]	103	16	NE	5/2	6.8	86	14	/	/
[b]Nadeau[47]	53	36	8/19	16/25.6	21/33.9	50	40	/	10
Clavier[33]	172	57	NE	6	15	31	54	15	/
[a]Sacco[48]	85	60	3.5/6.8	10.7/12	17.3/32.6	NE			
Kappelle[49]	1216	36	NE	3.6/3.6	8.8/9	28	49	11	12
Samuelson[50]	81	68	NE	6.8	27	65	20	15	/
Salgado[34]	145	60	NE	7	28	63	23	7	7
Yamamoto[35]	19	60	NE	NE	NE	48	48	3.5	/

Pairs of percent values separated by slash indicate recurrent rates in lacunar/non-lacunar infarcts.
LI = lacunar infarcts; NLI = non-lacunar infarcts; PH = parenchymal hemorrhage; UK = unknown.
NE = not evaluated.
[a]Recurrence rates of non-lacunar infarcts recalculated from original tables reporting atherothrombotic, cardioembolic and cryptogenic infarcts separately.
[b]Recurrence rates of non-lacunar infarcts recalculated from original table reporting thromboembolic and cardioembolic infarcts separately.
* Including 17% of non-further classified reversible ischemic attacks.

The hypothesis of a specific and unique pathogenetic mechanism for both the index and recurrent infarcts is undoubtedly simple and, hence, appealing. It is, unfortunately, applicable only to series in which recurrent stroke is more frequently lacunar,[31,34,46–48,50] and is contradicted by those in which recurrent lacunes are less frequent and the pattern of recurrence is somewhat more complex[27,33,35,45,49] and requires a more elaborate explanation. Recurrent infarcts of the lacunar type might be less frequently reported by patients because they are minimally disabling or even silent. Silent strokes are treated in another chapter of this book, and we limit ourselves to observing that in some series the impact of silent lacunes is not significant,[49] whereas in others their pathogenesis is believed to be cardioembolic.[56]

As reported in the first part of this chapter, patients with lacunar infarcts may have atherosclerotic lesions in large vessels as well,[15,16,23,27,29,32,36] and which of the two vessel types the disease manifests itself in may merely be a matter of chance. Moreover, atherosclerotic lesions may occur in the middle cerebral artery mainstem and block the origin of one or more small perforating arteries,[57] although studies have shown that atherothrombosis of intracerebral arteries is less likely in caucasians[58] and more frequent in orientals and blacks.[59] Recurrent infarcts may be cardioembolic in approximately one-fifth of cases[35] since lacunar infarcts themselves may be embolic,[60] but it remains to be defined why the same mechanism may first involve perforating and subsequently non-perforating arteries. The possibility of recurrent stroke being a parenchymal hemorrhage might be due to chance since the frequency of this occurrence is similar to that observed in the general population.[50] However, it has also been suggested that a more severe degree of leukoaraiosis, as may be observed in patients with lacunar infarcts, increases the risk of parenchymal hemorrhage.[50]

Finally, it is noteworthy that when predictors of stroke recurrence in patients with an index lacunar infarct were searched, only older age,[50] DM[35] and leukoaraiosis[31] were found to be related to the risk of recurrence. Age and DM are, however, predictors of stroke recurrence in general,[61,62] and, as mentioned above, DM may be associated more with non-lacunar than with lacunar infarcts,[36] while leukoaraiosis is not related to recurrence in other series.[33,34] Interestingly, the presence and duration of HT is never significantly associated with stroke recurrence.[33,34,45,50]

CONCLUSION: WHAT KIND OF PREVENTIVE TREATMENT?

We are unable to provide evidence-based indications on the best preventive treatment; while on the one hand, information on the pathogenesis of index and recurrent strokes is controversial, that on the efficacy of treatments, on the other, is scanty. Only six articles reported the treatment administered to patients, which consisted mainly of 30–283 mg/day aspirin,[33–35,49,50] while warfarin was given to a minority of patients.[34,35] The data showing that recurrent events are more frequently non-lacunar[33,35,49] would theoretically indicate that aspirin may prevent thrombosis more effectively in small rather than in large vessels,[49] as is also suggested by the observation that in patients taking aspirin, recurrent stroke is generally more often due to large vessel disease.[64] However, this does not apply to the studies in which recurrent events were more frequently lacunar.[34,50] Moreover, it is also contradicted by the results of the only study that has so far specifically attempted to evaluate the efficacy of antiplatelets in preventing recurrence in lacunar infarcts.[64] The comparison of 332 patients, with CT- or MRI-verified lacunar infarct, receiving aspirin or ticlopidine (the choice of drug and drug dose were left to each participant) with 278 patients not receiving antiplatelets, during 5 years of follow-up showed that recurrence rates were 4.7% per year and 4.1% per year, respectively, and parenchymal hemorrhages were 0.8% per year and 0.4% per year, respectively. In a larger series of lacunar infarcts diagnosed on clinical grounds in the context of the Chinese Acute Stroke Trial,[65] 2.6% of those receiving 160 mg/day aspirin and 2.9% of those taking placebo experienced the combined 1-month endpoint of death or recurrent non-fatal stroke. Moreover, blood pressure control might also be inadequate to prevent the development of new silent or symptomatic strokes.[66,67]

In conclusion, at present there is no definite answer to the question of what is the best preventive treatment for patients with index lacunar infarcts. It is likely that this answer could be obtained by enrolling CT- or MR-defined lacunar infarct patients in pharmacological trials using one or more of the antiplatelet agents which have so far shown the most promising risk/benefit profile.[68–70]

Therefore, for the time being we fully agree with the recommendation[1] that as complete as possible a diagnostic work-up be made in patients with lacunar infarct in order to identify the possible heterogeneous pathogenetic mechanisms other than hypertensive arteriolopathy, and to choose preventive treatments accordingly.

REFERENCES

1. Mohr JP, Marti-Vilalta JL. Lacunes. In: *Stroke. Pathophysiology, Diagnosis and Management* (Barnett HJM, Mohr JP, Stein BM, Yatsu FM, eds), 3rd edn, pp. 599–602. New York; Churchill Livingstone: 1998.
2. Fisher CM. Lacunes: small, deep infarcts. *Neurology* 1965; **17**:774–84.
3. Fisher CM. The arterial lesion underlying lacunes. *Acta Neuropathol* 1969; **12**:1–15.
4. Fisher CM. Lacunar infarcts—a review. *Cerebrovasc Dis* 1991; **1**:311–20.
5. Fisher CM. Pure motor hemiplegia of vascular origin. *Arch Neurol* 1965; **13**:130–40.
6. Fisher CM. Pure sensory stroke involving face, arm and leg. *Neurology* 1965; **15**:76–80.
7. Fisher CM. Homolateral ataxia and crural paresis. A vascular syndrome. *J Neurol Neurosurg Psychiatr* 1965; **28**:48–55.
8. Fisher CM. A lacunar stroke. The dysarthria clumsy hand syndrome. *Neurology* 1967; **17**: 614–7.
9. Mohr JP, Kase CS, Meckler RJ, Fisher CM. Sensorimotor stroke. *Arch Neurol* 1977; **34**:739–41.
10. Bamford JM, Warlow CP. Evolution and testing of the lacunar hypothesis. *Stroke* 1988; **19**: 1074–82.
11. Lodder J, Bamford J, Kappelle J, Boiten J. What causes false clinical prediction of small deep infarcts? *Stroke* 1994; **25**:86–91.
12. Toni D, Del Duca R, Fiorelli M *et al.* Pure motor hemiparesis and sensorimotor stroke: accuracy of the very early clinical diagnosis of lacunar strokes. *Stroke* 1994; **25**:92–6.
13. Bamford J, Sandercock P, Jones L, Warlow CP. The natural history of lacunar infarction: the Oxfordshire Community Stroke Project. *Stroke* 1987; **18**:545–51.
14. Norrving B, Cronqvist S. Clinical and radiologic features of lacunar versus nonlacunar minor stroke. *Stroke* 1989; **20**:59–64.
15. Lodder J, Bamford JM, Sandercock PAG, Jones LN, Warlow CP. Are hypertension or cardiac embolism likely causes of lacunar infarction? *Stroke* 1990; **21**:375–81.
16. Landi G, Cella E, Boccardi E, Musicco M. Lacunar versus non-lacunar infarcts: pathogenetic and prognostic differences. *J Neurol Neurosurg Psychiatr* 1992; **55**:441–5.
17. Tuszynski MH, Petito CK, Levy DE. Risk factors and clinical manifestation of pathologically verified lacunar infarctions. *Stroke* 1989; **20**:990–9.
18. Bamford J, Sandercock P, Dennis M, Burn J, Warlow C. Classification and natural history of clinically identifiable subtypes of cerebral infarction. *Lancet* 1991; **337**:1521–6.
19. Boiten J, Lodder J. Lacunar infarcts. Pathogenesis and validity of the clinical syndromes. *Stroke* 1991; **22**:1374–8.
20. Chimowitz MI, Furlan AJ, Sila CA, Paranandi L, Beck GJ. Etiology of motor or sensory stroke: a prospective study of the predictive value of clinical and radiological features. *Ann Neurol* 1991; **30**:519–25.
21. Arboix A, Marti-Vilalta JL. Lacunar syndromes not due to lacunar infarcts. *Cerebrovasc Dis* 1992; **2**:287–92.
22. Wrisberg LA. Computed tomography and pure motor hemiparesis. *Neurology* 1979; **4**:490–5.
23. Ghika J, Bogousslavsky J, Regli F. Infarcts in the territory of the deep perforators from the carotid system. *Neurology* 1989; **39**:507–12.
24. Melo TP, Bogousslavsky J, Van Melle G, Regli F. Pure motor hemiparesis: a reappraisal. *Neurology* 1992; **42**:789–98.
25. Toni D, Fiorelli M, De Michele M *et al.* Clinical and prognostic correlates of stroke subtype misdiagnosis within 12 hours from onset. *Stroke* 1995; **26**:1837–40.
26. Gandolfo C, Caponnetto C, Del Sette M, Santoloci D, Loeb C. Risk factors in lacunar syndromes: a case control study. *Acta Neurol Scand* 1988; **77**:22–6.
27. Sacco SE, Whisnant JP, Broderick JP, Phillips SJ, O'Fallon WM. Epidemiological characteristics of lacunar infarcts in a population. *Stroke* 1991; **22**:1236–41.
28. Chamorro A, Sacco RL, Mohr JP *et al.* Clinical-computed tomographic correlations of lacunar infarction in the stroke data bank. *Stroke* 1991; **22**:175–81.
29. Tegeler CH, Fenglin S, Morgan T. Carotid stenosis in lacunar stroke. *Stroke* 1991; **22**:1124–8.
30. Horowitz DR, Tuhrim S, Weinberger JM, Rudolph SH. Mechanisms in lacunar infarction. *Stroke* 1992; **23**:325–7.
31. Miyao S, Takano A, Teramoto J, Takahashi A. Leukoaraiosis in relation to prognosis for patients with lacunar infarction. *Stroke* 1992; **23**:1434–8.
32. Boiten J, Lodder J. Prognosis for survival, handicap and recurrence of stroke in lacunar and superficial infarction. *Cerebrovasc Dis* 1993; **3**:221–6.
33. Clavier I, Hommel M, Besson G *et al.* Long term

prognosis of symptomatic lacunar infarcts—a hospital-based study. *Stroke* 1994; **25:**2005–9.

34. Salgado AV, Ferro JM, Couveia-Oliveira A. Long term prognosis of first ever lacunar stroke. A hospital based study. *Stroke* 1996; **27:**661–6.
35. Yamamoto H, Bogousslavsky J. Mechanisms of second and further strokes. *J Neurol Neurosurg Psychiatr* 1998; **64:**771–6.
36. Schmal M, Marini C, Carolei A, Di Napoli M, Kessels F, Lodder J. Different vascular risk factor profiles among cortical infarcts, small deep infarcts, and primary intracerebral hemorrhage point to different types of underlying vasculopathy. A study from the L'Aquila Stroke Registry. *Cerebrovasc Dis* 1998; **8:**14–9.
37. Bogousslavsky J, Van Melle G, Regli F. The Laussane Stroke Registry: analysis of 1,000 consecutive patients with first stroke. *Stroke* 1988; **19:**1083–92.
38. Millikan C, Futrell N. The fallacy of the lacunar hypothesis. *Stroke* 1990; **21:**1251–7.
39. Kittner SJ, Sharkness CM, Price TR *et al.* Infarcts with a cardiac source of embolism in the NINCDS stroke data bank: historical features. *Neurology* 1990; **40:**281–4.
40. Albers GW, Comess KA, De Rook FA *et al.* Transesophageal echocardiographic findings in stroke subtypes. *Stroke* 1994; **25:**23–8.
41. Censori B, Colombo F, Valsecchi MG *et al.* Early transoesophageal echocardiography in cryptogenic and lacunar stroke and transient ischaemic attack. *J Neurol Neurosurg Psychiatr* 1998; **64:**624–7.
42. Futrell N, Watson BD, Dietrich WD, Prado R, Millikan C, Ginsberg MD. A new model of embolic stroke produced by photochemical injury to the carotid artery of the rat. *Ann Neurol* 1988; **23:**251–7.
43. Futrell N, Millikan C, Watson BD, Dietrich WD, Prado R, Ginsberg M. Embolic stroke from a carotid arterial source in the rat: pathology and clinical implications. *Neurology* 1989; **39:**1050–6.
44. Sacco R, Toni D, Mohr JP. Classification of ischemic stroke. In: *Stroke. Pathophysiology, Diagnosis and Management* (Barnet HJM, Mohr JP, Stein BM, Yatsu FM, eds), 3rd edn, pp. 341–54. New York; Churchill Livingstone: 1998.
45. Gandolfo C, Moretti C, Dall'Agata D *et al.* Long term prognosis of patients with lacunar syndromes. *Acta Neurol Scand* 1986; **74:** 224–9.
46. Hier DB, Foulkes MA, Swiotonowski M *et al.* Stroke recurrence within 2 years after ischemic infarction. *Stroke* 1991; **22:**155–61.
47. Nadeau SE, Jordan JE, Mishra SK *et al.* Stroke rates in patients with lacunar and large vessel cerebral infarction. *J Neurol Sci* 1993; **114:**128–37.
48. Sacco RL, Shi T, Zamanillo MC *et al.* Predictors of mortality and recurrence after hospitalized cerebral infarction in an urban community: the Northern Manhattan stroke study. *Neurology* 1994; **44:**626–34.
49. Kappelle LJ, van Latum JC, Algra A *et al.* Dutch Trial Study Group. Recurrent stroke after transient ischemic attack or minor ischemic stroke: does the distinction between small and large vessel disease remain true to type? *J Neurol Neurosurg Psychiatry* 1995; **59:** 127–31.
50. Samuelsson M, Lindell D, Norrving B. Presumed pathogenetic mechanisms of recurrent stroke after lacunar infarction. *Cerebrovasc Dis* 1996; **6:**128–36.
51. Jørgensen HS, Nakayama H, Raaschou HO, Olsen TS. Effect of blood pressure and diabetes on stroke in progression. *Lancet* 1994; **344:**156–9.
52. Lotz PR, Ballinger WE Jr, Quisling RG. Subcortical arteriosclerotic encephalopathy: CT spectrum and pathologic correlation. *Am J Necl Radiol* 1986; **7:**817–22.
53. Gupta SR, Naheedy MH, Young JC, Ghobrial M, Rubino FA, Hindo W. Periventricular white matter changes and dementia: clinical, neuropsychological, radiological and pathological correlation. *Arch Neurol* 1989; **46:**1124–8.
54. Kawamura J, Meyer JS, Terayama Y, Weathers S. Leukoaraiosis correlates with cerebral hypoperfusion in vascular dementia. *Stroke* 1986; **74:**224–9.
55. Herholz K, Heindel W, Rackl A *et al.* Regional cerebral blood flow in patients with leukoaraiosis and atherosclerotic carotid artery disease. *Arch Neurol* 1990; **47:**392–6.
56. Feinberg WM, Seeger JF, Carmody RF, Anderson DC, Hart RG, Pearce LA. Epidemiologic features of asymptomatic cerebral infarction in patients with nonvalvular atrial fibrillation. *Arch Intern Med* 1990; **150:**2340–4.
57. Caplan LR. Intracranial branch atheromatous disease: a neglected, understudied and underused concept. *Neurology* 1989; **39:**1246–50.
58. Fieschi C, Argentino C, Lenzi GL, Sacchetti ML, Toni D, Bozzao L. Clinical and instrumental evaluation of patients with ischemic stroke within the first six hours. *J Neurol Sci* 1989; **91:**311–21.
59. Caplan LR, Gorelick PB, Hier DB. Race, sex and occlusive cerebrovascular disease: a review. *Stroke* 1986; **17:**648–55.

60. Bogousslavsky J, Cachin C, Regli F *et al.* Cardiac sources of embolism and cerebral infarction—clinical consequences and vascular concomitants: the Lausanne Stroke Registry. *Neurology* 1991; **41:**855–9.
61. Jørgensen HS, Nakayama H, Reith J, Raaschou HO, Olsen TS. Stroke recurrence: predictors, severity and prognosis. The Copenhagen Stroke Study. *Neurology* 1997; **48:**891–5.
62. Hankey GJ, Jamrozik K, Broadhurst RJ *et al.* Long-term risk of first recurrent stroke in the Perth Community Stroke Study. *Stroke* 1998; **29:**2491–500.
63. Chimowitz ML, Furlan A, Nayak S, Sila CA. Mechanism of stroke in patients taking aspirin. *Neurology* 1990; **40:**1682–5.
64. Yamagucchi T for Japanese Antiplatelet Stroke Prevention Study Group. Effect of antiplatelet therapy on recurrent ischemic stroke and brain hemorrhage in lacunar stroke [Abstract]. *Stroke* 1994; **25:**272.
65. CAST (Chinese Acute Stroke Trial) Collaborative Group. CAST: randomised placebo-controlled trial of early aspirin use in 20000 patients with acute ischemic stroke. *Lancet* 1997; **349:**1641–9.
66. Watanabe N, Imai Y, Nagai K *et al.* Nocturnal blood pressure and silent cerebrovascular lesions in elderly japanese. *Stroke* 1996; **27:**1319–27.
67. Yamamoto Y, Akiguchi I, Oiwa K, Hayashi M, Kimura J. Adverse effect of nighttime blood pressure on the outcome of lacunar infarct patients. *Stroke* 1998; **29:**570–6.
68. CAPRIE Steering Committee. A randomised, blinded, trial of clopidogrel versus aspirin in patients at risk of ischemic events (CAPRIE). *Lancet* 1996; **348:**1329–39.
69. Tijssen JG. Low-dose and high-dose acetylsalicylic acid, with and without dipyridamole: a review of clinical trial results. *Neurology* 1998; **51**(Suppl 3):15–6.
70. Easton JD. What have we learned from recent antiplatelet trials? *Neurology* 1998; **51**(Suppl 3):36–8.

12

Silent infarcts: etiology, prognosis and therapy

François JG Vingerhoets and Julien Bogousslavsky

CONTENTS • **Definitions of silent infarcts** • **Prevalence and characteristics of silent infarcts** • **Prognosis and treatment of SI** • **Prognosis and treatment of SI associated with other diseases** • **Conclusions**

DEFINITIONS OF SILENT INFARCTS

Silent infarcts (SI) are brain infarcts that have not been noticed or recognized by the patient. This silence may be secondary to: (1) the size and/or location of the lesion which did not lead to symptoms;[1] (2) the symptoms produced by the SI which have been overlooked or forgotten by the patient. The latter category is related to the 'cerebral infarct with transient symptoms' (CITS),[2] where symptoms of a transient ischemic attack result from an infarct visible by neuroimaging. Reversible ischemic neurological symptoms (RINDS), where the neurological examination is back to normal within 6 weeks following the stroke, may also present later as an SI when the patient has forgotten the event. With such diversity, the absence of signs and symptoms of SI should be ascertained by careful examination of the patients and detailed analysis of their history, including a review of all available charts and an interview with the relatives. Unfortunately this is rarely done in studies and almost never achieved in daily practice. To avoid overlooking lesions being silent, just because of a poor history, SI should be managed in daily practice as a 'symptomatic' stroke (in this chapter we will call a stroke a symptomatic event).

Silent infarcts were first reported at necropsy.[3] Recent progress in neuroimaging has allowed their diagnosis during life, usually during the investigation of other, symptomatic, diseases. This peculiarity leads to an important problem of definition: how to ascertain the ischemic origin of an image of a sequellar lesion in the brain?

Currently, in studies using brain computed tomography (CT), the vascular distribution and the sharp delimitation of deep lesions are accepted criteria of their vascular origin. The two main uncertainties of this CT definition are: (1) the differentiation between the ischemic and hemorrhagic origin of a sequellar lesion; and (2) the poor definition of cortical lesions, especially when they are mixed with cortical atrophy in elderly patients. These uncertainties lead to underestimation of cortical SI and to some overestimation of deep lesions by CT studies.

Magnetic resonance imaging (MRI) has a higher sensitivity than CT but it is also less specific.[4–6] MRI criteria for the diagnosis of SI have therefore important effects on the results of studies using this technique. This has been exemplified by a study reporting an identical prevalence of unselected MRI signal hyperintensities in stroke patients (44% with hyperintensities) and normal volunteers (47.5%). When punctate MRI lesions were appropriately excluded, the same study reported a significant difference between the two groups (19.5% and 7.5%, respectively).[7] Current criteria for a vascular origin to an MRI lesion are: (1) a lesion visible in T1- (hypodensity) and T2- (hyperdensity) weighted images (this criterion excludes mainly the unidentified bright objects of unknown significance seen only in T2-weighted images); and (2) a lesion larger than 5 mm (this criterion prevents misclassification of the images secondary to the enlargement of the Virschow–Robin spaces—'état criblé').

PREVALENCE AND CHARACTERISTICS OF SILENT INFARCTS

Prevalence

The prevalence of SI in the normal population is estimated between 7.5 and 28% by neuroimaging.[7–13] In a series of 966 consecutive autopsies, the prevalence of SI was found to be 17.5%.[14]

In association with symptomatic brain infarcts, SI have been reported in 10–38% of cases (Table 12.1). A clinicopathological study gave an estimate of 22%.[15] These figures are usually higher than those found in the normal population or in control groups suggesting common mechanisms between symptomatic and silent infarcts. Differences between these two types of infarcts are probably explained by the characteristics of SI.

Characteristics

Silent infarcts are smaller than strokes. From 60% up to 93% of SI have a diameter smaller than 1.5 cm.[14,16–21] They tend to be unique and are located preferentially in deep, usually silent brain areas (e.g., basal ganglia, anterior arm of the internal capsule).[14,16–20,22,23] These characteristics explain these lesions being asymptomatic.[1,18] A similar absence of a clinical relationship is reported by pathological studies for 77% of the lacunar strokes[3] but only 34% of unselected strokes.[15]

When all SI are considered, they distribute equally in both cerebral hemispheres. However, when lesions involving the cortex are analyzed separately, involvement of the right hemisphere predominates.[1,24] This predominance, inverse to that of symptomatic infarcts, may be due to the higher frequency of heminegligect following the right hemisphere involvement.[1,24]

ETIOLOGIES OF SILENT INFARCTS

Risk factors

Risk factors are similar when comparing SI and other infarcts[1,18,25,26] except for age. The prevalence of SI increases with age, both in normal subjects and in patients with other diseases

Table 12.1 Prevalences of SI

Normal population[7–12]	7–28%
First stroke[1,9,16,23,28,29,39,40]	11–38%
Transient ischemic attack[4,19,27,32,37,63]	0–47%
Carotid stenosis[19–21,31,33–37,64]	13–42%
Atrial fibrillation[8–10,26]	13–58%

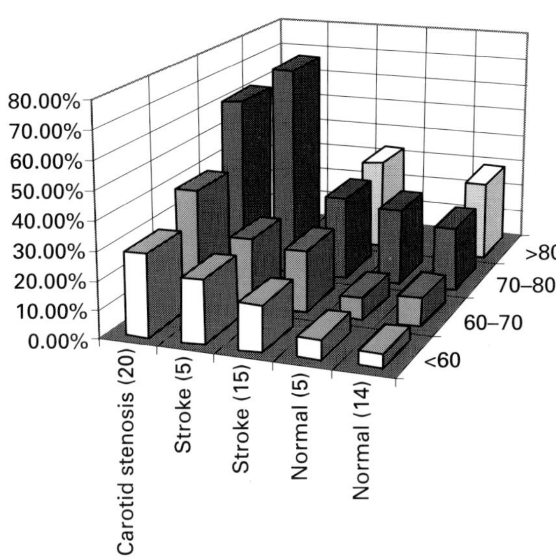

Figure 12.1 Age effect on the prevalence of silent infarcts.

(Fig. 12.1). Beside age, almost all cerebrovascular risk factors have been reported in association with SI, including hypertension,[14,16,17,19,27] male sex,[16,28,29] leukoaraiosis,[30] current cigarette smoking,[23,27] history of heart disease[12] and diabetes.[18] Among these risk factors, only hypertension has been regularly found to be independently associated with SI.[14,17,19] However, hypertension is also a predominant risk factor for lacunar strokes. This may suggest that the association of SI and hypertension merely reflects the increased representation of lacunar infarcts in the SI. This is further supported by the disappearance of the association between SI and hypertension when cortical vs. deep SI are considered.[17]

Association with carotid stenosis

In association with carotid stenosis, the prevalence of SI is estimated between 13 and 42% (Table 12.1)[19,21,31–36] and is related to the severity of the stenosis.[21,37,38] Some of the SI associated with carotid stenosis are preceded by transient ischemic attack (TIA), but the symptoms are not always related to the localization of the SI.[35]

Cardioembolic SI

The prevalence of SI is double to triple in patients with cardioembolic strokes compared to those with ischemic lesions from another etiology.[1,39,40] Multiple SI and SI involving the cortex (particularly right cortical SI) increase this trend.[1,18,24,40] The cortical distribution of SI of cardioembolic origin should be emphasized, as two studies showed that a cardioembolic origin of an index stroke in the presence of SI was significantly more frequent only when small deep SI were excluded from the analysis.[1,17] On the other hand, when all SI are considered, a cardioembolic origin is confirmed for the index stroke only in 18–30% of the cases (Table 12.2). These findings suggest that SI should be analyzed and subdivided in a similar way to ischemic strokes in general, and that considering SI as a single entity is not correct. Currently, it seems that a lacunar SI should be regarded as an index of small-vessel disease, while a territorial SI should lead to a cardiac work-up, especially when they are multiple, and involve a different vascular territory than the index stroke.

Careful, controlled studies have shown a two- to four-fold increase in the prevalence of the number of SI in patients with chronic AF compared to normal controls.[8–10,26,41] This association is further reinforced by a reduction of other cerebrovascular risk factors in the atrial fibrillation (AF) group.[26] Echocardiographic studies[30,41] found no particular anomaly related to SI. The discovery of SI in a patient with AF is therefore not a particular indication to perform echocardiography.

PROGNOSIS AND TREATMENT OF SI

Little is known about the prognosis of isolated SI. From the cross-sectional studies showing

Table 12.2 Etiology of the index stroke when associated with SI (control group: strokes without SI)

Study	*Cardioembolic (%)*	*Large-artery atherosclerosis (%)*	*Lacunes (%)*	*Others and undetermined (%)*
Kase[18]	30.8 (31.5)	46.2 (45.1)	7.7 (10.5)	15.3 (12.9)
Chodosh[1]	17.8 (4.3)	12.6 (20.0)	25.2 (22.3)	44.5 (53.4)
Boon[17]	21.4 (24.4)	20.8 (24.2)	41.7 (31.0)	16 (20.4)
Territorial SI[17]	37.8	27.2	18.9	16

that the number of these subclinical lesions increases with age, it may be inferred that SI represent a progressing disease. However, the clinical significance of this progression is still unknown. There are two domains where this question has been addressed. A prospective study showed that the annual risk of stroke (ischemic or hemorrhagic) in patients with deep SI was 10-fold the risk of those with normal imaging.[42] This suggests that SI should be considered as a preclinical marker of patients at risk of developing a stroke.

Another domain where the progression of SI may be of clinical significance is the development of dementia. As with other white matter or cortical lesions found on MRI in the elderly,[43] SI might be related to vascular dementia.[44] However, the definition of vascular dementia includes an association with clinical signs.[45] This contrasts with the a priori absence of clinical signs and symptoms in SI. It is therefore not surprising that the relationship between SI and dementia is controversial. Up to now, there has been no definite evidence to support the association of SI and dementia. In particular, absence of significant motor, cognitive or behavioral change in patients with SI has been shown repeatedly,[1,8,16,17,20,25,27] and SI do not predict the development of dementia after a stroke.[46] Some correlation between the degree of carotid stenosis and the severity of ipsilateral cerebral atrophy[47] and a high frequency of SI in patients with 'pre-senile' (51%) and 'senile' (93%) depression[48] have been reported. Similarly, a high prevalence of SI has been reported in late-onset mania (65%).[49] These findings may be regarded as confounding (e.g., depression may mimic dementia) or confirming (e.g., depression may precede dementia) information. This controversy will probably continue until a longitudinal comparison between matched patients with or without dementia and with or without SI is performed.

Despite these uncertainties, SI should be considered by the clinician as a preclinical marker of a potentially ongoing deleterious cerebrovascular process that deserves attention. While SI seem to progress despite current standard stroke treatments,[50] there is no specific treatment. However, as markers they should encourage the clinician to look actively for cerebrovascular risk factors, especially hypertension, and to treat them appropriately.

PROGNOSIS AND TREATMENT OF SI ASSOCIATED WITH OTHER DISEASES

Stroke and TIA

The short- and long-term outcome of a stroke is usually not affected by the presence of SI.[1,16,17,28,51] This might be explained by the fact that as SI are clinically silent before the stroke, they remain so after it. An alternative explanation is that SI could worsen the outcome, but not sufficiently to be demonstrated by the currently used rating scales.[17] It should be mentioned that in some situations, a previous SI may substantially modify the clinical presentation of a stroke, such as with acute pseudobulbar palsy secondary to sequential bilateral lesions of corticonuclear pathways, the first lesion having been silent.[52] Another example is the development of severe aphasia in a right-handed patient with a right-side stroke in the presence of an old SI on the left. The significance of SI in association with TIA is unsettled. The finding of a brain ischemic lesion in the work-up of the TIA (i.e., with symptoms lasting less than 24 h) led to a subclassification of the TIA some situations into a true TIA (without radiological lesions) and a CITS (with lesions).[5,23] CITS are intermediate between SI and RINDS (stroke with a symptom duration of less than 6 weeks). A higher risk of developing a future major vascular event has been shown for RINDS, as compared to TIA.[54] This risk increases gradually with the duration of symptoms. Similarly, it has been shown that the risk of CITS increases with the duration of symptoms in TIA. Better survival was also demonstrated for patients with TIA compared with those with CITS.[55] This suggests that CITS may worsen the usual prognosis of TIA.[19,32] It should be mentioned, however, that the North American Symptomatic Carotid Endarterectomy Trial (NASCET) group showed that the worse prognosis for patients with CITS vs. TIA[19,56] disappeared when other factors were accounted for on multivariate analysis: indeed, hypertension and contralateral carotid occlusion were the only independent factors for a poor prognosis.[19]

Carotid stenosis

The NASCET study concluded that patients with symptomatic carotid stenosis over 50% benefited from endarterectomy.[57,58] However, it was also shown that this should be tempered for moderate stenosis (50–70%). For these patients, risks of stroke recurrence on medical treatment should be particularly balanced against the risk of a perioperative event. Men vs. women, stroke vs. TIA, and hemispheric vs. retinal events increase the risk of recurrence, while diabetes, hypertension, contralateral occlusion, left-sided disease and a visible lesion on imaging increase the risk of a perioperative event. In addition, it has been shown that the finding of a SI in the preoperative investigation does not change the prognosis of carotid endarterectomy,[34,35,56] but worsens it in the case of an emergency procedure (e.g., crescendo TIA, fluctuating neurological deficit).[35] From these results it may be reasonably concluded that SI should not influence the decision plan of patients with symptomatic carotid stenosis.

In asymptomatic carotid stenosis, the presence of SI may be of importance as the prognosis of patients with carotid stenosis has been reported to be worse for those having SI.[56] However, in the Asymptomatic Carotid Atherosclerosis Study (ACAS),[20] the baseline analysis of 848 completely asymptomatic patients with carotid stenosis greater than 60% showed neither a relationship between the degree of stenosis and the occurrence of SI, nor a higher distribution of SI on the side of the stenosis. The beneficial effect of surgery in these patients with asymptomatic stenosis led to an interruption of the ACAS.[59,60] Therefore, the significance of SI in the management of asymptomatic carotid stenosis might be limited to mild stenosis, although this has not been formally studied yet.

Atrial fibrillation

It has been shown that stroke risk in patients with AF depends on the association of various features, such as history of hypertension, diabetes, coronary artery disease, congestive heart failure, left ventricular dysfunction, age, and previous stroke or TIA.[61] The presence of one of these factors in addition to AF puts the patients at a high risk of stroke and is an indication for anticoagulation in patients under the age of 75. It may therefore be useful in patients with AF and without any of these features to look for a SI on imaging before labeling them as being at low risk and leaving them untreated or on aspirin. It should, however, be emphasized that the studies leading to guidelines in patients with AF did not differentiate between SI and other strokes. Further studies are needed to confirm the assumption that SI, as other TIA or stroke, indicate anticoagulation in patients with AF.[62]

CONCLUSIONS

SI are only diagnosed in vivo with the help of modern neuroimaging techniques. Their prevalence in the general population increases with age. SI are associated with hypertension, and in the majority of cases they appear as a lacunar lesion on CT or MRI. This lesion is probably often secondary to fibro-hyalinosis of small penetrating arteries. However, when SI involve the cortex, a cardioembolic origin is more probable and should be looked for, especially when multiple vascular territories are involved. Prognosis of SI is still unsettled but SI do increase in number with time. Patients with SI are more prone to develop a stroke later than those without SI. In addition, a potential role of SI in the etiology of vascular dementia has been suggested, although this remains controversial. For these reasons, SI should be considered as a preclinical marker of cerebrovascular disease and should stimulate careful search and treatment of risk factors, particularly hypertension. When found in the work-up of a stroke, SI do not usually change the immediate outcome of stroke. In association with a carotid stenosis, SI seem to be of marginal significance, while an association with AF reinforces the indication for anticoagulant therapy.

REFERENCES

1. Chodosh EH, Foulkes MA, Kase CS *et al.* Silent stroke in the NINCDS stroke data bank. *Neurology* 1988; **38:**1674–9.
2. Bogousslavsky J, Regli F. Cerebral infarct in apparent transient ischemic attack. *Neurology* 1985; **35:**1501–3.
3. Fisher CM. Lacunes: small deep cerebral infarcts. *Neurology* 1965; **15:**774–84.
4. Awad I, Modic M, Little JR *et al.* Focal parenchymal lesions in transient ischemic attacks: correlation of computed tomography and magnetic resonnance imaging. *Stroke* 1986; **17:**399–402.
5. Salgado E, Weinstein M, Furlan AJ. Proton magnetic resonance imaging in ischemic vascular disease. *Ann Neurol* 1986; **20:**502–7.
6. Arboix A, Marti V, Pujol J, Sanz M. Lacunar cerebral infarct and nuclear magnetic resonance. A review of sixty cases. *Eur Neurol* 1990; **30:**47–51.
7. Hedershee D, Hijdra A, Algra A. Silent stroke in patients with transient ischemic attack or minor ischemic stroke. *Stroke* 1992; **23:**1220–4.
8. Petersen P, Madsen EB, Brun B, Pedersen F, Gyldensted C, Boysen G. Silent cerebral infarction in chronic atrial fibrillation. *Stroke* 1987; **18:**1098–100.
9. Petersen P, Pedersen F, Johnson A. Cerebral computed tomography in paroxysmal atrial fibrillation. *Acta Neurol Scand* 1989; **79:**482–6.
10. Sasaki W, Yanagisawa S, Maki K *et al.* High incidence of silent small cerebral infarction in the patients with atrial fibrillation [Abstract]. *Circulation* 1987; **76:**104.
11. Kobayashi S, Okada K, Yamashita K. Incidence of silent lacunar lesion in normal adults and its relation to cerebral blood flow and risk factors. *Stroke* 1991; **22:**1379–83.
12. Lindgren A, Roijer A, Rudling O *et al.* Cerebral lesions on magnetic resonance imaging, heart disease, and vascular risk factors in subjects without stroke. *Stroke* 1994; **25:**929–34.
13. Price TR, Manolio TA, Kronmal RA *et al.* Silent brain infarction on magnetic resonance imaging and neurological abnormalities in community-dwelling older adults. The Cardiovascular Health Study. CHS Collaborative Research Group. *Stroke* 1997; **28:**1158–64.
14. Shinkawa A, Ueda K, Kiyohara Y *et al.* Silent cerebral infarction in a community-based autopsy series in Japan: the Hisayama study. *Stroke* 1995; **26:**380–5.
15. De Reuk J, Sieben G, De Coster W, Vander E. Stroke pattern and topography of cerebral infarcts: a clinicopathological study. *Eur Neurol* 1981; **20:**411–5.
16. Jorgensen HS, Nakayama H, Raaschou HO, Olsen GJ. Silent infarction in acute stroke patients. Prevalence, risk factors, and clinical

significance: The Copenhagen Stroke Study. *Stroke* 1994; **25:**97–104.
17. Boon A, Lodder J, Heuts-van Raak L, Kessels F. Silent brain infarcts in 755 consecutive patients with a first-ever supratentorial ischemic stroke. *Stroke* 1994; **25:**2384–90.
18. Kase CS, Wolf PA, Chodosh EH *et al.* Prevalence of silent stroke in patients with initial stroke: the Framingham study. *Stroke* 1989; **20:**850–2.
19. Eliasziw M, Streifler JY, Spence JD, Fox AJ, Hachinski VC, Barnett HJ. Prognosis for patients following a transient ischemic attack with and without cerebral infarction on brain CT. *Neurology* 1995; **45:**428–31.
20. Brott T, Tomsick T, Feinberg W *et al.* Baseline silent cerebral infarction in the Asymptomatic Carotid Atherosclerosis Study. *Stroke* 1994; **25:**1122–9.
21. Hougaku H, Matsumoto M, Handa N *et al.* Asymptomatic carotid lesions and silent cerebral infarction. *Stroke* 1994; **25:**566–70.
22. Lindgren A, Norrving B, Rudling O, Johansson BB. Comparison of clinical and neuroradiological findings in first-ever stroke. *Stroke* 1994; **25:**1371–7.
23. Loeb C, Gandolfo C, Del Sette M, Conti M, Finocchi C, Calautti C. Asymptomatic cerebral infarctions in patients with ischemic stroke. *Eur Neurol* 1996; **36:**343–7.
24. Norrving B, Bogousslavsky J. Side asymmetries in hemispheric stroke [Abstract]. *J Neurol* 1991; **238:**121.
25. Feinberg WM, Seeger JF, Carmody RF, Anderson DC, Hart RG, Pearce LA. Epidemiologic features of asymptomatic cerebral infarction in patients with nonvalvular atrial fibrillation. *Arch Intern Med* 1990; **150:**2340–4.
26. Kempster PA, Gerraty RP, Gates PC. Asymptomatic cerebral infarction in patients with chronic atrial fibrillation. *Stroke* 1988; **19:**955–7.
27. Herderschee D, Hijdra A, Algra A, Koudstaal PJ, Kappelle LJ, van Gijn J, for the Dutch TIA Trial Study Group. Silent stroke in patients with transient ischemic attack or minor ischemic stroke. *Stroke* 1992; **23:**1220–4.
28. Ricci S, Celani MG, La Rosa F, Righetti E, Duca E, Caputo N. Silent brain infarctions in patients with first-ever stroke. *Stroke* 1993; **24:**647–51.
29. Davis PH, Clarke WR, Bendixen BH, Adams HPJ, Woolson RF, Culebras A. Silent cerebral infarction in patients enrolled in the TOAST Study. *Neurology* 1996; **46:**942–8.
30. Mounier-Vehier F, Leys D, Rondepierre P, Godefroy O, Pruvo JP. Silent infarcts in patients with ischemic stroke are related to age and size of the left atrium. *Stroke* 1993; **24:**1347–51.
31. Berguer R, Sieggreen MY, Lazo A, Hodakowski GT. The silent brain infarct in carotid surgery. *J Vasc Surg* 1986; **3:**422–7.
32. Dennis M, Bamford J, Sandercock P, Molyneux A, Warlow C. Computed tomography in patients with transient ischaemic attacks: when is a transient ischaemic attack not a transient ischaemic attack but a stroke? *J Neurol* 1990; **237:**257–61.
33. Graber JN, Vollman RW, Johnson WC *et al.* Stroke after carotid endarterectomy: risk as predicted by preoperative computerized tomography. *Am J Surg* 1984; **147:**492–7.
34. Ricotta JJ, Ouriel K, Green RM, Deweese JA. Use of computerized tomography in selection of patients for elective and urgent carotid endarterectomy. *Ann Surg* 1985; **202:**783–7.
35. Sise MJ, Sedwitz MM, Rowloy WR, Shackford SR. Prospective analysis of carotid endarterectomy and silent cerebral infarction in 97 patients. *Stroke* 1989; **20:**329–32.
36. Street DL, O'Brien MS, Rocotta JJ *et al.* Observations on cerebral computed tomography in patients having carotid endarterectomy. *J Vasc Surg* 1988; **7:**798–801.
37. Norris JW, Zhu CZ. Silent stroke and carotid stenosis. *Stroke* 1992; **23:**483–5.
38. Nicolaides A, Kalodiki A, Ramaswami G *et al.* The significance of cerebral infarcts on CT scans in patients with transient ischaemic attack. In: *Cerebral Revascularization* (Bernstein EF, Callow AD, Nikolaides AN. eds.), pp. 159–78. London; Med-Orion: 1993.
39. Bogousslavsky J, Cachin C, Regli F, Despland PA, Van Melle G, Kappenberger L. Cardiac sources of embolism and cerebral infarction—clinical consequences and vascular concommitants: The Lausanne Stroke Registry. *Neurology* 1991; **41:**855–9.
40. Harrison MJ. Silent infarcts on computed tomography scans are more common in cardiogenic stroke. *Stroke* 1991; **22:**693.
41. Peterson P, Pedersen F, Madsen EB, Brun B, Gyldensted C, Boysen G. Echocardiography and cerebral computed tomography in chronic atrial fibrillation. *Eur Heart J* 1989; **10:**1101–4.
42. Kobayashi S, Okada K, Koide H, Bokura H, Yamaguchi S. Subcortical silent brain infarction as a risk factor for clinical stroke. *Stroke* 1997; **28:**1932–9.

43. Longstreth WTJ, Manolio TA, Arnold A *et al.* Clinical correlates of white matter findings on cranial magnetic resonance imaging of 3301 elderly people. The Cardiovascular Health Study [see comments]. *Stroke* 1996; **27:**1274–82.
44. Hachinski VC, Lassen NA, Marshall J. Multi-infarct dementia a cause of mental deterioration in the elderly. *Lancet* 1974; **ii:**207–10.
45. Roman GC, Tatemichi TK, Erkinjutti T *et al.* Vascular dementia. Diagnostic criteria for research studies: Report of the NINDS-AIREN international workshop. *Neurology* 1993; **43:**250–60.
46. Bornstein NM, Gur AY, Treves TA *et al.* Do silent brain infarctions predict the development of dementia after first ischemic stroke? *Stroke* 1996; **27:**904–5.
47. Grigg MJ, Papadakis K, Nicolaides AN *et al.* The significance of cerebral infarction and atrophy in patients with amaurosis fugax and transient ischemic attacks in relation to internal carotid artery stenosis: a preliminary report. *J Vasc Surg* 1988; **7:**215–22.
48. Fujikawa T, Yamawaki S, Touhounda Y. Incidence of silent cerebral infarction in patients with major depression. *Stroke* 1993; **24:**1631–4.
49. Fujikawa T, Yamawaki S, Touhouda Y. Silent cerebral infarctions in patients with late-onset mania. *Stroke* 1995; **26:**946–9.
50. van Zagten M, Boiten J, Kessels F, Lodder J. Significant progression of white matter lesions and small deep (lacunar) infarcts in patients with stroke. *Arch Neurol* 1996; **53:**650–5.
51. Brainin M, McShane LM, Steiner M, Dachenhausen A, Seiser A. Silent brain infarcts and transient ischemic attacks. A three-year study of first-ever ischemic stroke patients: the Klosterneuburg Stroke Data Bank. *Stroke* 1995; **26:**1348–52.
52. Besson G, Bogousslavsky J, Regli F, Maeder P. Acute pseudobulbar or suprabulbar palsy. *Arch Neurol* 1991; **48:**501–7.
53. Waxman SG, Toole JF. Temporal profile resembling TIA in the setting of cerebral infarction. *Stroke* 1983; **14:**433–7.
54. The Dutch TIA Trial Study Group. Predictors of major vascular events in patients with transient ischemic attack or nondisabling stroke. *Stroke* 1993; **24:**527–31.
55. Evans GW, Howard G, Murros KE, Rose LA, Toole JF. Cerebral infarction verified by cranial computed tomography and prognosis for survival following transient ischemic attack. *Stroke* 1991; **22:**431–6.
56. Streifler JY, Fox AJ, Wong CJ *et al.* Importance of "silent" brain infarctions in TIA patients with high-grade carotid stenosis: Results from NASCET [Abstract]. *Neurology* 1992; **42**(Suppl 3):204.
57. NASCET Collaborators. Beneficial effect of carotid endarterectomy in symptomatic patients with high grade stenosis. *N Engl J Med* 1991; **325:**445–53.
58. Barnett HJM, Taylor DW, Eliasziw M *et al.* Benefit of carotid endarterectomy in patients with symptomatic moderate or severe stenosis. *N Engl J Med* 1998; **339:**1415–25.
59. Moore WS, Barnett HJ, Beebe HG *et al.* Guidelines for carotid endarterectomy. A multi-disciplinary consensus. *Stroke* 1995; **26:**188–201.
60. Asymptomatic Carotid Atherosclerosis Study Group Committee. Endarterectomy for asymptomatic carotid artery stenosis. *J Am Med Assoc* 1995; **273:**1421–8.
61. Hart RG, Sherman DG, Easton JD, Cairns JA. Prevention of stroke in patients with nonvalvular atrial fibrillation. *Neurology* 1998; **51:**674–81.
62. Ezekowitz MD, James KE, Nazarian SM *et al.* Silent cerebral infarction in patients with non-rheumatic atrial fibrillation. The Veterans Affairs Stroke Prevention in Nonrheumatic Atrial Fibrillation Investigators. *Circulation* 1995; **92:**2178–82.
63. Bogousslavsky J, Hachinski VC, Boughner DR, Fox AJ, Vinuela F, Barnett JM. Clinical predictors of cardiac and arterial lesions in carotid transient ischemic attacks. *Arch Neurol* 1986; **43:**229–33.
64. Asymptomatic Carotid Atherosclerosis Study Group. Silent cerebral infarction in the asymptomatic carotid atherosclerosis study (ACAS) [Abstract]. *Stroke* 1991; **22:**147.

13

Prophylactic neuroprotection

Michel Torbey and Marc Fisher

CONTENTS • **Introduction** • **Review of pathophysiology of stroke** • **Available neuroprotective agents** • **Short-term prophylactic neuroprotection** • **Long-term neuroprotection** • **Concomitant prophylactic neuroprotection** • **Neuroprotective agent trials** • **Suggestions for future clinical trials** • **Conclusion**

INTRODUCTION

Stroke is the leading cause of disability in the United States and continues to have an enormous socioeconomic impact on public health systems worldwide. Each year 550 000 Americans experience a stroke at a rate of one stroke every 53 s and 150 000 deaths.[1,2] The annual costs of this devastating disease have been estimated at $20–40 billion with an average cost per case of approximately $50 000.[3] Therapies for acute ischemic stroke have progressed to a great extent over the past decade. According to market research, approximately 6000 patients with stroke in the United States were treated with iv tissue-type plasminogen activator (tPA) in the 12 months since its approval suggesting that only 1.5% of patients who might be candidates for tPA are receiving it. The major reasons cited for this underutilization are short time window (<3 h), physicians' concerns about the efficacy and safety of tPA, and lack of infrastructure for administration of the medication.[4] Animal studies showed that neuroprotective agents are more effective when given prior to the ischemic event. It is unrealistic to treat prophylactically a large group of people for an extended period of time to afford an opportunity for beneficial prophylaxis in a select few. The risk–benefit ratio under such conditions is likely to be narrow at best. However, some groups of patients are at increased risk for ischemic stroke during either a short or extended time period. It is for these subgroups that prophylactic neuroprotection might offer an attractive treatment approach.

REVIEW OF PATHOPHYSIOLOGY OF STROKE

Ischemia results in increased extracellular glutamate, which induces postsynaptic activation of N-methyl-D-asportate, alpha-amino-3-hydroxy-5-methylisoxazole-4-propionate (AMPA) and metabatropic channels.[5,6] This results in an increase in intracellular water, calcium, sodium, chloride, and diacylglycerol. The inward flux of calcium is further amplified by release of intracellular stores, triggering the release of endonucleases and proteases, such as calmodulin and calpain.[7] Reperfusion of the ischemic brain is associated with an increase of free radical production and nitric oxide.[8] Peri-infarct depolarizing events (SD), spreading over the ipsilateral cortex, are associated with a larger stroke size in animals.[9] Several glutamate receptor antagonists reduced the number of peri-infarct SD events and infarct size.[10] Maxi-K channels may also play a neuroprotective role by hyperpolarizing ischemic cells. Gamma aminobutyric acid

(GABA) and 5-HT agonists also hyperpolarize the cells, limiting the number of depolarizing events and thus having a potential neuroprotective effect.

Polymorphonuclear leukocytes (PMN) contribute to the evolution of ischemic injury by obstructing the microvasculature, contributing to the 'no reflow' phenomenon of large vessel recanalization.[11–13] PMN also enhance tissue injury by inducing vasoconstriction and releasing cytokines such as interleukin 1 (IL-1) and tumor necrosis factor alpha (TNF-α). Cell adhesions molecules, such as intercellular adhesion molecule 1 (ICAM-1) and CD11b/CD18, play an important role in mediating the interactions between circulating PMN and endothelial cells.[13]

AVAILABLE NEUROPROTECTIVE AGENTS

Several classes of neuroprotective agents have been investigated in animal stroke models and clinical trials (Table 13.1 and 13.2). Nimodipine, a voltage-sensitive calcium-channel antagonist, was one of the first agents to be evaluated in large clinical trials of acute ischemic stroke. The results of phase III clinical trials were negative with the majority of patients treated 6 h after stroke onset. A post hoc meta-analysis suggested that treatment within 12 h of stroke onset might be effective.[14] Competitive and non-competitive antagonists of the NMDA-mediated calcium channel, such as dextrorphan, CGS-19755, MK-801, CNS-1102 (cerestat), and selfotel, reduce ischemic lesion size in animal stroke models when initiated up to 1 h after stroke onset.[15] The results with these NMDA antagonists in clinical trials were disappointing because of their unfavorable risk–benefit ratios.[16,17] Magnesium, a non-competitive NMDA antagonist, demonstrated neuroprotective effects in animal stroke models.[18] A multinational study of iv magnesium in acute ischemic stroke is underway.[19] Several new NMDA antagonists are currently being evaluated, including NPS1506 and ARL15896AR.[20,21] Memantine is an available non-competitive NMDA antagonist that can be given orally and has a tolerable side-effect profile.[22]

Table 13.1 Classes of neuroprotective agents for consideration of prophylactic neuroprotection

Calcium channel antagonists
Voltage regulated
Receptor mediated
N-methyl-D-aspartate antagonists
Competitive
Non-competitive
Modulatory glutamate, glycine and polyamine site antagonists
Presynaptic release inhibitors
Postsynaptic antagonists
Synaptic modulators
Sodium channel antagonists
AMPA antagonists
GABA agonists
Calpain antagonists
Calmodulin antagonists
Nitric oxide antagonists
nNOS antagonists
eNOS upregulators
Serotonin agonists
Maxi-K channel agonists
Endothelin antagonists
Adenosine enhancers
Neurotrophic growth factors
Anti-adhesion molecules
Apoptosis inhibitors
Antioxidants
IL-1 antagonists

Several antagonists of the obligatory glycine and polyamine modulatory sites demonstrated neuroprotective effects in animal stroke models. GV150526A, a glycine antagonist, is in advanced clinical trial.[23] A clinical trial with eliprodil, a polyamine site antagonist, failed to show any efficacy hence development was halted. AMPA antagonists have shown efficacy

Table 13.2 Current status of neuroprotective agents

Drug	*Status*	*Side-effects*
Non-competitive NMDA antagonist		
MK801	Discontinued	Cerebellar vacuolar changes in dogs
Dextrorphan	Discontinued after phase II trial	Somnolence, vomiting, hypotension
Cerestat	Phase III stopped	Safety concerns and drug company decision. Transient catatonia reported
Magnesium	Multinational study of IV form is underway	Reasonable safety demonstrated
Competitive NMDA antagonist		
Selfotel	Phase III trial terminated prematurely	Increased mortality in treated patients
Glycine site antagonist	Phase III trials / No oral preparation	
GV150526A		
Polyamine site antagonist		
Eliprodil	Phase III trial halted No efficacy seen	QT prolongation
AMPA antagonist		
NBQX	Clinical development halted	Renal toxicity
Na channel blockers		
BW619C89	Phase II trial halted	High side-effect profile
Fos-phenytoin	Phase III trial negative	Reasonable safety profile
Lipid peroxidation inhibitors		
Trilazad	Phase III trial. No detectable treatment effect seen within 6 h of stroke onset	
Ebselen	Phase IIb trial. Improved clinical outcome at 30 days Oral form available	
Nitric oxide synthase (NOS) inhibitors		
Lubeluzole	Decreased mortality after stroke in phase II. Recent phase III trial results were negative. No oral preparation	
GABA agonist		
Clomethiazol	Phase III trial completed. Results were encouraging in a subgroup with large strokes	
5-HT agonists		
Bay-3702	Phase II completed	Reasonable safety
Antiadhesion molecules		
Enlimolab	Discontinued. Worse outcome than placebo	High risk of infections
Growth factors		
bFGF	American phase III trial halted European phase III trial stopped	Phase II trial had reasonable safety profile
Membrane repair		
Citicoline	Phase II trial showed favorable outcome at day 9. Phase III trial completed. Better outcome in patients with NIH score >7	
Voltage sensitive calcium channel antagonist	Phase III completed	Efficacy in 12 h subgroup
Nimodipine	Discontinued	

in animal stroke models. A prototype, NBQX, had disturbing renal toxicity and clinical development was stopped.[24]

Presynaptic inhibition of excitatory amino acid release is another approach to inhibiting the exitotoxic cascade at an early stage. Animal studies of sodium-channel blockers such as BW619C89, lamotrigine and fos-phenytoin, demonstrated neuroprotective effects.[24] Fosphenytoin recently completed an apparently negative phase III trial. Potassium channels inhibit presynaptic release of excitatory amino acids hence maxi-K channel activation may limit ischemic injury by reducing postsynaptic calcium entry and hyperpolarizing neurons.[25] Pharmacologically relevant maxi-K channel agonists are being developed for application in stroke trials.

Tirilazad, a 21-aminosteroid lipid peroxidation inhibitor, was successfully tested in animal stroke models.[26] In a phase III clinical trial, no detectable treatment effect was observed in stroke patients who began tirilazad within 6 h of stroke onset.[27] Ebselen, another lipid peroxidation inhibitor, reduced infarct size in rats subjected to temporary focal ischemia. Oral ebselen, in a phase II trial, given twice daily for 2 weeks within 48 h after stroke onset improved the outcome at 30 days.[28]

Alpha-phenyl-N-butyl nitrone (PBN), a spin trap of oxygen free radicals, reduced infarct size when initiated 1 h after reperfusion. No active clinical trials have yet been initiated.[29] nNOS inhibitors, such as ARL17477 and 7-nitroindazole, reduce infarct size in rat temporary and permanent focal ischemia models.[30] Lubeluzole inhibits NO-mediated toxicity.[31] Initial optimism was generated by a phase II trial of lubeluzole that demonstrated reduced mortality and better functional outcome with only a moderate dose. An initial 1 year suggestive phase III trial with lubeluzole led to a further trial.[32] However, the results were apparently negative because further development of lubeluzole has been halted.[33] Trifluorperazine, a calmodulin antagonist, reduced infarct size when initiated 5 min after the onset of 2 h of temporary focal ischemia, but was not effective when therapy began at either 1 or 2 h after the onset of ischemia. AK275 and AK295, calpain inhibitors, reduced infarct size in an animal model. A neuroprotective effect was observed with initiation of treatment up to 3 h after stroke onset. Another calpain antagonist, MDL28,170 significantly reduced infarct size in a 3-h temporary occlusion model when initiated 6 h after stroke onset, but not with an 8-h delay.[34]

Muscimol and clomethiazole, both GABA agonists, effectively reduced infarct size in animal stroke models.[35,36] One 5-HT agonist, Bay-3702, is currently being assessed in a clinical, acute stroke trial. Enlimolab, an anti-ICAM murine monoclonal antibody, had a very discouraging clinical trial result.[37] The enlimolab-treated group did worse than the placebo group regarding functional outcome, mortality and hemorrhagic transformation. The rate of fever and serious infection was also increased in the enlimolab group. Basic fibroblast growth factor (bFGF) reduced infarct size in animal models.[38] The drug is currently in a phase III trial.[39] Citicoline or CDP-choline, a membrane repair enhancer, had a favorable functional outcome at day 90 in a phase II trial;[40] the results of a phase III trial were negative.[41]

SHORT-TERM PROPHYLACTIC NEUROPROTECTION

Patients undergoing cardiac or neurovascular procedures have an elevated risk of stroke during the periprocedure period (Table 13.3). With the aim of reducing the morbidity and disability related to that risk, a short treatment period before and after the procedure with a neuroprotective agent might be effective.

More than 800 000 patients a year undergo myocardial revascularization procedures throughout the world. These patients are prone to marked hemodynamic fluctuations, cerebral embolization of atherosclerotic plaque, air, fat, and platelet aggregates. This makes them prone to develop stroke, encephalopathy, and other neurological types of dysfunction. The perioperative stroke-related mortality rates have not decreased over the past decade. It was 7.2%

Table 13.3 Short-term prophylactic candidates and specific predictive factors

Type of surgery	*Predictors of high risk patients*
Cardiac surgery	
Coronary artery bypass graft Left ventricular assist device Heart transplant	Urgent operation, recent MI, unstable angina, hypertension, low ejection fraction, old age, renal function, obesity, alcohol intake, previous CABG, PVD, postoperative fibrillation, carotid stenosis, bypass time, aortic atheromas
Neurovascular procedures	
Carotid endarterectomy	Females, age, hypertension, PVD, contralateral carotid disease, cerebral events on presentation
Carotid angioplasty and stents	Age >80 years, long or multiple area of stenosis
Cardiac catherization Percutaneous transluminal coronary angioplasty Percutaneous transluminal valvuloplasty Neurovascular embolization	Atherosclerosis

in the late 1970s and almost 20% by mid-1980 and it continues to increase. This is due to the older higher risk population undergoing the procedure.[42] The total costs accumulated from post-coronary artery bypass graft (CABG) surgery complications are about $2–4 billion annually.[43] Therefore it is of economic interest to identify these high-risk patients early in the process. Adverse cerebral outcomes occurred in 6.1% of patients undergoing CABG surgery: type I (3.1%) which is focal injury, stupor or coma at discharge; and type II (3%) which is deterioration in intellectual function, memory deficit or seizures. Patients with type I neurological outcome had a higher in-hospital mortality (10-fold) increase compared to type II (5-fold), longer hospitalization in the ICU and ward service, and a higher rate of discharge to facilities for intermediate or long-term care.[44]

Since this is a controlled and timed situation, it is important to identify patients who may have the periprocedure complications for optimal use of available resources. Epidemiological studies demonstrated clearly that the most powerful factors predicting post-CABG complications are: emergency CABG operation, recent myocardial infarction (MI), unstable angina, antihypertensive therapy, low ventricular ejection fraction (<0.49), age greater than 70 years, decreased renal function, obesity, use of intra-aortic balloon pump, diabetes mellitus, history of pulmonary disease and excessive consumption of alcohol, systolic blood pressure >180 mmHg at admission, history of previous CABG, prior stroke or transient ischemic attack (TIA), peripheral vascular disease (PVD), postoperative atrial fibrillation, carotid stenosis greater than 50%, cardiopulmonary bypass time, significant aortic atherosclerosis, postoperative amrinone, or epinephrine use.[44,45] Central nervous system (CNS) complications occur much more frequently after heart transplantation than elective CABG and valve surgery. The overall incidence of CNS complications was 51.3% in emergency valve surgery, 19.8% in heart transplantation; 10.3% in emergency CABG, 9.5% in elective valve surgery, 7.6% combined procedures (valves and coronary artery surgery), and 3.1% in elective CABG.[46] The highest risk of complication with valvular surgery is during aortic cannulation, the release of aortic clamps, and weaning from bypass secondary to macroembolization of air or particulate matter as measured with transcranial Doppler studies (TCD).[47–49] Atheromatous disease of the descending aorta is a strong predictor of stroke and death after CABG with a 1 week stroke rate of 5.5, 10.5, 45.5% corresponding to grades III, IV, and V, respectively.[50]

Newman *et al.* developed a model that allows the prediction of potential CNS injury rate associated with CABG by the patient's age and the number of additional risk factors.[51] They projected a normogram (Fig. 13.1) where risk is determined by assigning points for each risk factor. After the total points are computed, the risk of CNS injury can be determined by plotting the total points received against the risk score at the bottom of the normogram. For example, consider a 75-year-old woman with unstable angina, diabetes, a history of neurological disease, prior CABG and a history of vascular disease and pulmonary disease. Assigning the appropriate point scores from the index (75 years old, 72 points; history of vascular disease, 18 points; diabetes, 17 points; history of neurological disease, 18 points; history of pulmonary disease, 15 points) yields a total point score of 140 points which correlates with a predicted risk of CNS injury of nearly 22%. These predictive models help us to identify these high-risk patients and treat them prophylactically for stroke prevention.

Early trials of carotid endarterectomy were controversial because of major morbidity and mortality rates of 11–35%. There is now a clear benefit of relieving high-grade symptomatic stenosis and asymptomatic carotid stenosis by surgical endarterectomy. The risk of procedural stroke or death with surgery was 5.8% in NASCET and 2.3% in ACAS. However, in high-risk patients undergoing endarterectomy, morbidity and mortality rates as high as 18% have been reported.[52,53] The majority of the intraoperative events are related to embolism of atherosclerotic debris or platelet–fibrin aggregates and hypoperfusion from carotid clamping.

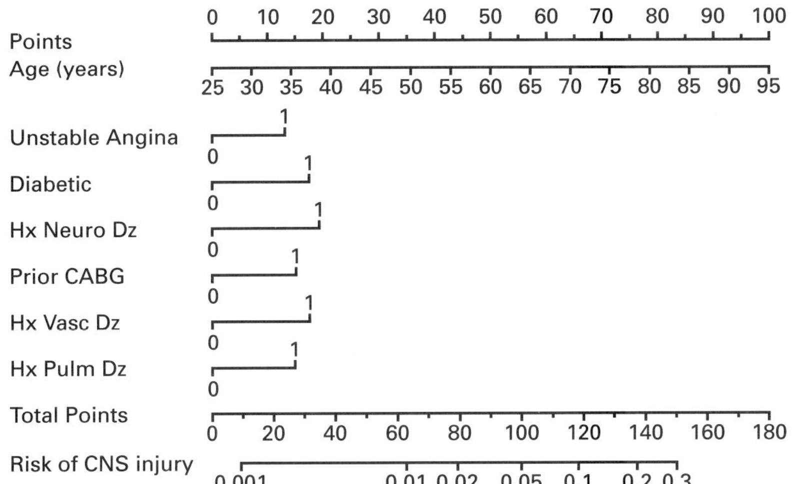

Figure 13.1 Normogram for computing risk of central nervous system (CNS) injury. Neurological risk is determined by assigning points for age and positive history of the predictors listed. (From Rosenthal *et al.*[54])

Postoperative events are also predominantly ischemic and related to thrombosis or thromboembolism of the newly debrided arterial surface or dissection of an intimal flap.[54] Predictive factors associated with a higher surgical risk are: female sex, subject age ⩾75 years, systolic blood pressure >180 mmHg, peripheral vascular disease, occlusion of the contralateral internal carotid artery, stenosis of the ipsilateral internal carotid siphon, stenosis of the ipsilateral external carotid artery, and cerebral versus ocular events at presentations.[55] These high-risk patients could potentially benefit the most from prophylactic neuroprotection.

Carotid angioplasty has been slowly evolving since 1980. About 2048 cases of endovascular carotid stent procedures have been reported worldwide to date.[56] This procedure is complicated by a 5% rate of dissection, 8% embolism, and 15% restenosis rate.[57] With the addition of stents, the rates of dissection and restenosis have been reduced to less than 5%. Although case series of 100–250 patients reported good success rates of 89–99%, perioperative rates of major stroke ranged from 0.5% to 6.4%; minor stroke 1–7%; and mortality rate less than 1%.[58] The only predictors of procedural stroke in carotid stenting were advanced age >80 years and long or multiple stenosis.[59] These patients are also potential candidates for prophylactic neuroprotection.

Percutaneous transluminal valvuloplasty emerged as a non-surgical treatment for valvular stenosis in adults and children. The risk of embolic stroke ranges from 1.4% to 11% for aortic valvuloplasty and from 3.2% to 4.2% for mitral valvuloplasty.[60] Embolic events during aortic valvuloplasty are often mild suggesting small calcific emboli. During mitral valvuloplasty, the guidewires puncture the intra-arterial septum. Hemodynamically significant mitral stenosis is commonly associated with abnormal atrial flow and tendency for thrombus formation that may be released during the procedure. Transesophageal echocardiography (TEE) and anticoagulation before the procedure have been recommended to reduce the risk of cerebral embolism. Prophylactic neuroprotective agents might also be useful to decrease the consequences of cerebral emboli in this setting.

The morbidity resulting from perioperative endovascular embolization varied between 1.98 and 6.9%. The most common cause of complications related to embolization was ischemia due to occlusion of a normal vessel. The neurological deficit was severe in 5.9% of patients, hence prophylactic neuroprotection should be considered for evaluation.[61]

LONG-TERM NEUROPROTECTION

The cornerstone of long-term neuroprotection strategies is to identify subjects who are at an increased risk of stroke and treat them prophylactically (Table 13.4). Epidemiological studies have identified several modifiable and non-modifiable risk factors (Table 13.3). Men over the age 65, African-Americans, and hypertensive individuals have a higher risk of stroke than the rest of the population.[62] These patients could be potential candidates for prophylactic neuroprotection trials.

Cardiac risk factors for stroke include atrial fibrillation, previous myocardial infarction, low ejection fraction, and valvular disease. Chronic artial fibrillation accounts for 7–30% of all strokes in patients over the age of 60.[63] Atrial fibrillation patients with high side-effect risks secondary to anticoagulation are usually left untreated. These individuals have a stroke risk of 3–7% per year and could constitute another important group in whom prophylactic neuroprotection might be considered. Even atrial fibrillation patients who are treated with anticoagulants or aspirin still have a stroke risk of 2–3% per year and may also be candidates for prophylactic neuroprotection.[64] Patients with asymptomatic cerebral embolic signals in the right middle cerebral artery, as detected by transcranial Doppler (TCD) in 87% of patients with the carbomedics bileaflet valve, are also potential candidates for neuroprotective agents.[65] Patients with low ejection fraction have a substantial risk of stroke. For every decrease of 5 percentage points in the ejection fraction there was an 18% increase in the risk of stroke. Patients with ejection fraction of ≤28% after MI had a relative risk of stroke of 1.86 as compared with patients with ejection fraction of >35%.[66] These findings suggest the idea of neuroprotection in the subset of patients with very low ejection fraction.

With the recent technological advances in imaging studies, more risk factors such as aortic plaques and intimal thickness have been identified. Aortic plaques ≥4 mm thick (including the thickness of the aortic wall) are a very strong independent predictor of recurrent brain infarction (relative risk = 3.8).[67] Intima–media thickness also has a positive association with stroke risk.[68] These patients might be candidates for prophylactic neuroprotection.

Table 13.4 Risk factors for ischemic stroke

Non-modifiable
Age
Gender
Family history
Race
Modifiable
Hypertension
Cardiac disease
Atrial fibrillation
Valvular disease
Low ejection fraction ≤28%
Recent MI
Diabetes
Hyperlipidemia
Vascular disease
Asymptomatic carotid stenosis
Intimal–medial thickness
Aortic plaques ≥4 mm thick
Ankle–brachial blood pressure ratio
Smoking
Hypercoagulability
Oral contraceptive use
Alcohol
Obesity
Transient ischemic attacks

Conditions such as diabetes, abnormal serum lipids, triglyceride, cholesterol, low-density lipoprotein (LDL), and high-density lipoprotein (HDL), are regarded as atherosclerosis risk factors.[69] The relative risk for ischemic stroke secondary to diabetes ranges from 1.5 to 3.0.[62] Cigarette smoking has been established as an independent determinant of stroke.[70] Stroke risk was increased two-fold in heavy smokers (more than 40 cigarettes/day) compared to light smokers (less than 10 cigarettes/day) and was reduced among those who quit smoking within 5 years of stroke onset compared to those who continued to smoke.[71] Alcohol has a J-shaped dose-dependent relationship to stroke, with an elevated stroke risk for moderate to heavy alcohol consumption and a protective effect in light drinkers compared to non-drinkers.[72] Patients with such a risk factor profile could be considered candidates for neuroprotection trials.

Another potential high-risk group are patients with asymptomatic carotid stenosis. Among this group, the annual stroke risk was 1.3% in those with less than 75% stenosis and 3.3% in those with stenosis of more than 75%.[73] Since carotid endarterectomy showed only a 55% relative risk reduction, patients with asymptomatic carotid stenosis may be another group to consider for prophylactic neuroprotection.[53]

Patients who have already developed symptoms of cerebral ischemia are at highest risk for stroke. The greatest risk occurs during the first 30 days after ischemic stroke.[74] The aggregate risk of stroke recurrence per year has been estimated at 6.1% after minor stroke and 9% after major stroke.[75] Antiplatelet agents such as aspirin, ticlopidine and clopidogrel can reduce this risk by only 20–30%.[76] Therefore non-surgical TIA patients might be appropriate candidates for prophylactic neuroprotection trials.

Using data from the Framingham study, a stroke probability can be estimated based on an individual's risk profile.[77] A 5 or 10 year probability of stroke can be estimated based on the sum of points that are given secondary to the presence or absence of various risk factors. Therefore individuals with a probability greater than a predefined acceptable risk may be potential candidates for long-term prophylactic neuroprotection.

CONCOMITANT PROPHYLACTIC NEUROPROTECTION

Several medications have proven efficacy in the reduction of stroke among high-risk patients. These agents include antihypertensives, platelet antiaggregants, anticoagulants, antiatherogenic and lipid lowering agents. If a drug used to treat a concurrent medical condition has neuroprotective potential then a concomitant effect might limit mortality and morbidity among patients who develop focal cerebral ischemia during treatment. In this case neuroprotection is provided as a secondary benefit. Voltage-sensitive calcium-channel antagonists, such as nifedipine, nicardipine, isradipine, diltiazem and others were shown to retard atherogenesis.[78] They would be potential candidates for concomitant neuroprotection. Another example is the beta-blocker carvedilol, which is an antihypertensive drug that has antioxidant and neuroprotective qualities.[79] An antithrombotic drug with neuroprotective qualities would be particularly attractive for many of the potential treatment populations. An antioxidant with neuroprotective potential that impedes foam cell formation and plaque development in an animal atherosclerosis model would be an attractive combination.

NEUROPROTECTIVE AGENT TRIALS

GM1 ganglioside study

GM1 ganglioside[80] is a complex sialic acid that has been shown to exert an acute neuroprotective effect. This was a double-blind, placebo-controlled, parallel group pilot study of 30 patients with the main objective to investigate the acute prophylactic neuroprotective effect of GM1 ganglioside in reducing CNS dysfunction from cardiac surgery under cardiopulmonary bypass (CS-CPB) and to estimate population sizes for potential confirmatory tests.[81] Candidates were adult men and women who were scheduled for non-emergency CABG surgery for either coronary vessels or valvular disease. All patients had a baseline neurological examination and neuropsychological testing, 1 day preoperatively, before receiving any test medications. Eighteen GM1 and 11 controls patients received two doses of intravenous study medications (300 mg GM1 or placebo): one the evening before and one the day of surgery. An acute post-neurological examination was scheduled for the day after surgery. Early and long-term follow up neurological examinations and neuropsychological testing were performed approximately 1 week and ≥6 months postoperatively, respectively. They used Clinical Change Scores (CCSs) to quantify neurological cerebral, neurological non-cerebral, and neuropsychological performance changes. Treatment with GM1 ganglioside (two 300 mg iv doses, preoperatively) was associated with a statistically non-significant benefit compared with control in the neurologist's mean cerebral CCSs at the acute postoperative assessment and in the neuropsychologist's mean CCS at an early follow up. The observed treatment differences suggest that an acute dosing higher than that used in stroke trials (100 or 200 mg initial dose, then 100 mg daily) would be appropriate. A recent study of Parkinson's disease[82] showed the safety and tolerance of a loading dose of 1000 mg, followed by daily dosing of 200 mg. Sample size estimation indicates that 150 patients per treatment arm would be needed (with $\alpha = 0.05$ and $\beta = 0.20$) to demonstrate a statistically significant effect on the acute postoperative cerebral CCS.

Nimodipine trial

This randomized, double-blind, single center, placebo-controlled trial was initiated to test whether nimodipine reduced the incidence of new neurological, neuro-ophthalmological, and neuropsychological deficits within the first week after cardiac valve replacement surgery.[83] Secondary aims were to assess the prevalence of deficits at 1 and 6 months after surgery. Nimodipine was given 12 h before surgery at an initial dose of 60 mg and two other preoperative doses of 30 mg were given 6 h later and just before the surgery. Postoperatively, within 1 h of arrival in the intensive care unit, nimodipine was restarted at 30 mg every 6 h for the first 5 days after surgery. Standardized neurological assessments were done preoperatively, 1 week, 1 month and 6 months after surgery. These included the US National Institutes of Health Stroke Scale, neuro-ophthalmological examination, and 11 neuropsychological tests. This trial was halted after enrolment of only 150 of the planned 400 patients because of a statistically significant increased mortality rate in the treated group and no beneficial effect in terms of neurological complications. The mortality rate was 10.7% in the nimodipine and 1.3% in the placebo group (hazard ratio of 8.0, $P = 0.02$). Major bleeding occurred in 13.3% of the nimodipine group and only 4.1% of the placebo group (odds ratio = 3.6, $P = 0.04$). Overall, new neurological deficits after surgery were observed in 72% of the placebo group and 7% of the nimodipine group at 1 week, 46% and 50% at 1 month, and 44% and 26% at 6 months, respectively. This trial failed because of a side-effect of the calcium-channel blocker used, but it did show the feasibility of such a trial design.

The dextromethorphan trial

Dextromethorphan, a non-competitive antagonist of the NMDA receptor, was used in a pilot study to assess possible neuroprotective effect. Children with congenital heart disease were randomly assigned to treatment or placebo. Inclusion criteria were age 3–36 months and expected cardiopulmonary bypass of at least 60 min duration. Solutions containing either dextromethorphan hydrobromide for oral administration or placebo were numbered in random order. Administration started 24 h before surgery with 2 mg/kg/day (0.5 mg/kg every 6 h). A dose of 10 mg/kg was administered after intubation but before surgery, and immediately after the end of surgery by nasogastric tube. Thereafter, 8 mg/kg was administered every 6 h until 48 h postsurgery, followed by stepwise weaning over another 48 h. During the first postoperative days a daily questionnaire was compiled on the clinical conditions, the use of drugs, communication skills, neurological symptoms and other events. A neurological examination and a developmental test were done before surgery, at hospital discharge and at least 3 months after surgery by one of two pediatric neurologists who were blind to the EEG and MRI results. MRI examination of the brain was performed before surgery and after clinical recovery.

Thirteen children were enrolled. Dextromethorphan was absorbed well and reached putative therapeutic levels in the blood and cerebrospinal fluid. Adverse effects were not observed. Sharp waves were recorded in postoperative continuous EEG in all placebo ($N = 7$) but only two of six treated children ($P = 0.02$). Pre- and postoperative MRI revealed less pronounced ventricular enlargement in the treated group without statistical significance. No elevation in CSF neuron-specific enolase levels was noted in both groups. Although there was a trend favoring a protective effect, the investigators could not conclude that there was a possible protective effect of dextromethorphan.[84]

SUGGESTIONS FOR FUTURE CLINICAL TRIALS

In spite of our refined understanding of stroke pathophysiology and the success of several animal trials, the clinical use of neuroprotective agents has been very limited. The most important explanation for this disparity of outcomes is the presence of major side-effects associated with these drugs. A neuroprotective agent should fulfil several criteria before being considered for a clinical trial. The drug needs to have a low side-effect and drug–drug interaction profile to warrant prolonged intake. It should also be available in oral forms. If all these criteria are met then the efficacy of the drug should be tested in a randomized clinical trial. For the design of such a trial, several steps need to be followed. A target population should be determined with very clear inclusion and exclusion criteria. The primary and secondary endpoints of the study should be prespecified. The length of follow-up should also be predetermined.

The safety of these neuroprotective drugs can be assessed by small pilot studies. The target population should have a high risk of stroke to warrant prolonged treatment with neuroprotective agents. Patients undergoing cardiac and neurovascular procedures would be potential candidates for such therapy. The duration over which the drug will be given and the length of the follow-up period is different for short-term and long-term neuroprotection. In short-term prophylactic neuroprotection studies, the drug can be administered 6–24 h prior to and after the surgery. Only three pilot studies have been initiated so far. The follow-up time could be set at 3–6 months. In order to have a statistically significant benefit in long-term neuroprotection trials, the drug should be given for a longer period of time. The follow-up time should be at least 2 years and can be as long as 5 years.

In order to estimate sample size in a randomized clinical trial, the investigator should specify the difference in response rates to be detected. The level of statistical significance and power desired should be made clear. They should also decide whether the test should be one-sided or two-sided. If a difference in cure rate in either direction is of interest then a two-sided test is used. If the investigator is interested in detecting only a cure rate, then a one-sided test can be used. Almost all clinical trials use an 80% power, two-tailed tests, and $\alpha = 0.05$. The advantage of short-term neuroprotection trials is the small number of subjects needed for the study. This is based on the fact that the risk of stroke is high in these individuals and that conventional therapy was not very successful. For example in a short-term prophylaxis trial with CABG, a sample size of 188 patients, who receive drug or placebo preoperatively, can detect a 40% improvement in outcome with 80% power and $\alpha = 0.05$. For long-term neuroprotection trials, the sample size is much larger and varies with the risk of stroke and the length of follow-up desired in the target population. Assuming that the target population had a stroke risk of 3% per year (14% over 5 years), a trial would require from 678 to 1618 individuals, depending on the relative improvement desired. To assess the effect of stroke recurrence among survivors of initial stroke with a 25% risk, 508 to 1214 volunteers may be required. The lower the risk of stroke and the shorter the follow-up period, the larger the sample size will be.[64]

The primary endpoints in these studies can include mortality rates, TIA attacks, neuropsychological deficits, and functional outcome. Secondary endpoints will include quality of life measurement, cost–benefit analysis, and use of health resources. A few pilot studies have supported the idea that such a trial design is feasible when patients are carefully selected.

CONCLUSION

In order to be efficient in stroke prevention we have to understand its complex pathophysiology. A large number of clinical trials failed to show any benefit from neuroprotection in contrast to animal trials because of the unacceptably high side-effect profile and the inability to start the medication on time. Based on previous epidemiological studies, patients with high-risk factors for stroke can now be easily identified and their stroke probability can be estimated. The concept of using a prophylactic neuroprotective agent in these groups is very appealing. Few pilot studies have proven that the design of such trials could be done although their results were not statistically significant. Prophylactic neuroprotection could be looked at as an adjuvant therapy for stroke prevention in a high-risk population.

REFERENCES

1. Sacco RL, Benjamin EJ, Broderick JP *et al.* Risk factors. *Stroke* 1997; **28:**1507–17.
2. American Heart Association. *1999 Heart and Stroke Statistical update.* Dallas, Texas; American Heart Association: 1998.
3. Matchar DB, Samsa GP, Matthews RJ *et al.* The stroke prevention policy model: linking evidence and clinical decisions. *Ann Intern Med* 1997; **127:**704–11.
4. Alberts MJ. tPA in acute ischemic stroke: United States experience and issues for the future. *Neurology* 1998; **51**(Suppl 3):53–5.
5. Sharp RS, Honkaniemi J, Massa S. Molecular approaches to therapy of stroke. In: *Molecular Neurology* (Martin JB, ed.). New York; Scientific American, Inc: 1998.
6. Choi DW, Lobner D, Dugan LL. Glutamate receptor-mediated neuronal death in the ischemic brain. In: *Ischemic Stroke: From Basic Mechanisms to New Drug Development* (Hsu C, ed.). Basel; Karger: 1998.
7. Bartus RT. The calpain hypothesis of neurodegeneration: evidence for a common cytotoxic pathway. *Neuroscientist* 1997; **3:**314–27.
8. Dalkara T, Moskowitz MA. The complex role of nitric oxide in the pathophysiology of focal cerebral ischemia. *Brain Pathol* 1994; **4:**49.
9. Hossmann KA. Periinfarct depolarizations. *Cerebrovasc Brain Metab Rev* 1996; **8:**195–208.
10. Tatlisumak T, Takano K, Meiler MR, Fisher M. A glycine site antagonist, ZD9379, reduces the number of spreading depressions and infarct size in rats with permanent middle cerebral artery occlusion. *Stroke* 1998; **29:**190–5.
11. Garcia JH, Liu KF, Yoshida Y *et al.* Influx of leukocytes and platelets in an evolving brain infarct (wistar rat). *Am J Pathol* 1994; **144:**188–99.
12. Clark RK, Lee EV, White RF *et al.* Reperfusion following focal stroke hastens inflammation and resolution of ischemic injury. *Brain Res Bull* 1994; **35:**387–92.
13. Pantoni L, Sarti C, Inzitari D. Cytokines and cell adhesion molecules in cerebral ischemia: experimental basis and therapeutic perspectives. *Arteriorscler Thromb Vasc Biol* 1998; **18:**503–13.
14. Mohr JP, Orgogozo JM, Harrison MJG *et al.* Meta analysis of oral nimodipine in acute ischemic stroke. *Cerebrovasc Dis* 1994; **4:**197–203.
15. Baron JC, von Kumar R, del Zoppo GJ. Treatment of acute ischemic stroke: challenging the concept of a rigid and universal time window. *Stroke* 1995; **26:**2219–21.
16. Muir KW, Lees KR. Clinical experience with excitatory amino acid antagonist drugs. *Stroke* 1994; **25:**1755–99.
17. Edwards K for the CNS 1102-008 Study Group. Cerestat (aptiganel hydrochloride) in the treatment of acute ischemic stroke [Abstract]. *Neurology* 1996; **48**(Suppl 1): 424.
18. Izumi Y, Roussel S, Pinard E, Seylaz J. Reduction of infarct volume by magnesium after middle cerebral artery occlusion in rats. *J Cereb Blood Flow Metab* 1991; **11:**1025–30.
19. Muir KW, Lees KR. Dose optimization of intravenous magnesium sulfate after acute stroke. *Stroke* 1998; **29:**918–23.

20. Cregan EF, Peeling J, Corbett D *et al.* S-alpha-phenyl-2-pyridine-ethanamine dihydrochloride, a low affinity uncompetitive n-methyl-d-aspartatic acid antagonist is effective in rodent models of global and focal ischemia. *J Pharm Exp Ther* 1997; **283:**1412–24.
21. Brady EM, Wells DS, Kierstead AE *et al.* Ascending dose safety and pharmacokinetic study of NPS 1506, a novel NMDA antagonist, in normal male volunteers [Abstract]. *Neurology* 1998; **50**(Suppl 4): 346.
22. Chen HSV, Pellegrini JW, Aggarwal SK *et al.* Open channel block of NMDA responses by memantine: therapeutic advantage against NMDA receptor-mediated neurotoxicity. *J Neurosci* 1992; **12:**4427–36.
23. GAIN Investigators. Phase 2 studies of the glycine antagonist, GV150526, in acute stroke. *Stroke* 1998; **29:**304.
24. Onal MZ, Fisher M. Acute stroke therapy: a clinical overview. *Eur Neurol* 1997; **38:**141–54.
25. Gribkoff VK, Starrett JE, Dworetzky SI. The pharmacology and molecular biology of large conductance calcium-activated (BK) potassium channels. *Adv Pharm* 1997; **37:**319–47.
26. The RANTTAS Investigators. A randomized trial of trilizad mesylate in patients with acute ischemic stroke (RANTTAS). *Stroke* 1996; **27:**1453–8.
27. Hall ED, Pazara KE, Braughler JM. The 21-aminosteroid lipid peroxidation inhibitor U74006F protects against cerebral ischemia in gerbils. *Stroke* 1988; **18:**997–1002.
28. Yamaguchi T, Sano K, Takakura K *et al.* Ebselen in acute ischemic stroke: a placebo-controlled, double blind clinical trial. *Stroke* 1998; **29:**12–7.
29. Zhao Q, Pahlmark K, Smith M-L *et al.* Delayed treatment with the spin trap alpha-phenyl-N-butyl nitrone (PBN) reduced infarct size following temporary transient middle cerebral artery occlusion in rats. *Acta Physiol Scand* 1994; **152:**349–50.
30. Dalkara T, Moskowitz MA. Nitric oxide in cerebrovascular regulation. In: *Ischemic Stroke: From Basic Mechanisms to New Drug Development* (Hsu CY, ed.), pp. 28–47. Basel, Karger: 1998.
31. Maiese K, Tenbroeke M, Kue I. Neuroprotection of lubeluzole is mediated through the signal transduction pathways of nitric oxide. *J Neurochem* 1997; **68:**710–4.
32. Diener HC, for the European and Australian Lubeluzole Ischemic Stroke Study Group. Multinational randomized controlled trial of lubeluzole in acute ischemic stroke. *Cerebrovasc Dis* 1998; **8:**172–81.
33. Diener HC. Lubeluzole in acute ischemic stroke treatment: lack of efficacy in a large phase III study with an 8-hour window. *Stroke* 1999; **30:**234.
34. Markgraf CG, Velayo NL, Johnson MP *et al.* Six hour window of opportunity for calpain inhibition in focal cerebral ischemia in rats. *Stroke* 1998; **29:**152–8.
35. Mies G, Kohno K, Hossmann KA. Prevention of peri-infarct DC shift with glutamate antagonist NBQX following occlusion of the middle cerebral artery in rats. *J Cereb Blood Flow Metab* 1994; **14:**802–7.
36. Wahlgren NG, for the Clomethiazole Acute Stroke Study (CLASS). Efficacy results in a subgroup of 545 patients with total anterior circulation syndrome. *Stroke* 1998; **29:**287.
37. Sherman DG, for the Enlimolab Acute Stroke Trial Investigators. The Enlimolab acute stroke trial: final results [Abstract]. *Neurology* 1997; **48:**270.
38. Fisher M, Meadows ME, Weise J *et al.* Delayed intravenous administration of basic fibroblast growth factor reduces infarct size following permanent focal cerebral ischemia in rats. *J Cereb Blood Flow Metab* 1995; **15:**953–9.
39. The FIBLAST safety study group. Clinical safety trial of intravenous basic fibroblast growth factor (bFGF, FIBLAST) in acute stroke. *Stroke* 1998; **29:**287.
40. Clark WM, Warach SJ, Pettigrew LC *et al.* A randomized dose–response trial of citicoline in acute ischemic stroke patients. *Neurology* 1997; **49:**671–8.
41. Clark WM, Williams BJ, Selzer KA *et al.* Randomized efficacy trial of citicoline in acute ischemic stroke. *Stroke* 1998; **29:**287.
42. Gardner TJ, Horneffer PJ, Manolio TA *et al.* Stroke following coronary artery bypass grafting: a ten-year study. *Ann Thorac Surg* 1985; **40:**574–81.
43. Mangano DT. Cardiovascular morbidity and CABG surgery—a perspective: epidemiology, costs, and potential therapeutic solutions. *J Card Surg* 1995; **10**(Suppl):336–8.
44. Roach GW, Kanchuger M, Mangano CM *et al.* Adverse cerebral outcomes after coronary bypass surgery. *N Engl J Med* 1996; **335:**1857–63.
45. Kurki TS, Kataja M. Preoperative prediction of postoperative morbidity in coronary artery bypass grafting. *Ann Thorac Surg* 1996; **61:**1740–5.

46. Inoue K, Luth JU, Pottkamper D *et al.* Incidence and risk factors of perioperative cerebral complications. Heart transplantation compared to coronary artery bypass grafting and valve surgery. *J Cardiovasc Surg* 1998; **39:**201–8.
47. Nussmeier NA. Adverse neurologic events: risks of intracardiac versus extracardiac surgery. *J Cardiothorac Vasc Anesth* 1996; **10:**31–7.
48. Ahlgren E, Aren C. Cerebral complications after coronary artery bypass and heart valve surgery: risk factors and onset of symptoms. *J Cardiothorac Vasc Anesth* 1998; **12:**270–3.
49. Dashe JF, Pessin MS, Murphy RE, Payne DD. Carotid occlusive disease and stroke risk in coronary artery bypass surgery. *Neurology* 1997; **49:**678–86.
50. Hartman GS, Yao FS, Bruefach M 3rd *et al.* Severity of aortic atheromatous disease diagnosed by transesophageal echocardiography predicts stroke and other outcomes associated with coronary artery surgery: a prospective study. *Anesthes Analg* 1996; **83:**701–8.
51. Newman Mark F, Wolman R, Kanchuger M *et al.* Multicenter preoperative risk index for patients undergoing coronary artery bypass graft surgery. *Circulation* 1996; **94**(Suppl II):74–80.
52. North American Symptomatic Carotid Endarterectomy Trial Collaborators. Beneficial effect of carotid endarterectomy in symptomatic patients with high grade carotid stenosis**.** *N Engl J Med* 1991; **325:**445–53.
53. Executive Committee for the Asymptomatic Carotid Atherosclerosis Study. Endarterectomy for asymptomatic carotid artery stenosis. *J Am Med Assoc* 1995; **273:**1421–8.
54. Rosenthal D, Zeichner WD, Lamis PA *et al.* Neurologic deficit after carotid endarterectomy: pathogenesis and management. *Surgery* 1983; **94:**776–80.
55. Rothwell PM, Slattery J, Warlow CP. Clinical and angiographic predictors of stroke and death from carotid endarterectomy: systematic review. *Br Med J* 1997; **315:**1571–7.
56. Sila CA. Neurologic complications of vascular surgery. *Neurol Clin N Am* 1998; **16:**9–20.
57. Kachel R. Results of balloon angioplasty in the carotid arteries. *J Endovasc Surg* 1996; **3:**22–30.
58. Wholey MH, Wholey M, Bergeron P *et al.* Current global status of carotid artery stent placement. *Cathet Cardiovasc Diagn* 1998; **44:**1–6.
59. Marthur A, Roubin GS, Iyer SS *et al.* Predictors of stroke complicating carotid artery stenting. *Circulation* 1998; **97:**1239–45.
60. Nishimura RA, Holmes DR, Reeder GS. Percutaneous balloon valvuloplasty. *Mayo Clin Proc* 1990; **65:**198–220.
61. Vinuela F, Dion JE, Duckwiler G *et al.* Combined endovascular embolization and surgery in the management of cerebral arteriovenous malformations: experience with 101 cases. *J Neurosurg* 1991; **75:**856–64.
62. Sacco RL, Lipset CH. Stroke risk factors: identification and modification. In: *Stroke Therapy,* (Fisher M, ed.), pp. 1–28. Stoneham MA: Butterworth-Heinemann, Inc.: 1995.
63. Wolf PA, Abbott RD, Kannel WB. Atrial fibrillation as an independent risk factor for stroke: The Framingham Study. *Stroke* 1991; **22:**983–8.
64. Fisher M, Jones S, Ralph LS. Prophylactic neuroprotection for ischemia. *Stroke* 1994; **25:**1075–80.
65. Braekken SK, Russell D, Brucher R *et al.* Incidence and frequency of cerebral embolic signals in patients with a similar bileaflet mechanical heart valve. *Stroke* 1995; **26:**1225–30.
66. Loh E, Sutton MS, Wun CC *et al.* Ventricular dysfunction and the risk of stroke after myocardial infarction. *N Engl J Med* 1997; **336:**251–7.
67. The French Study of Aortic Plaques in Stroke Group. Atherosclerotic disease of the aortic arch as a risk factor for recurrent ischemic stroke. *N Engl J Med* 1996; **334:**1216–21.
68. O'Leary DH, Polak JF, Kronmal RA *et al.* Carotid artery intima and media thickness as a risk factor for myocardial infarction and stroke in older adults. *N Engl J Med* 1999; **340:**14–22.
69. Summary of the National Cholesterol Education Program (NCEP) Adult Treatment Panel II Report. *J Am Med Assoc* 1993; **269:**3015–23.
70. Shinton R, Beevers G. Meta-analysis of relation between cigarette smoking and stroke. *Br Med J* 1989; **298:**789–94.
71. Fine-Edelstein JS, Wolf PA, O'Leary DH *et al.* Precursors of extracranial carotid atherosclerosis in the Framingham study. *Neurology* 1994; **44:**1046–50.
72. Sacco RL. Risk factors, outcomes, and stroke subtypes for ischemic stroke. *Neurology* 1997; **49**(Suppl 4):39–44.
73. Norris JW, Zhu CZ, Bornstein NM *et al.* Vascular risks of asymptomatic carotid stenosis. *Stroke* 1991; **22:**1485–90.
74. Sacco RL, Foulks MA, Mohr JP *et al.* Determinants of early recurrence of cerebral infarction: Stroke Data Bank. *Stroke* 1989; **20:**983–9.
75. Witterdink JL, Easton JD. Vascular events rates

in patients with atherosclerotic cerebrovascular disease. *Arch Neurol* 1992; **49:**626–34.

76. Easton JD. Antiplatelet therapy for prevention of ischemic stroke. *Cerebrovasc Dis* 1992; **2**(Suppl 1):6–13.
77. Wolf PA, D'Agostino RB, Belanger AJ *et al.* Probability of stroke: a risk profile from the Framingham study. *Stroke* 1991; **22:**312–8.
78. Hossman KA. Viability thresholds and the penumbra of focal ischemia. *Ann Neurol* 1994; **36:**557.
79. Yue TL, Cheng HY, Lysko PG *et al.* Carvelidol, a new vasodilator and beta adrenoreceptor antagonist, is an antioxidant and free radical scavenger. *J Pharm Exp Ther* 1992; **263:**92–8.
80. Ferrari G, Fabris M, Gorio A. Gangliosides enhance neurite outgrowth in PC12 cells. *Dev Brain Res* 1983; **8:**215–21.
81. Grieco G, d'Hollosy M, Culliford A *et al.* Evaluating neuroprotective agents for clinical anti-ischemic benefit using neurological and neuropsychological changes after cardiac surgery under cardiopulmonary bypass: methodological strategies and results of a double-blind, placebo-controlled trial of GM_1 ganglioside. *Stroke* 1996; **27:**858–74.
82. Schneider JS, Roeltgen DP, Rothblat DS *et al.* GM_1 ganglioside treatment of Parkinson's disease: an open pilot study of safety and efficacy. *Neurology* 1995; **45:**1149–54.
83. Legault C, Furberg CD, Wagenknecht LE *et al.* Nimodipine neuroprotection in cardiac valve replacement—a report of an early terminated trial. *Stroke* 1996; **27:**593–8.
84. Schmitt B, Bauersfeld U, Fanconi S *et al.* The effect of the N-methyl-D-aspartate receptor antagonist Dextromethorphan on perioperative brain injury in children undergoing cardiac surgery with cardiopulmonary bypass: results of a pilot study. *Neuropediatrics* 1997; **28:**191–7.

14

Carotid plaques and stenosis: molecular mechanisms affecting the development of symptomatic lesions

Petri T Kovanen, Olli Carpén, Riitta Lassila and Markku Kaste

INTRODUCTION

Cerebrovascular disorders (CVD) are the third largest cause of death and the single most important cause of disability and loss of quality-adjusted years of life in the world.[1] The burden of stroke continues despite improved identification and medical care of hypertension, hypercholesterolemia, and other risk factors of the cerebrovascular disorders, adoption of healthier dietary habits, and reduced smoking. The most common type of cerebrovascular disorder, up to 80%, is ischemic brain infarction. Twenty to thirty per cent of ischemic brain infarctions are caused by atherothrombotic disease of the internal carotid arteries either through recurrent thromboembolism or through hemodynamic impairment and secondary intracranial thrombosis.[2] Progress has been made in the medical secondary prevention of ischemic stroke but, in skilled hands, surgery of symptomatic severe carotid stenosis (equal to or more than 70%) is superior to medical therapy. Accordingly, patients with this condition obtain longlasting benefit from endarterectomy whereas, in patients with moderate carotid stenosis of 50–69%, endarterectomy results in only a moderate reduction in the risk of stroke.[3] Surgical treatment of asymptomatic moderate to severe stenosis (over 60%) is now considered a safe form of primary prevention of stroke[4], but requires exceptional surgical skills.

Lesions of the carotid bifurcation remain silent in some individuals for years, while in others they turn into clinically active lesions causing TIAs and strokes. Yet, radiologically, these lesions may appear to be quite similar. Why, then, do some carotid lesions become active and begin to send emboli into the cerebral circulation? Does it depend on the cellular architecture and the chemical composition of the plaque? We have, as yet, no definite answers to these questions. We discuss here the pathophysiological processes that could be involved in transforming asymptomatic atherosclerotic lesions into symptomatic ones, and endeavor to shed some light on the important question of which of the unique characteristics of stenosis or of carotid plaques are critical.

ROLE OF ATHEROSCLEROSIS IN CEREBRAL ISCHEMIA

The usual disease process underlying ischemic stroke is atherosclerosis, a disease of large- and medium-sized arteries. In autopsy studies, 80–90% of patients with a cerebral infarct also have more or less advanced atherosclerosis of the extra- and intracranial arteries.[5] Indeed, the infarct has usually occurred in the area supplied by the artery found to be most severely occluded.[6] Accordingly, a frequent cause of an ischemic stroke is atherosclerosis of a large extracranial or intracranial artery. Likewise, thromboembolic strokes, in which the embolus originates in the heart or in the ascending aorta, are usually related to atherosclerosis. Thus, 25% of cerebral emboli of cardiac origin are due to myocardial infarction with accompanying left ventricular aneurysm. Emboli originating in the ascending aorta are practically always due to local atherosclerotic changes. Finally, local processes occluding small intracranial arteries, and causing about 15% of ischemic strokes[7], may also be related to atherosclerosis. Although the underlying pathology of these 'lacunar infarcts' is usually fibrinoid necrosis or lipohyalinosis, the changes in the small arteries may resemble those found in the earliest stages of atherosclerosis, i.e. those found in fatty streaks (see below).

LIPID ACCUMULATION DURING ATHEROGENESIS

Development of the arterial intima, the site of atherogenesis

The innermost layer of the arterial wall, that is, the arterial intima, is the site of atherogenesis, i.e., the tissue site in which lipids accumulate. The intima is composed of an endothelial layer with underlying stromal tissue, the intima proper. The intima is separated from the medial layer by an internal elastic lamina. At birth, the intima is extremely thin, and the endothelium lies directly upon the internal elastic lamina in most areas of the arterial tree; however, at the outer curvatures of both the intra- and the extracranial arteries, the intima is already thick at birth. These physiological 'eccentric thickenings' are called polsters, pads, or cushions, since they are adaptations to the turbulent flow at the branch sites, and absorb the shocks created during systole.[8,9] The bigger the artery and the more severe the hemodynamic forces, the thicker the intima will grow. Accordingly, among the cerebral arteries, the intima is thickest in the outer curvatures of the carotid bifurcation.

The stromal cells of the intima are smooth muscle cells. Even during fetal life, medial smooth muscle cells migrate through the intimal elastic layer into the subendothelial space, where they start to divide and secrete the various components of the extracellular matrix: collagen, elastin, and proteoglycans. When the thickness of the intima has reached a level that is physiologically meaningful, the intimal smooth muscle cells stop dividing and secreting the matrix components.[10]

In general, the thicker the intima, the more likely it is that atherosclerosis will develop. Therefore, it is not surprising that the topography of the intimal thickenings resembles that of atherosclerosis. Moreover, in thick intimas, atherosclerosis tends to develop earlier and at a faster rate than in thin intimas. Thus, ischemic infarctions due to large-artery atherosclerosis are caused by the lesions found in the internal carotid artery or siphon, basilar artery, or the major cerebral artery stem. Yet, among the cerebral arteries, the areas that are most prone to atherosclerosis are the eccentric intimal thickenings at the carotid bifurcations.

Macroscopic changes during lipid accumulation

Macroscopically, lipid accumulations can be divided into two types: fatty streaks and atheromas. The first changes that are visible to the naked eye are fatty streaks, and these start to develop in the carotid arteries even during the first decade of life. Fatty streaks are found in all populations, including those without any ischemic complications of the cerebral arteries.[11] Fatty streaks are flat, and do not cause local obstruction of the blood flow. It is not known whether they are thrombogenic, and, consequently, their clinical significance remains to be determined.

As atherosclerosis advances, fatty streaks are converted into atheromas. Indeed, systematic autopsy studies have revealed that atheromas develop only in areas in which fatty streaks are usually present.[11] In populations in which ischemic cerebral diseases are prevalent, the carotid arteries may show atheromas as early as the third decade of life.[12] An atheroma differs in its anatomy from a fatty streak, for it contains a lipid core and a fibrous cap which separates the core from the circulating blood.[13,14] It is this peculiar anatomical structure that makes the atheroma a clinically significant lesion. Thus, in terms of clinical significance, the key process in the development of atherosclerosis is the conversion of fatty streaks into atheromas.

The advanced raised lesions or atheromas are also called atherosclerotic plaques. If they contain predominantly fibrous material, the term fibrous plaque is preferable, and if, in addition to fibrous material, they also contain substantial amounts of lipid, the term fibro-fatty plaque (or atheroma) can be used. In this chapter, all these terms are used.

Microscopic changes during lipid accumulation: clues to the mechanisms of accumulation

Development of a fatty streak

The lipids that accumulate in the arterial intimal tissue during atherogenesis are derived from plasma lipoproteins, notably from low density lipoproteins (LDL) which carry the majority (about 75%) of plasma cholesterol.[15] In other tissues, LDL lipids do not accumulate even if the concentration of LDL particles in the blood plasma is high (with the notable exceptions of skin and tendons, in which xanthomas may develop). What may be the factors leading to the accumulation of LDL lipids in the arterial intima, and the factors preventing other tissues from such accumulation?

The LDL circulate as distinct particles with diameters of about 20 nm, their physiological role being to deliver cholesterol to cells.[16,17] In most extrahepatic tissues, some of the circulating LDL particles cross the capillary endothelium by a process known as transcytosis and enter the extracellular fluids. These particles then bind to the LDL receptors on the surfaces of the extrahepatic parenchymal cells, and become endocytosed along with the LDL receptors. From the endosomes, the LDL receptors return to the cell surface to pick up new LDL particles, while the LDL particles enter the lysosomal compartment, where they are degraded. The cholesterol released by LDL particle degradation becomes available to the cells for use as the building blocks of their membranes. Any LDL particles that are not bound by the receptors are rapidly drained from the interstitial fluid by the local lymphatic capillaries and returned to the circulation.

Once the cells have obtained enough cholesterol, they cease to produce LDL receptors and, accordingly, the LDL particles in the extracellular fluid are no longer taken up by the cells, and will be returned to the circulation. As a result of this feedback regulation of the LDL receptor system, LDL cholesterol does not accumulate inside cells. Importantly, because of the efficient system for removal of excess LDL particles from the extracellular fluid by the lymphatic capillaries, LDL particles do not accumulate outside cells either. Indeed, the concentration of LDL in the extracellular fluid is much lower than in the corresponding blood plasma (only 1/10).[18]

Some of the circulating LDL particles cross the arterial endothelium and enter the arterial intima (Fig. 14.1). There, however, their fate differs dramatically from that in other extrahepatic tissues. Perhaps the most important difference is the long residence time of the LDL particles in the extracellular spaces of the intima. This phenomenon is known as retention of LDL.[19] Retention of LDL is a consequence of the peculiar structure of the intima. For one thing, the intima lacks both blood capillaries and lymphatic capillaries, the nearest of these latter capillaries originating in the medial layer. Accordingly, the LDL particles that have crossed the arterial endothelium and entered the intimal space have to move through the intimal layer to be drained by the lymphatic system: the thicker the intima, the longer the passage. It is also difficult for the LDL particles to leave the intima, since the internal elastic lamina that separates it from the media acts as a barrier.[19] A third factor that increases the residence time of LDL particles is their slow move-

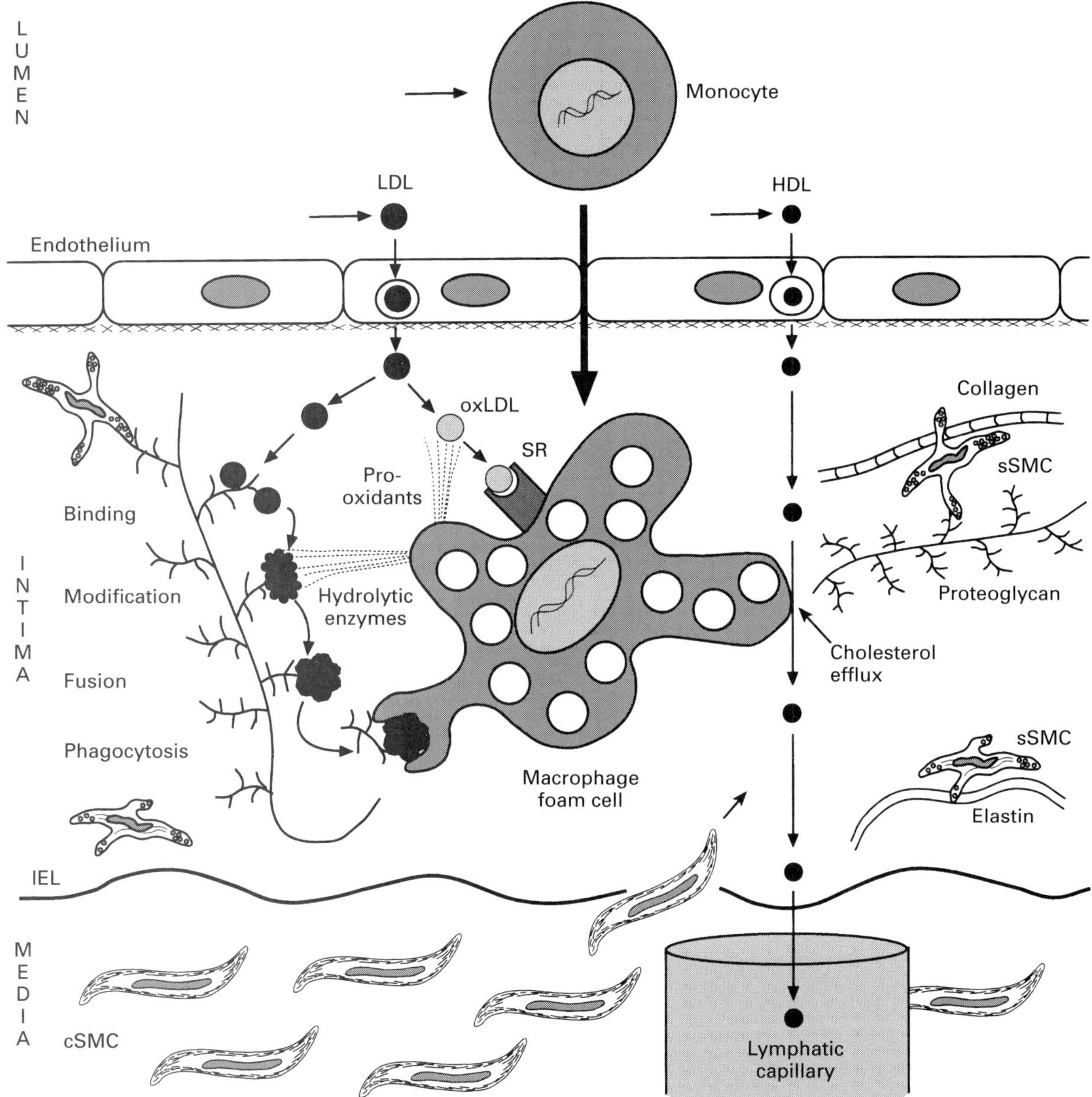

Figure 14.1 Formation of a fatty streak
Contractile smooth muscle cells (cSMCs) have migrated from the media through the internal elastic lamina (IEL) into the intimal space. In the intima, their phenotype is changed and they are converted into synthesizing smooth muscle cells (sSMCs). The sSMCs synthesize and secrete the various components of the extracellular matrix, notably collagen, proteoglycans, and elastin (right). Monocytes enter the intima from the circulation and are converted into tissue macrophages (middle). LDL particles cross arterial endothelial layer by transcytosis and enter the intima. In the subendothelial layer, they bind to proteoglycans (left). This binding is weak and short-lived, and the particles are released from the proteoglycan to be bound again. Along their way towards the medial layer, the LDL particles become modified when cell-derived proteolytic and lipolytic enzymes attack them. The LDL particles become unstable and fuse to form large lipid droplets, which bind tightly to the proteoglycans. Ultimately, a macrophage phagocytoses the proteoglycan-bound lipid droplets. If LDL particles become oxidized,

ment through the proteoglycan matrix of the intima.[20,21] The proteoglycans form a close network that is negatively charged. An LDL particle binds to the network via ionic interactions when the positively charged lysine residues of its apolipoprotein B-100 component interact with the negatively charged sulfate groups of the glycosaminoglycan component of a proteoglycan. After a while, the bound LDL particle is released, only to be bound again later in its passage through the intima. This repetitive cycle of binding and release retards the movement of the LDL particles.

The retention of LDL particles results in a dramatic increase in their concentration in the intimal fluid, which normally reaches a value equaling or even exceeding that in the corresponding blood plasma, and, accordingly, is at least 10 times as high as in the extracellular fluids of other extrahepatic tissues.[19] Indeed, the concentration of LDL particles in the intima is about 100–fold that found in the adjacent medial tissue. When compared with other plasma-derived molecules, such as α_1-antitrypsin and albumin the retention of LDL in the arterial intima is much higher, so emphasizing the uniqueness of LDL among the plasma-derived components present in the intimal fluid.

The high concentration of the LDL particles in the intimal fluid inhibits synthesis of LDL receptors by intimal cells. In contrast to other extrahepatic tissues, LDL receptors are not expressed in the intimas of normal or atherosclerotic arteries.[22] Accordingly, this pathway of cellular uptake and degradation of LDL particles is blocked, and consequently, the concentration of the particles in the intimal fluid tends to still increase. The high local concentration of the LDL particles also favors their binding to the extracellular matrix.

During their long residence in the intima, the LDL particles are modified by the various enzymes and oxygen radicals secreted by the cells of the intima. Such modified LDL particles are removed from the intimal fluid by intimal macrophages (Fig. 14.1). On their surfaces, the macrophages express scavenger receptors which bind the negatively charged oxidatively modified LDL particles, and carry them into the macrophages like the LDL receptors carry unmodified LDL particles into other types of cells.[23–25] However, in contrast to the LDL receptors, the scavenger receptors are not downregulated by the incoming cholesterol, and their continuing activity leads to progressive uptake of modified LDL particles by the macrophages. This, again, fills the macrophages with cholesterol and so converts them into foam cells. In addition to the oxidative processes, proteolytic and lipolytic enzymes also modify the LDL particles in the intima.[26] Importantly, these two latter changes render the LDL particles unstable, trigger their fusion, and strengthen their binding to arterial proteoglycans.[27] Such fused particles may consist of several hundred LDL particles and have diameters of up to several hundred micrometers. Under the microscope they appear as lipid droplets.

At the prelesional stage, when the intimal thickenings of the carotid arteries still appear normal to the naked eye, the lipid droplets are distributed diffusely in the subendothelial extracellular space and form perifibrous droplets mainly on the surfaces of collagen bundles.[28] When fatty streaks develop, the

---

they will not bind to proteoglycans. Such oxidized LDL particles (oxLDL) bind with high affinity to the scavenger receptors (SR) on the surface of macrophages. The macrophage then ingests the receptor-bound oxidized LDL particles. The role of the macrophage is to clean the intima of modified LDL particles. In doing so, it becomes filled with LDL-derived cholesterol, which is stored as cytoplasmic cholesteryl ester droplets. A cholesterol-filled macrophage is called a foam cell. HDL particles also enter the intima (right). They do not bind to proteoglycans. Once they encounter a foam cell, they induce efflux of cholesterol from the foam cell, and pick up the released cholesterol. The cholesterol-filled HDL particles then move to the medial layer and enter the lymphatic vessels and ultimately return to the circulation. Thus, cholesterol entering the intima in LDL particles leaves the intima in HDL particles through the action of macrophages.

perifibrous lipid droplets disappear, and foam cells are formed in the subendothelial space. This switch appears to reflect the phagocytotic or scavenger receptor-mediated uptake of the perifibrous droplets by macrophages and also by smooth muscle cells. These cells, when stuffed with ingested lipid droplets, are converted into foam cells. When numerous foam cells form clusters, these have a yellow appearance visible to the naked eye and the area is called a fatty streak.

High density lipoprotein (HDL) particles also enter the intima from the circulation. These HDL particles are smaller than LDL particles, and their apolipoprotein component (apoA) does not contain positively charged domains. Therefore, they are likely to traverse the intima easily and find their way into the lymphatic vessels of the next layer of the arterial wall, the media. If the HDL particles encounter a subendothelial foam cell, they pick up cholesterol from it, and carry it back into the circulation (Fig. 14.1). Thus, the role of foam cells is to clear modified (e.g. oxidized) LDL particles from their surroundings and transfer LDL-derived cholesterol to HDL particles. Granted this 'balance concept' of atherogenesis, it is reasonable that the concentration of LDL in the intimal fluid should be low, and that of HDL high.[29] Since the concentrations of LDL and HDL in the intima reflect the values in the blood, the LDL/HDL ratio in blood plasma should also remain low. This conclusion is supported by the clinical data available, which confirm that this ratio is a good predictive indicator of the development of carotid atherosclerosis,[30] although not as strong as in the case of coronary atherosclerosis.

Development of an atheroma

In atheromas, in sharp contrast to the early lipid-containing lesions, the lipids are stored both intra- and extracellularly (Fig. 14.2). The extracellular lipid deposits are located deep in the intima, where they are usually bound to elastin fibers.[31] The fate of the lipid droplets in the deep intima is different from that of the droplets in the subendothelial layer. Instead of being taken up by cells, the droplets remain in the extracellular space. The reasons for this may be the paucity of macrophages in the deep intimal layers, and the inability of the local smooth muscle cells to compensate for this absence of droplet ingestion. Moreover, some of the foam cells may undergo a necrotic death and extrude their lipids into the extracellular space.[32]

If the process of droplet formation continues in the deep layers of the intima, the droplets coalesce into larger lipid lakes, and more foam cells die. Then a 'lipid core' or a 'necrotic core' visible to the naked eye is formed.[31,32]

Lipid accumulation in carotid arteries – a postprandial process?

After a fat-containing meal, the gut synthesizes and secretes triglyceride-rich chylomicrons.[16] These giant lipoprotein particles cannot pass through the endothelium. However, in the capillary circulation, they are converted into smaller particles called chylomicron remnants. The liver also synthesizes and secretes into the circulation triglyceride-rich lipoproteins, the very low density lipoproteins (VLDL). These particles are produced even during the fasting state. However, like the chylomicrons, they are converted into smaller particles in the capillary beds of the tissues, and are then called VLDL remnants. Recent experimental evidence suggests that the remnants of triglyceride-rich particles are small enough to pass through the endothelium and enter the arterial intima, where they become trapped to at least the same extent as LDL.[33] Increased plasma levels of triglyceride-rich lipoproteins in the postprandial state (chylomicron remnants) and in the fasting state (VLDL remnants) predict increased plaque lipid content.[34] Thus, whereas the plasma level of LDL cholesterol is the best lipid predictor for the extent of carotid atherosclerosis, the level of triglyceride-rich lipoproteins in plasma predicts an echolucent lipid-rich plaque prone to rupture and associated with a high risk of neurological events. The new results on carotid plaques give support to the old, but recently revived, hypothesis that atherosclerosis is at least to some extent a postprandial phenomenon.[35]

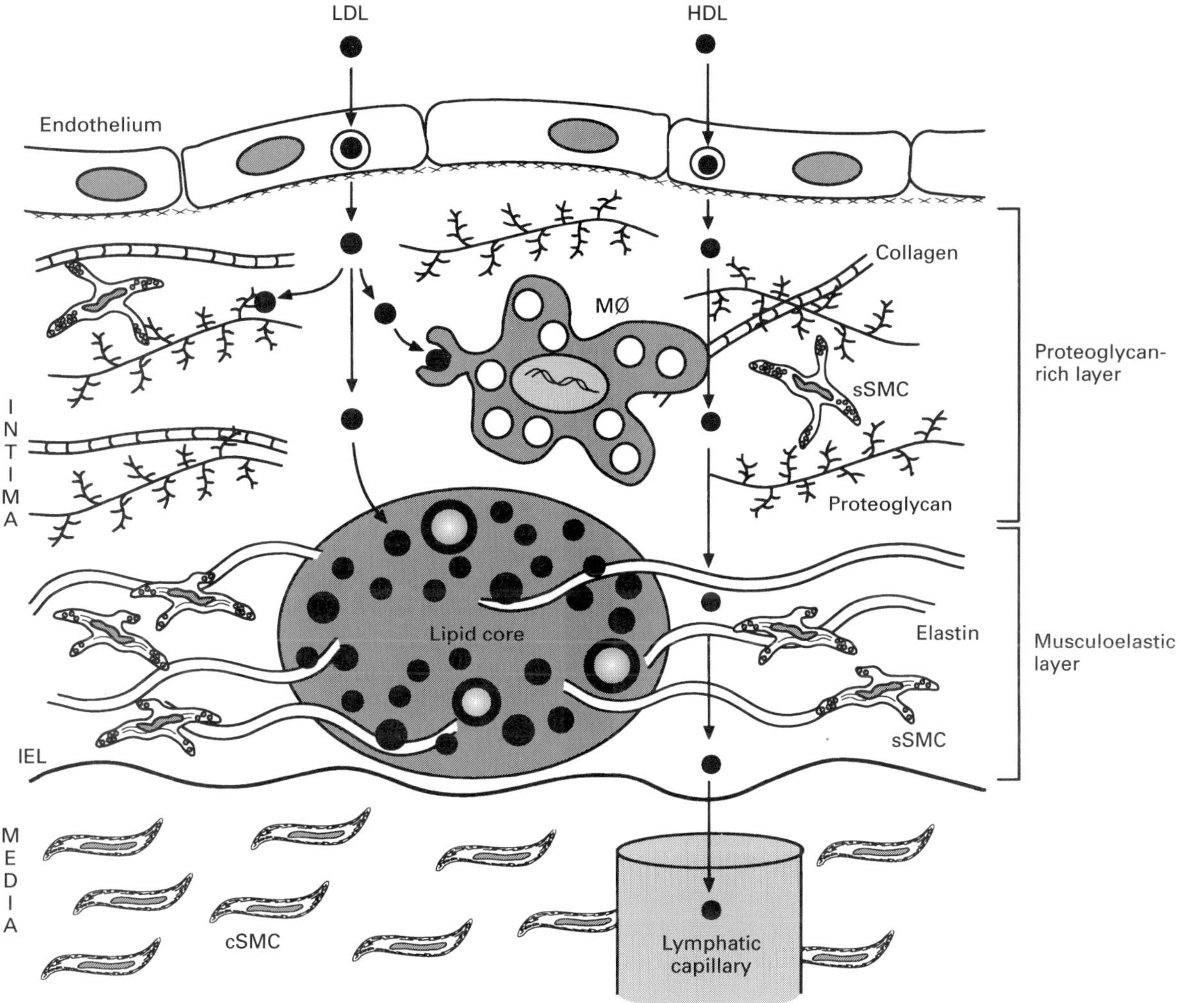

Figure 14.2 Formation of an atheroma
An excess of LDL particles enters the intima. A fraction of them are not cleared by the macrophages (Mø), which are present in the subendothelial proteoglycan-rich layer, but enter the deep musculoelastic layer of the intima. Here, in between elastic fibers, the particles are modified by proteolytic, lipolytic, and oxidative agents, and are converted into lipid droplets and vesicles. Progressive growth of the size and the number of the extracellular lipid droplets and vesicles leads to formation of an extracellular lipid core. In very advanced lesions, such a core may also contain lipids derived from dead foam cells. An intimal area with a lipid core tends to bulge into the arterial lumen.

Cellular and molecular mechanisms converting a stable atheroma into an unstable one: role of inflammation

The layer overlying the lipid core and separating it from the circulation is called the fibrous cap of the atheroma. The fibrous cap is characterized by a dense extracellular matrix, of which the major component is collagen (types I and III).

In their architecture, advanced atherosclerotic plaques vary from a solid fibrous lesion with a small lipid core and a thick cap (also called a 'fibrous plaque') to a lipid-rich lesion with a large lipid core and a thin cap ('fibro-fatty plaque').[36–38] An atheroma with a thick cap is considered to be essentially stable, whereas an atheroma with a thin cap is prone to rupture (Fig. 14.3). Of the components of the fibrous cap, the most abundant is collagen, which makes the greatest contribution to the structural integrity of the cap and accounts for its strength. Mechanical tests have shown that forces concentrate on the fibrous cap, and that only a thick cap can resist the high stresses and avoid rupture.

As the lipid core grows, it pushes the cap toward the lumen of the artery, and finally the lesion may occlude the lumen. This occluding tendency is counteracted by 'remodeling' of the atheroma, a process that allows maintenance of blood flow, the lesion expanding outward and the cap becoming thinner. But, as the lipid core grows and the cap thins, the stable fibrous lesion is converted into an unstable lipid-rich lesion. Even lesions with 'stable morphology' can become thrombogenic when the surface of a thick cap is eroded and subendothelial thrombogenic structures are exposed.[39]

Data emerging from clinical and pathological studies on coronary arteries have led to a new dogma, which states that inflammatory mechanisms modulate the morphology of an atheroma by promoting synthesis (strengthening) and/or lysis (weakening) of the fibrous cap.[40] The key elements in the production of local inflammation in an atherosclerotic plaque are (1) the inflammatory cells, notably macrophages, T lymphocytes, and mast cells; (2) the inflammatory mediators secreted by these cells, e.g. the proinflammatory cytokines interfereron-γ (INF-γ), tumor necrosis factor-α (TNF-α), and interleukin-1β (IL-1β), and growth factors such as transforming growth factor-β (TGF-β); and (3) the complement system.

It is important to note that, in the cap, only the smooth muscle cells produce the various structural components of the extracellular matrix, whereas all the cell types found in the cap participate in degradation of the matrix components. Lesions whose tensile strength is diminished by mechanical stress and regions of the fibrous cap particularly prone to disruption contain relatively few smooth muscle cells, but increased numbers of inflammatory cells of three types: macrophages,[41] T lymphocytes,[42] and mast cells.[43] Of these three cell types, the macrophages are by far the most numerous, followed by the T lymphocytes, the mast cells displaying the smallest numbers. Accordingly, plaque cap remodelling, i.e. alteration in cap thickness and in the density of the cap matrix, is orchestrated by the interplay between these three cell types and the smooth muscle cells. Importantly, the actual sites of atheromatous ulceration, either rupture or erosion, have invariably shown the presence of inflammatory infiltrates (Fig. 14.3).[44,45] It appears that the intensity of the inflammatory reaction is less severe at sites of superficial ulceration (erosion) than at sites where the cap shows deep ulceration (rupture) extending to the lipid core.[39] In the latter case, a few subendothelial inflammatory cells, most of which appear to be macrophage foam cells, may be sufficient to cause ulceration of the plaque. Taken together, irrespective of the structure of the atherosclerotic plaque, the actual site of atheromatous ulceration (erosion or rupture) with ensuing local thrombus formation is characterized by an inflammatory process. The dominant role of inflammation in the conversion of an asymptomatic lesion into a symptomatic one seems also to apply to plaques of the carotid artery.[46]

In view of the importance of the fibrous matrix in determining plaque stability, it is essential to understand the factors that regulate the rates of synthesis of the various matrix components by the smooth muscle cells (SMCs) of the cap, and also the factors that regulate the degradation of the matrix components. The net production of matrix components depends on the number of matrix-producing SMCs and the ability of the individual cells to produce such components (Fig. 14.3). The number of SMCs, in turn, depends on the balance between cell replication and cell death. In atherosclerotic lesions, the rate of cell replication is very low, and so is the rate of cell death. Therefore, changes in the total cell mass of the tissue must be due to very

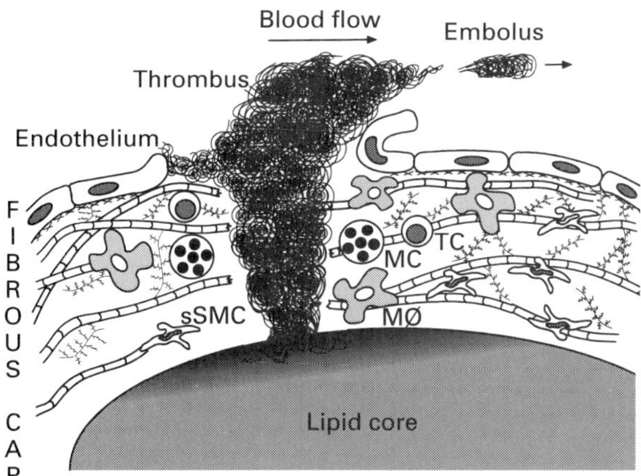

Figure 14.3 Rupture of an atheroma
The lipid core of an atheroma is separated from the circulating blood by a fibrous layer called the cap of the atheroma. The cap is produced when smooth muscle cells of the synthesizing phenotype (sSMCs) are stimulated to produce the various components of the extracellular matrix, notably collagen. Small repetitive endothelial erosions with ensuing platelet aggregation and release of growth factors (e.g. platelet derived growth factor, PDGF) is thought to be a common cause of such stimulation of the sSMCs. The strength of the cap depends on its collagen content and on its thickness. An infiltrate of inflammatory cells is present in the cap. The infiltrate consists of macrophages (Mø), T lymphocytes (TC), and mast cells (MC). These cells tend to weaken the cap by rendering it thinner and more fragile. They do this by secreting eg. cytokines which induce apoptosis of the sSMCs and inhibit their ability to secrete components of the extracellular matrix. In addition, both macrophages and mast cells produce enzymes which degrade the various components of the extracellular matrix. Shown is a deep rupture of the cap which extends into the lipid core. The subendothelial structures, notably collagen are thrombogenic. Also tissue factor is produced by the macrophages, which renders an inflamed tissue very thrombogenic. An intramural thrombus has formed and covers the thrombogenic surface. Depending on its growth potential, it may block partially or totally block the arterial lumen. Also a non-occluding thrombus of a carotid atheroma is clinically significant, since it usually seeds emboli into the cerebral circulation (right).

small changes in the subtle balance between growth and death. SMCs in the inflammatory cap areas express human leukocyte antigen DR. These antigens are induced by interferon gamma (INF-γ), which is a product of activated T cells.[47] Cell culture studies have shown that, in HLA-DR-positive SMCs, the capacity to form collagen is reduced. A reduction in the number of SMCs would also reduce the total capacity of SMCs to produce matrix components. In vitro studies of cultured SMCs have revealed that INF-γ markedly decreases the ability of human arterial SMCs to express the interstitial collagen genes. In addition, cell culture studies have shown that INF-γ can inhibit proliferation of SMCs and, in combination with other proinflammatory cytokines, such as TNF-α and IL-1β, contribute to their apoptotic death. In advanced human carotid plaques, the plaque-infiltrating lymphocytes are of the Th1 subpopulation of CD4+ cells, and the proinflammatory (Th1) cytokines dominate.[48] This finding points to INF-γ as the major T cell-specific cytokine released by the plaque-infiltrating lymphocytes.[47] Indeed, among the cells present in human atherosclerotic plaques, so far only T lymphocytes have been found to secrete INF-γ. Thus, activation of T lymphocytes, due to chronic immune stimulation within the cap of an atheroma, could lower the rate of collagen production both by lowering the number of collagen-producing SMCs and by inhibiting the rate of synthesis of those SMCs that survive.

Not only impaired synthesis of collagen, but also accelerated degradation of collagen and other matrix components, could contribute to the weakening of the fibrous cap.[38] The various components of the extracellular matrix, such as collagen, can be degraded by members of the superfamily of matrix metalloproteinases (MMPs). Notably, interstitial collagenase (MMP-1) can degrade the otherwise protease-resistant fibrillar collagen fibers into fragments, and another member of the family, 92–kD gelatinase (MMP-9), can extend the breakdown of the collagen fragments. Finally, a third member of the MMP family, stromelysin (MMP-3), has a broad spectrum, and can degrade other components of the extracellular matrix as well, including proteoglycans and elastin.

The potential of the MMPs for degrading the extracellular matrix is controlled at three levels: (1) transcriptional control of MMP synthesis; (2) activation of the secreted proenzyme forms of MMPs in the extracellular space; and (3) inhibition of the MMPs by specific molecules known as tissue inhibitors of metalloproteinases (TIMPs). In human carotid plaques, MMPs are expressed by SMCs, T lymphocytes, and macrophages.[49] Moreover, interstitial collagenase (MMP-1) is expressed by the endothelial cells that overlie carotid atheromas, but not by those that overlie normal vessels. Of special interest is the finding that the endothelial cells of the carotid plaque's rich microvasculature express this metalloproteinase.[49] In coronary atheromas, mast cells accompany such microvessels.[50] Such mast cells also contain chymase capable of activating MMP-1. Taken together, the above observations suggest a role for mast cells in facilitating the formation of new neovascular sprouts and perhaps increased susceptibility to intraplaque hemorrhage.

In vitro experiments with cultured cells have indicated that exposure to one or other of the potent proinflammatory cytokines, IL-1β and TNF-α, induces smooth muscle cells[51] and macrophages[52] to express MMPs. Moreover, animal experiments have revealed that macrophage-derived foam cells are induced to express these matrix-degrading enzymes, providing an interesting link between intracellular cholesterol accumulation and plaque vulnerability.[53] Regarding MMP activation in atherosclerotic plaques, it is likely that the plasmin produced by intimal macrophages is an important MMP-activating enzyme. MMP-3 may also play an important role by activating other members of the MMP family. Currently, emerging data are pointing to the importance of TIMP regulation in the delicate balance between MMP activation and inactivation, providing new therapeutic targets for the pharmacological control of plaque stabilization.[54]

Mast cells also appear to participate in the orchestration of matrix remodeling. These cells differ from the other cells of the intima in their very high content of neutral proteases.[55] The cytoplasmic secretory granules of mast cells store these proteases (chymase and tryptase) which, upon mast cell activation and ensuing degranulation, are released into the extracellular fluid. In contrast to the MMPs, chymase and tryptase are secreted as active enzymes, and are likely to act in the microenvironment of their parent cells. In addition to the enzymes, the cytoplasmic secretory granules contain macromolecular heparin and histamine, which are released from the activated mast cells along with the proteases. Experimental studies have shown that mast cell heparin proteoglycans can reduce the replication rate of SMCs, and that mast cell chymase can promote apoptosis of SMCs in vitro.[56] In addition, both chymase[57] and tryptase[58] can activate MMPs. TNF-α, which is capable of stimulating MMP synthesis by SMCs and macrophages, is also synthesized and secreted by the activated mast cells present in atherosclerotic lesions.[59] Support for the notion that mast cell proteases play a role in enhancing MMP activity in advanced atherosclerotic lesions of the carotid arteries was obtained recently, when stimulation of mast cells in fresh carotid endarterectomy samples led to increased MMP activity.[60] Thus, activated mast cells may trigger several mechanisms that tend to weaken the cap of a carotid atheroma and so predispose to a greater risk of plaque thrombosis. Mast cells are the major source of tissue heparin, and recent data imply that activation of vascular mast cells with ensuing secretion of heparin (macromolecular heparin) may locally attenuate the thrombogenicity of matrix collagen.[61] Thus, mast cells in atherosclerotic lesions appear not only to be involved in the pathogenesis of vascular injury but also to exert a physiological function by regulating hemostasis (local inhibition of platelet aggregation, but not adhesion) in the injured vascular wall.

Infection has been suggested to be one of the etiological factors causing plaque inflammation and predisposing to a greater risk of thrombotic complications in the plaques.[62,63] Indeed, seroepidemiological evidence links *Chlamydia pneumoniae* with the pathogenesis and natural history of coronary atherosclerosis.[64] More recent histopathological studies have revealed the presence of these micro-organisms in atherosclerotic plaques, and it is possible that the plaques become secondarily infected when they are invaded by circulating monocytes carrying within them infectious material such as *Chlamydia pneumoniae*.[65] Persisting infection within the plaque may then lead to persisting inflammation, and even weakening of the fibrous cap when macrophages become stimulated to synthesize and secrete MMPs. Recently, the heat shock protein (Hsp) component of *Chlamydia pneumoniae* was found to be present in human coronary atheromas, where it may induce macrophages to secrete MMP-9.[66] This new observation links Hsp with the late events of atherogenesis, and so extends an earlier hypothesis that Hsp is an early inductor of atherogenesis.[67] According to this interesting hypothesis, atherogenesis is a 'primary immunological reaction', in which hemodynamic, toxic, or viral stress to endothelial cells leads to expression of Hsp60 in the stressed endothelial cells and to an autoimmune reaction against the Hsp60. Such immune reactions to heat shock proteins could then participate in the initiation of atherogenesis, and act as a possible link between infection and atheroslerosis.[68] Indeed, antibodies against Hsp60 have been found in the sera of clinically healthy subjects with atherosclerotic lesions in their carotid arteries as measured by ultrasound.[67] Interestingly, the viral pathogenesis of atherosclerosis was proposed more than 20 years ago,[69] and further evidence was recently presented that infectious agents play a role in atherosclerosis of the carotid artery. Thus, in a study by Chiu and coworkers,[70] *Chlamydia pneumoniae*, cytomegalovirus, and herpes simplex virus were commonly detected in atherosclerotic plaques of the carotid arteries.

The immunological activation of a plaque is a complex phenomenon that also involves the complement system. Increased levels of serum immunoglobulins predict ruptures of coronary atherosclerotic plaques,[71] and circulating immunoglobulins are known to be deposited as immune complexes in atherosclerotic lesions, in which local activation of the complement system also takes place.[72] The complement system, again, can contribute significantly to the development and maintenance of the inflammatory response in the atherosclerotic lesions. Taken together, immunological activation of a plaque, involving both infection and inflammation, is the key element in converting a stable plaque into an unstable one.

INFLAMMATORY CELLS AND ADHESION MOLECULES IN CAROTID PLAQUES

As indicated above, inflammatory cells participate in the initiation and progression of atherosclerotic lesions. In regions where the adhesive properties of endothelial cells have been modified, circulating inflammatory cells adhere to the vessel wall and migrate into the subendothelial space. Several factors, including the presence of infectious agents in the atherosclerotic lesion, may induce emigration of inflammatory cells.[73] These cells, monocytes/macrophages, lymphocytes, and mast cells, are assumed to contribute to the initiation and progression of atherosclerotic plaques by secreting a variety of inflammatory mediators, e.g., cytokines and growth factors.

The general mechanisms that guide extravasation and accumulation of inflammatory cells in several diseases are also to be found in developing carotid plaques. Experimental studies and *in situ* analyses of human carotid artery plaques have revealed increased accumulation of inflammatory cells in the intimal space,[74] and several studies have shown that the severity of carotid artery disease in general correlates with the extent to which inflammatory cells accumulate.

An *in situ* analysis of high-grade stenosis in carotid arteries has revealed a correlation between the percentage of macrophage-rich areas and the presence of intimal T cells with clinical features of plaque destabilization.[46,74] Both recent ischemic symptoms and the occurrence of cerebral microembolization clinically verified by Doppler ultrasound monitoring are more frequent in plaques containing large numbers of inflammatory cells. Infiltration by macrophages and T cells is more pronounced in plaques that are predominantly lipid-rich (atheromatous) than in those that are fibrotic, and there is some correlation between the presence of inflammatory cell infiltration and surface ulceration and luminal thrombosis.

The distribution of macrophages within the carotid plaques is interesting. Significantly larger numbers of macrophages are detected in the proximal upstream parts of the plaques, whereas more SMCs are present in the downstream areas.[75] These cell types have been suggested to have opposite effects on plaque stability, regions with a high macrophage content being more prone to erosion and rupture. In line with this hypothesis, the sites of breakdown in ruptured plaques are more frequent in the upstream part. Thus, the progression of the plaques appears to be regulated not only by the total number of inflammatory cells, but also by their topological organization. Why the macrophages preferentially collect in the upstream part of the plaque is not entirely clear. Possibly, adhesion molecules in the vessel wall, which are required for transendothelial migration of inflammatory cells, are differently distributed within the plaque. The proximal region of a plaque is under high shear stress, whereas, at distal sites, low shear stress prevails. It is known that high shear stress upregulates the expression of some adhesion molecules, particularly ICAM-1, which is crucial for leukocyte emigration.[76] Also, thrombi preferentially develop in areas exposed to high stress (see later).

Adhesion of leukocytes to endothelial cells, followed by transendothelial migration, is a strictly controlled multistep process. It requires the interplay of adhesion molecules of several different types (Fig. 14.4).[77] The initial phase of adhesion is mediated by adhesion molecules of the selectin family (E-selectin and P-selectin on endothelial cells), which bind to fucosylated carbohydrate determinants on leukocytes. In the resting state, endothelial cells express negligible amounts of selectins, but their expression is upregulated by various cytokines, and also by thrombin. The selectin-mediated adhesion of circulating leukocytes occurs under high shear-stress, but is weak. It provides a high on-and-off rate, the results being that leukocytes roll along the endothelial surface. During this rolling stage, the leukocytes are activated by inflammatory mediators typically secreted by subendothelially located inflammatory cells, including macrophages and mast cells. This activation changes the functional state (low vs. high avidity) of the integrin receptors on the circulating leukocytes. Thus, an increase in the avidity state of the β2–integrins (CD11a/CD18 or LFA-1, CD11b/CD18 or Mac-1, CD11c/CD18 or p150/95) or the VLA-4 integrin (CD29d/CD49 or α4/β1) enables the leukocytes to bind to counter-receptors on the endothelial surface. The counter-receptors, which belong to the immunoglobulin superfamily, are ICAM-1 and ICAM-2 for LFA-1 and Mac-1, ICAM-1 for p150/95, and VCAM-1 for VLA-4. Mac-1 can also bind fibrin(ogen), which may be deposited on the endothelial surface (see Fig. 14.6b). The avidity of ICAMs and VCAM-1, unlike that of integrins, is not regulated. However, the ICAM and VCAM-1 adhesion pathways can be modulated by transcriptional control of the level of receptor expression. The adhesion between integrins and receptors belonging to the immunoglobulin family is stronger than between selectins and carbohydrates, and allows firm attachment of the leukocytes, providing a foothold for migration to intercellular junctions and, ultimately, for transendothelial migration, i.e. extravasation.

Immunohistochemical analysis of human carotid plaques and studies of animals have indicated that the general pattern of expression of the adhesion molecules required for leukocyte adhesion and extravasation takes place in carotid atherosclerotic lesions.[78,79] Analysis of the various endothelial cell adhesion molecules has indicated the presence of ICAM-1 in low-grade atherosclerotic lesions. On the other hand, only weak immunoreactivity for E-selectin and VCAM-1 has been detected. Normal arteries are negative for E-selectin and VCAM-1 staining. In fatty streaks and fibrofatty plaques (atheromas), some intimal VCAM-1 staining can be detected but endothe-

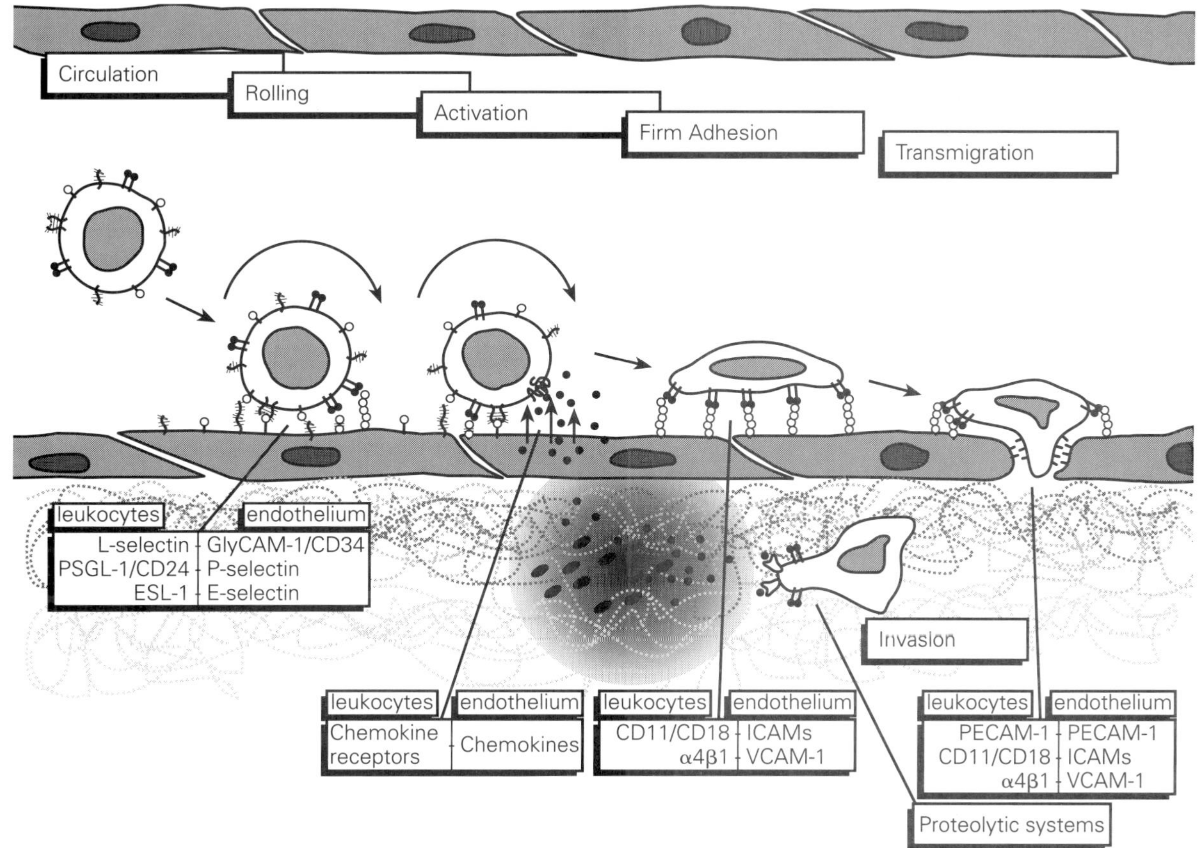

Figure 14.4 The model of sequential adhesion and extravasation of inflammatory cells
Initially, circulating leukocytes adhere to endothelial cells only transiently and roll down the endothelium. This stage involves an interaction between selectins and selectin ligands. During the rolling stage, inflammatory cells are activated by cytokines and/or chemokines, which leads to conformational activation of their integrin receptors CD11/CD18 and $\alpha4\beta1$. Expression on endothelial cells of the integrin counter receptors, ICAMs and VCAM-1, is regulated by shear stress and/or inflammatory mediators. The integrins provide a mechanism for firm adhesion and migration across the endothelium towards the intimal space of the carotid plaques. The molecules involved in each step are depicted in boxes.
The figure was kindly provided by Dr Leena Valmu, University of Helsinki.

lial reactivity is sparse. In contrast to VCAM-1 and E-selectin, some focal ICAM-1 immunoreactivity can be demonstrated in morphologically unaltered carotid bifurcations. In early lesions the expression is increased. The expression shows anatomical predilection, the lateral wall of the internal carotid artery expressing the most intense immunoreactivity and the lateral wall of the external carotid artery having weaker expression. ICAM-1 expression is present on the endothelial lining and also on the intimal smooth muscle cells.

In advanced plaques, expression of all three of the adhesion molecules mentioned above can be detected. However, the level of ICAM-1 is much higher than that of VCAM-1 or E-selectin.

Both ICAM-1 and E-selectin are present on the endothelial cells, whereas the expression of VCAM-1 is very weak. Smooth muscle cells express ICAM-1 and VCAM-1. Maximal ICAM-1 staining is present in macrophage-rich regions, a finding which is in line with the idea of an interplay between inflammatory cells and adhesion molecules. Endothelial cells overlying advanced atherosclerotic plaques show increased expression of ICAM-1.

The expression of ICAM-1 is increased at the carotid bifurcation, the predilection site of carotid atherosclerosis, a fact that is of special interest. The increased expression may be due, at least in part, to the strong shear force, a special feature of ICAM-1 being that it is upregulated under conditions of high shear stress.[76] This is understandable, since the promoter region of the ICAM-1 gene contains a transcriptional control element, the so-called shear stress element, which is responsive to shear stress. Thus, it is possible that the increased expression of ICAM-1, induced by shear stress, is one of the factors that initiate the atherosclerotic cascade which, by altering the properties of the endothelial surface, render it suitable for inflammatory cells to adhere and then emigrate into the intimal space. In more advanced stages, the expression of VCAM-1 and E-selectin, whose genes do not contain a shear response element, is increased, presumably by some other mechanism, such as increased local concentration of the inflammatory mediators IL-1, TNF-α, and IFN- γ, which are known to upregulate the expression of all three of these adhesion molecules.

An experimental animal model, in which the carotid artery shear stress was manipulated by surgically altering the diameter of the vessel lumen, has further verified the role of shear stress alterations in the expression of carotid artery adhesion molecules and in the endothelial adhesion of circulating monocytes.[80] In this model, the shear rate is reduced distal to the ligated carotid segment, and simultaneously, an increased flow rate is detected in the contralateral carotid artery. Since luminal narrowing occurs at sites of carotid plaques, the animal model has relevance to the atherosclerotic disease. It was observed that, expression of both VCAM-1 and ICAM-1 is sensitive to shear stress, although in different ways. Low shear stress upregulates VCAM-1 and downregulates ICAM-1, whereas both molecules are upregulated when shear stress is elevated.

Several studies have analyzed the alterations in adhesion molecule expression after carotid endarterectomy and the effect of anti-adhesion therapy with monoclonal antibodies in preventing the development of postoperative intimal hyperplasia.[81–83] These studies have shown that ICAM-1 expression is upregulated on regenerating vascular smooth muscle cells and on regenerating endothelial cells. Prevention of the β2–integrin/ICAM-1 interaction by a monoclonal antibody capable of blocking the function of ICAM-1 resulted in significant attenuation of intimal hyperplasia, although the study did not clarify the mechanism of inhibition. Similarly, inhibition of β2–integrin or VLA-4 function has been shown to reduce intimal thickening. The treatments also resulted in decreased accumulation of mononuclear leukocytes (monocytes and lymphocytes) and completely abolished the minimal influx of basophils and eosinophils.

The level of circulating adhesion molecules has been found to correlate with the severity of several diseases. The source and role of circulating adhesion molecules is poorly understood, but they may provide a mechanism for controlling adhesive events. Two recent studies have established a correlation between serum adhesion molecule levels and the severity of carotid atherosclerosis.[84,85] In one study, elevated levels of E-selectin expression were correlated with the acute stage of ischemic stroke and symptomatic carotid atherosclerosis, whereas no fluctuations were detected in serum ICAM-1 and serum VCAM-1 levels. Another study indicated a relationship between serum ICAM-1 and serum E-selectin and the degree of asymptomatic carotid atherosclerosis. The relatively small increase in serum levels and the poor specificity make it unlikely that circulating adhesion molecules could be used for clinical purposes to predict the outcome or severity of carotid atherosclerotic disease.

THROMBOSIS ON CAROTID PLAQUES

Thrombosis is a dynamic process. Platelets, by adhering to the surfaces of eroded or ruptured vessels, assemble the coagulation cascade on their membranes and effectively increase thrombus growth. Platelets and thrombin, the end product of coagulation activity, both proceed to stabilize the formed thrombus by converting soluble fibrinogen into insoluble fibrin, which rapidly binds plasminogen to its strands (Fig. 14.5). Simultaneously, in response to thrombin, the endothelial cells initiate fibrinolysis by liberating the tissue-type plasminogen activator, tPA. In turn, tPA activates fibrin-bound plasminogen, turning it into plasmin which degrades the fibrin strands unless they have been strongly cross-linked. This cross-linkage, with subsequent resistance to fibrinolysis, is also provided by the platelets. Thus, there are two interrelated but opposing mechanisms: first, the prothrombogenic and antifibrinolytic interphase excited by the platelets and the coagulation cascade; and second, the anticoagulant and fibrinolytic actions exerted by the adjacent endothelium.

These above interactions take place under considerable forces exerted by the arterial blood stream. Indeed, fluid dynamics play a crucial role in dictating the morphology of the forming thrombus.[86] Thus, in stasis or at low flow rates, such as occur in venous thrombosis, the prevailing activity is coagulation. In contrast, in the arterial lumen, thrombus formation is initially driven by platelets, and then also by markedly enhanced coagulation activity, as the flow becomes compromised by the growing thrombus. As a result, a thrombus tail develops with a high content of fibrin.[87] The shear forces also tend to break up the forming thrombus, and the stability of the clot depends on both thrombin generation and fibrinolytic activity exerted by the surrounding endothelial cells. Embolization occurs, leaving a highly thrombogenic surface on the initial breakage site,[88] while the embolized thrombus fragments cause further damage and even occlusion downstream. As an example, emboli causing stroke originate not only from carotid lesions but also from the atheromatous aortic arch.[89] At the site of injury, new platelets rapidly adhere to the clot, become activated, and lead to continuing coagulation activity. This may be a repetitive process: dynamic embolization and regrowth of the thrombus continue for long periods.

The three phases of thrombosis, i.e., platelet adhesion, triggering of the coagulation system, and activation of fibrinolysis, will be discussed separately below.

Platelet adhesion, activation, and aggregation

Within a few seconds of the erosion or rupture of an atheromatous plaque, platelets adhere with their specific adhesion receptors to the damaged vascular wall, which is normally sealed off beneath the endothelium.[90] The most thrombogenic elements of the wall are collagen, vonWillebrand factor, and fibrin(ogen).[91] In a superficial erosion, the platelets recognize type IV collagen in the basal lamina, and in deeper damage extending to the intima and media they adhere to type I and type III collagen, where smooth muscle cells have synthesized these matrix components. The vonWillebrand factor, which is the carrier of coagulation factor VIII, is deposited on collagen from plasma and is also secreted in abluminal sites by endothelial cells. Finally, fibrinogen has affinities for both the matrix and the forming clot, where active thrombin rapidly converts it into fibrin.

Flow characteristics affect platelet adhesion – the higher the shear forces, the more platelets initially adhere and then rapidly aggregate further platelets upon themselves, again shear-dependently.[86] The thrombogenicity of a high-grade (>50%) stenotic arterial tissue was demonstrated both in experimental models of thrombosis and in carotid lesions.[92] In extracorporeal circulation platelets, when subjected to stenotic flow chambers with an exposed medial aortic layer, accumulated in response to increasing severity of the stenosis (up to 80%) and seeded emboli which left the highly thrombogenic surface.[88] Furthermore, in patients with ulcerated carotid plaques, deposition of ^{111}indium-labeled platelets on plaques correlated

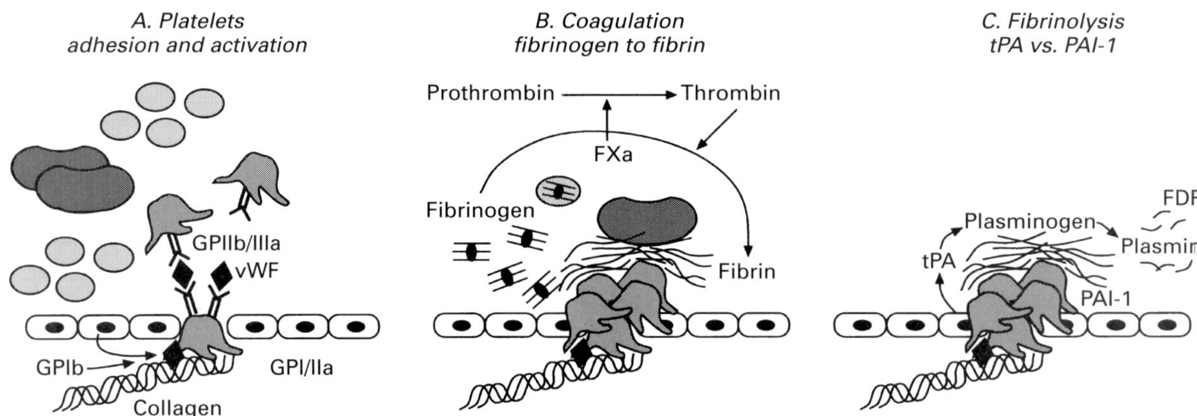

Figure 14.5 The three phases of arterial thrombosis.

(a) Mainly with the help of their adhesion receptors, glycoprotein (GP) Ia/IIa and GPIb, platelets adhere to exposed subendothelial collagen and von Willebrand factor (vWF), respectively. Adhesion triggers platelet activation and a conformational change in GPIIb/IIIa, the integrin receptor for soluble or immobilized von Willebrand factor and fibrinogen. Upon activation, this receptor becomes competent to bind these ligands and thus bridges platelets together to form platelet aggregates.

(b) Adherent platelets direct coagulation activity on the site of the vessel injury. The procoagulant alteration of the adherent platelet membranes enables sequential activation of the coagulation cascade, where activated factor X (FXa) cleaves prothrombin into thrombin, the key enzyme of the coagulation cascade. Thrombin turns soluble fibrinogen into insoluble fibrin, thus stabilizing the thrombus.

(c) In the presence of fibrin, plasminogen immediately binds to fibrin strands, rendering it susceptible to conversion into plasmin. Both fibrin and thrombin stimulate the endothelium to release tissue-type plasminogen activator (tPA), which cleaves plasminogen into plasmin. Plasmin degrades fibrin into soluble fibrin degradation products (FDP). Plasminogen activator inhibitor (PAI-1), the controller of tPA, also has a high affinity for fibrin, and so will regulate fibrinolysis in the vicinity. Platelets in the thrombus provide a rich source of PAI-1 and contribute significantly to the resistance to fibrinolysis.

positively with the severity of carotid stenosis.[93] Also, ulceration of a plaque with luminal thrombosis and stenosis of the internal carotid artery exceeding 70% seeds cerebral microemboli at high frequency.[94,95] The results of carotid artery surgery are beneficial especially in this group of patients with a high degree of carotid stenosis.[3]

At high shear rates, platelets, by adhering to the damaged vascular wall, orchestrate the subsequent sequences. These flow conditions and adhesive events activate other platelets and render them capable of recruiting new platelets from the blood stream to form a platelet-rich clot typical for arterial thrombi. Thus, platelet adhesion regulates the affinity state of platelet glycoprotein (GP) IIb/IIIa (integrin $\alpha_{IIb}\beta_3$) so that normally platelets and their ligands, namely vonWillebrand factor and fibrinogen, do not recognize each other, but after activation, the luminal face of the platelet attaches to these local ligands, which subsequently bridge several platelets to the injury site.[96] The resulting platelet aggregate grows rapidly by the action of local platelet activators, such as thrombin, adenosine diphosphate, platelet-activating factor, adrenaline, thromboxane A_2, and serotonin. The two latter, in addition to being platelet activators, also cause local vasoconstriction, which enhances the shear forces and activates the platelets still further.

Triggering of the coagulation cascade

The basic function of platelets is to transport the coagulation system to the site of vascular injury. By providing anionic phospholipids on their membrane surface after strong activation, such as is induced by collagen and thrombin together, or the final complement complex C5b-9, platelets become procoagulant and assemble the factors of the coagulation cascade on their surfaces in a coordinated fashion.[97] There are always trace amounts of thrombin available, and one of the crucial functions of thrombin is to activate anticoagulant mechanisms. Thus, thrombin regulates its own generation via three different mechanisms provided by endothelial cells, namely by binding to thrombomodulin and activating protein C, by binding to antithrombin III tethered by heparan sulfate, and by releasing the tissue factor pathway inhibitor, and inhibiting tissue factor–factor VIIa complex or even factor Xa directly[98,99] (Fig. 14.6).

These anticoagulant mechanisms are easily overcome during vascular injury, where in addition to the adherent platelets and their procoagulant membrane surface, large amounts of tissue factor are also exposed. Tissue factor is the membrane-bound accelerator of the extrinsic coagulation pathway, and the deeper the damage, the more tissue factor will be present. Finally, hemostasis is secured by the abundance of tissue factor in the adventitia.[100] Tissue factor binds to factor VIIa, which then activates both factors IX and X. Factor IXa is the necessary component of the tenase complex together with factor VIIIa to further amplify thrombin generation. Under the inflammatory conditions which prevail in atheromas, tissue factor generation is significantly enhanced. Finally, tissue macrophages markedly upregulate the synthesis of tissue factor during inflammation, rendering inflammatory states prothrombogenic. Furthermore, during inflammation, several of the anticoagulant mechanisms on the endothelium are downregulated, and thus thrombin generation predominates. Thrombin expresses P-selectin on endothelial cells and the leukocytes start to roll (Figs. 14.4 and 14.6b).[101,102] The fibrin formed offers a permanent specific attachment surface for leukocytes, thus further linking inflammation with coagulation.

Generation of thrombin from prothrombin is triggered by activated factor Xa in the prescence of a cofactor, factor V (the prothrombinase complex). In all, in the presence of prothrombin and factor Va, phospholipids accelerate the speed of thrombin generation 300 000–fold. The phospholipids are mainly provided by the platelets, but activated endothelial cells and leukocytes are also competent to maintain coagulation activity on their surfaces.[98] During thrombosis, thrombin acts mainly on fibrinogen and platelets. However, thrombin also induces endothelial cells and smooth muscle cells to participate in wound healing.

Thrombin tends to rapidly stabilize the clot by activating platelets. These mainly provide more clot-generating material and a greater catalyzing surface, and thereby further accelerate the generation of thrombin by positive feedback activation via cofactors VIII and V. Moreover, thrombin activates factor XIII, which cross-links the forming fibrin and provides resistance to fibrinolysis.

Fibrinolysis—the regulator of the thrombotic process

In arterial thrombi, the platelets provide strong resistance to fibrinolysis by their capacity to retract the clot, to cross-link fibrin via localizing active factor XIII and inactivate both tPA and plasmin with secreted plasminogen activator inhibitor-1 (Fig. 14.5) and α2-antiplasmin, respectively. Thus, when thrombin and fibrin are formed, tPA is released from the endothelium to initiate fibrinolysis,[103] but the more platelets the thrombus in question contains, the less susceptible it is to fibrinolysis. However, the fibrin component may be lysed, and the dynamic blood flow tends to seed emboli into the distal circulation. The tighter the stenosis, when exceeding 50%, the greater the number of emboli that will be seeded.[88,94,95]

The surfaces of the emboli themselves and the surfaces they leave behind are rough and contain high concentrations of active thrombin

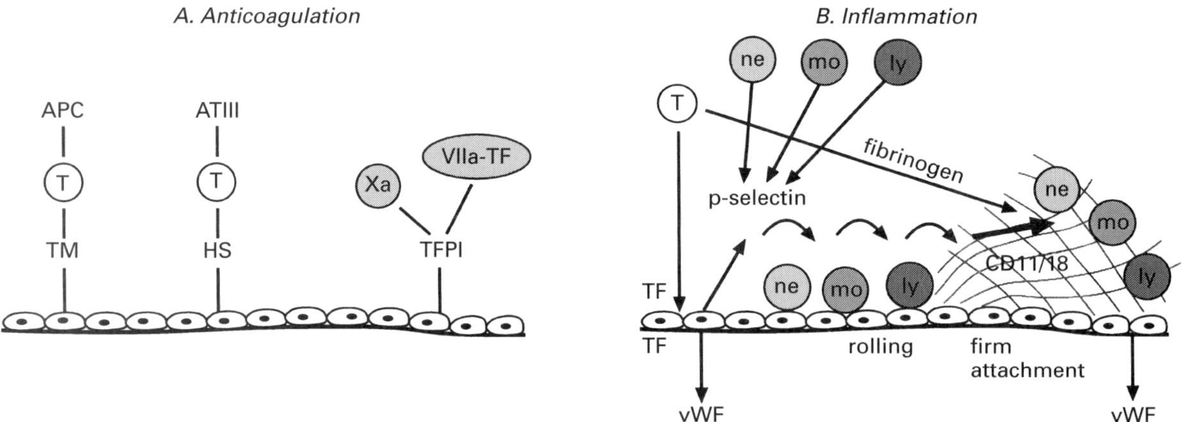

Figure 14.6 The opposite roles of endothelium: normally anticoagulant, but procoagulant during inflammation.

(a) Upon activation of the coagulation cascade and formation of thrombin, normal endothelial cells are anticoagulant and tend to inhibit thrombin formation. The endothelium is responsible for the control of the coagulation activity and thrombin formation by at least three different mechanisms.
   1. The thrombin (T) formed binds to thrombomodulin (TM) and this complex activates protein C (aPC). APC inactivates factors Va and VIIIa, thus inhibiting the formation of new thrombin.
   2. Locally, heparan sulfate proteoglycans (HS) on the endothelial surface enhance the inactivation potential of antithrombin III (AT III) towards thrombin and factor Xa, in the same way as systematically administered commercial heparins.
   3. The powerful tissue factor (TF)-induced extrinsic pathway of coagulation, including both the complex between TF and activated factor VII (TF–VIIa) and the subsequently activated factor X (Xa), is inhibited by the tissue factor pathway inhibitor (TFPI), which endothelial cells release.

(b) During inflammation, the anticoagulative capacity of the endothelium is reduced when both TM and HS are downregulated or shed. Endothelial cells also respond to inflammation by initiating synthesis of tissue factor. Secretion of vonWillebrand factor and P-selectin from the endothelial Weibel–Palade bodies induces adhesive cascades, not only for platelets, but also for inflammatory cells, neutrophils (ne), monocytes (mo), and lymphocytes (ly). These inflammatory cells start to roll on the endothelium. In this interphase between coagulation and inflammation, the fibrin strands formed provide firm attachment sites for the inflammatory cells. These cells have specific binding receptors, CD11/18 or Mac-1, which recognize fibrin. Furthermore, the inflammatory cells are competent to support thrombin generation on their membrane phospholipids. During inflammation, at least monocytes/macrophages add their synthesis of tissue factor, thus providing an additional positive feedback loop for the ongoing coagulation.

which, when in the fibrin mesh, is protected from its natural inactivator, i.e., antithrombin III. This thrombin activates platelets, and so supports thrombus growth and further generation of thrombin. Furthermore, after adhesion- and activation-triggered (costimulation with collagen and thrombin) alteration of the membrane, the platelets become procoagulant, and this is followed by microvesiculation associated with additional stimulation by shear forces, and also complement activation. Microvesicles derived from aggregating platelets contain P-selectin and they expose negatively charged phospholipids with procoagulant activity. Since these highly procoagulant and proinflammatory particles bind locally to clots exerting ongoing coagulative and inflammatory activity, they may well be linking coagulation and inflammation together.[104]

CONCLUSIONS

There are several overlapping pathobiological mechanisms which would explain how an obliterative lesion of the carotid artery can actually precipitate TIAs and strokes. When an asymptomatic plaque turns into a symptomatic one, the process involves not only the factors within the plaque, but also those of the circulating cells and factors of coagulation and the fibrinolytic system acting on the plaque. Importantly, the inflammatory cells of the plaque originate in the circulation and, when in the plaque, contribute to the initiation and progression of the plaque by secreting a variety of inflammatory mediators, cytokines, and growth factors. These agents may promote the pathogenetic cascade in multiple ways, such as modifying lipoproteins, stimulating smooth muscle cell growth, and altering the properties of the overlying endothelium. The cells also release matrix-degrading enzymes and thrombogenic substances, which may participate in the disruption of plaques and promote local thrombosis. Thus, the inflammation caused by circulatory blood cells that have migrated into the plaques may be critical in plaque destabilization, which manifests clinically as transient ischemic attacks and strokes.

In summary, insults to the endothelium resulting in its dysfunction are likely to be key factors in the initiation of the long term process eventually leading to clinically significant atherosclerosis.[105] Early changes in the endothelium lead to increased permeability to lipoproteins, and adherence and migration of monocytes and lymphocytes. In the subendothelial space, the monocytes are converted into macrophages, which then become lipid-laden and turn into foam cells. Some of these cells die and, with the extracellularly generated lipid droplets and lipid lakes, form a lipid core, also known as a necrotic core. Around the core, smooth muscle cells form a fibrous cap that separates the core from the lumen of the artery. This represents a type of healing process of the vessel wall injury.

Indeed, recent molecular and cell biology studies on the inflammatory processes continuously present in the lesions have revealed that one critical local process contributing to the pathogenesis of clinically significant carotid atherosclerosis is the release of metalloproteinases by macrophages, and of other proteolytic enzymes by mast cells. These enzymes cause degradation of the matrix, which can lead to hemorrhage from the vasa vasorum, causing intraplaque hemorrhage and softening of the plaque. Erosion of the endothelial lining or deep fissuring (rupture) of the plaque may then result, because it can no longer resist the shear force of the blood flow. Exposure of the thrombogenic subendothelial structures leads to thrombus formation and shedding of emboli, and sometimes even to local occlusion of the artery.

Hypercholesterolemia is an important risk factor for atherosclerosis, and the role of cholesterol as an essential component of atherosclerotic plaques was emphasized in this chapter. Indeed, the cholesterol-rich and the triglyceride-rich lipoproteins, when combined with ultrasound analysis, are good predictors of lipid-rich, rupture-prone plaques in the carotid artery.[34] However, lipid accumulation alone is insufficient to explain fully the long atherosclerotic process in the arteries and, as is well known, patients with severe carotid atherosclerosis and stenosis are often not hypercholesterolemic, yet they suffer TIAs and strokes.[106] Recently, reduction of stroke incidence was reported in a placebo-controlled trial in a large group of patients with a recent history of myocardial infarctions and moderately elevated LDL cholesterol, and who were treated with statins.[107] Interestingly, 85% of the subjects also used antiplatelet drugs. The statins are lipid lowering drugs, but their beneficial effects, which may potentially alter the natural course of cerebrovascular disease, are likely to be multimodal, some directly and others indirectly related to lipid lowering.[108] Properties of the latter type include plaque stabilization, suppression of inflammation, improvement of endothelial function, and reduced procoagulant platelet activation.

A challenge for future studies is to unravel the molecular mechanisms that explain the connection between certain risk factors and carotid atherosclerosis. The most important risk factors for cerebral ischemia include hypertension, cigarette smoking, and diabetes. These factors may well exert their harmful effects via the inflammatory mechanisms described in this chapter. Indeed, the results reported in this chapter support the concept that the key factor in the conversion of a stable atheroma into a labile, clinically significant atheroma is the strong inflammatory component typical of advanced carotid plaques. However, it should also be noted that inflamed atherosclerotic plaques may remain silent even until an advanced age.[109] Therefore, for atherosclerosis to turn into a clinically significant atherothrombotic disease, many still unknown factors must also play a role. Whether some of them are aggravating, and some protecting from, the potentially deleterious effects of systemic or local inflammation, remains to be discovered.

ACKNOWLEDGMENTS

We wish to thank Mrs. Jean Margaret Perttunen for editing the English of the manuscript.

REFERENCES

1. World Bank. *World Bank Development Report 1993. Investigating Health.* New York; Oxford University Press; 1993.
2. Timsit SG, Sacco RL, Mohr JP *et al.* Early clinical differentiation of cerebral infarction from severe atherosclerotic stenosis and cardioembolism. *Stroke* 1992; **23:**486–91.
3. Barnett HJM, Taylor DW, Aliasziw M *et al.* Benefit of carotid endarterectomy in patients with symptomatic moderate or severe stenosis. *N Engl J Med* 1998; **339:**1415–25.
4. Executive committee for the Asymptomatic Carotid Atherosclerosis Study. Endarterectomy for asymptomatic carotid artery stenosis. *J Am Med Assoc* 1995; **273:**1421–8.
5. Millikan CH, McDowell F, Easton JD. General pathophysiology and neuropathology of stroke. In: *Stroke* (Millikan CH, McDowell F, Easton JD, eds), pp. 33–61. Philadelphia; Lea & Febiger: 1987.
6. Baker AB, Dahl E, Sandler B. Cerebrovascular disease. Etiologic factors in cerebral infarction. *Neurology* 1963; **13:**445–54.
7. Mohr JP, Caplan LR, Melski JW *et al.* The Harvard cooperative stroke registry: a prospective registry. *Neurology* 1978; **28:**754–62.
8. Stehbens WE. Structure and pathophysiology of cerebral blood vessels. In: *Pathology of the Cerebral Blood Vessels,* (Stehbens WE, ed.) pp. 60–97. St. Louis; Mosby: 1972.
9. Stehbens WE. Localization of atherosclerotic lesions in relation to haemodynamics. In: *Atherosclerosis, Biology and Clinical Science,* (Olsson AG, ed.), pp. 175–82. Edinburgh; Churchill Livingstone: 1987.
10. Mosse PRL, Campbell GR, Campbell JH. Smooth muscle phenotypic expression in human carotid arteries. II. Atherosclerosis–free diffuse intimal thickenings compared with the media. *Arteriosclerosis* 1986; **6:**664–9.
11. Solberg LA, Eggen DA. Localization and sequence of development of atherosclerotic lesions in the carotid and vertebral arteries. *Circulation* 1971; **43:**711–24.
12. Solberg LA, McGarry PA, Moossy J *et al.* Distribution of cerebral atherosclerosis by geographic location, race and sex. *Lab Invest* 1968; **18:**604–12.
13. Stary HC, Chandler AB, Glagov S *et al.* A definition of initial, fatty streak, and intermediate lesions of atherosclerosis. A report from the Committee on Vascular Lesions of the Council on Arteriosclerosis, American Heart Association. *Arterioscler Thromb* 1994; **14:**840–56.
14. Stary HC, Chandler AB, Dinsmore RE *et al.* A definition of advanced types of atherosclerotic lesions and a histological classification of atherosclerosis. A report from the Committee on Vascular Lesions of the Council on Arteriosclerosis, American Heart Association. *Circulation* 1995; **92:**1355–74.
15. Smith EB. The relationship between plasma and tissue lipids in human atherosclerosis. *Adv Lipid Res* 1974; **12:**1–49.
16. Brown MS, Kovanen PT, Goldstein JL. Regulation of plasma cholesterol by lipoprotein receptors. *Science* 1981; **212:**628–35.

17. Brown MS, Goldstein JL. A receptor-mediated pathway for cholesterol homeostasis. *Science* 1986; **232:**34–47.
18. Reichl D, Postiglione A, Myant NB, Pflug JJ, Milis GL. The lipids and lipoproteins of human peripheral lymph, with observations on the transport of cholesterol from plasma and tissues into lymph. *Clin Sci Mol Med* 1973; **49:**419–26.
19. Smith EB. Transport, interactions and retention of plasma proteins in the intima: the barrier function of the internal elastic lamina. *Eur Heart J* 1990; **11**(Suppl E):72–81.
20. Camejo G, Hurt-Camejo E, Wiklund O, Bonjers G. Association of apo B lipoproteins with arterial proteoglycans: pathological significance and molecular basis. *Atherosclerosis* 1998; **139:**205–22.
21. Williams KJ, Tabas I. The response-to-retention hypothesis of atherogenesis reinforced. *Curr Opin Lipidol* 1998; **8:**471–4.
22. Ylä-Herttuala S, Rosenfeld ME, Parthasarathy S *et al.* Gene expression in macrophage-rich human atherosclerotic lesions. 15-lipoxygenase and acetyl low density lipoprotein receptor messenger RNA colocalize with oxidation specific lipid–protein adducts. *J Clin Invest* 1991; **87:**1146–52.
23. Brown MS, Goldstein JL. Lipoprotein metabolism in the macrophage: implications for cholesterol deposition in atherosclerosis. *Ann Rev Biochem* 1983; **52:**223–61.
24. Steinberg D, Parthasarathy S, Carew TE, Khoo JC, Witztum JL. Beyond cholesterol. Modifications of low-density lipoprotein that increase its atherogenicity. *N Engl J Med* 1989; **320:**915–24.
25. Krieger M, Hertz J. Structures and functions of multiligand lipoprotein receptors: macrophage scavenger receptor and LDL receptor-related protein (LRP). *Ann Rev Biochem* 1994; **63:**601–37.
26. Kruth HS. Cholesterol deposition in atherosclerotic lesions. In: *Subcellular Biochemistry, Vol. 28: Cholesterol: its Functions and Metabolism in Biology and Medicine* (Bittman R, ed.), pp. 319–62. New York; Plenum Press: 1997.
27. Paananen K, Saarinen J, Annila A, Kovanen PT. Proteolysis and fusion of low density lipoprotein particles strengthen their binding to aortic proteoglycans. *J Biol Chem* 1995; **270:**12257–62.
28. Pasquinelli G, Preda P, Vici M *et al.* Electron microscopy of lipid deposits in human atherosclerosis. *Scan Micros* 1989; **3:**1151–9.
29. Kovanen PT. Atheroma formation: defective control in the intimal round-trip of cholesterol. *Eur Heart J* 1990; **11** (Suppl E):238–46.
30. Tell GS, Crouse JR, Furberg CD. Relation between blood lipids, lipoproteins, and cerebrovascular atherosclerosis. *Stroke* 1988; **19:**423–30.
31. Guyton JR, Klemp KF, Black BL, Bocan TMA. Extracellular lipid deposition in atherosclerosis. *Eur Heart J* 1990; **11**(Suppl E):20–8.
32. Stary HC. The sequence of cell and matrix changes in atherosclerotic lesions of coronary arteries in the first forty years of life. *Eur Heart J* 1990; **11**(Suppl E):3–19.
33. Nordestgaard BG. The vascular endothelial barrier-selective retention of lipoproteins. *Curr Opin Lipidol* 1996; **7:**269–73.
34. Gronholdt M-LM. Ultrasound and lipoproteins as predictors of lipid-rich, rupture-prone plaques in the carotid artery. *Arterioscler Thromb Vasc Biol* 1999; **19:**2–13.
35. Zilversmit D. Atherogenesis—a postprandial phenomenon. *Circulation* 1979; **60:**473–85.
36. Mann JM, Davies MJ. Vulnerable plaque: relation of characteristics to degree of stenosis in human coronary arteries. *Circulation* 1996; **94:**928–31.
37. Falk E, Shah PK, Fuster V. Coronary plaque disruption. *Circulation* 1995; **92:**657–71.
38. Libby P, Molecular bases of the acute coronary syndromes. *Circulation* 1995; **91:**2844–50.
39. Farb A, Burke AP, Tang AL *et al.* Coronary plaque erosion without rupture into a lipid core. A frequent cause of coronary thrombosis in sudden cardiac death. *Circulation* 1996; **93:**1354–63.
40. van der Wal AC, Becker AE, van der Loos CM, Tigges AJ, Das PK. Fibrous and lipid-rich atherosclerotic plaques are part of interchangeable morphologies related to inflammation: a concept. *Coron Artery Dis* 1994;**5:**463–9.
41. Davies MJ, Richardson PD, Woolf N, Katz DR, Mann JM. Risk of thrombosis in human atherosclerotic plaques: role of extracellular lipid, macrophage and smooth muscle cell content. *Br Heart J* 1993; **69:**377–81.
42. Jonasson L, Holm J, Skalli O, Bondjers G, Hansson GK. Regional accumulation of T cells, macrophages, and smooth muscle cells in the human atherosclerotic plaque. *Arteriosclerosis* 1986; **6:**131–8.
43. Kaartinen M, Penttilä A, Kovanen PT. Accumulation of activated mast cells in the shoulder region of human coronary atheroma, the predilection site of atheromatous rupture. *Circulation* 1994; **90:**1669–78.
44. van der Wal AC, Becker AE, van der Loos CM,

Das PK. Site of intimal rupture or erosion of thrombosed coronary atherosclerotic plaques is characterized by an inflammatory process irrespective of the dominant plaque morphology. *Circulation* 1994; **89:**36–44.

45. Kovanen PT, Kaartinen M, Paavonen T. Infiltrates of activated mast cells at the site of coronary atheromatous erosion or rupture in myocardial infarction. *Circulation* 1995; **92:** 1084–8.
46. Carr SC, Farb A, Pearce WH, Virmani R, Yao JS. Activated inflammatory cells are associated with plaque rupture in carotid artery stenosis. *Surgery* 1997; **122:**757–63.
47. Hansson GK. Cell-mediated immunity in atherosclerosis. *Curr Opin Lipidol* 1997; **8:**301–11.
48. Frostegård J, Ulfgren A–K, Nyberg P *et al.* Cytokine expression in advanced human atherosclerotic plaques: dominance of proinflammatory (Th1) and macrophage-stimulating cytokines. *Atherosclerosis* 1999, in press.
49. Galis ZS, Sukhova GK, Lark MW, Libby P. Increased expression of matrix metalloproteinases and matrix degrading activity in vulnerable regions of human atherosclerotic plaques. *J Clin Invest* 1994; **94:**2493–503.
50. Kaartinen M, Penttilä A, Kovanen PT. Mast cells accompany microvessels in human coronary atheromas: implications for intimal neovascularization and hemorrhage. *Atherosclerosis* 1996; **123:**123–31.
51. Galis Z, Muszynski M, Sukhova G *et al.* Cytokine-stimulated human vascular smooth muscle cells synthesize a complement of enzymes required for extracellular matrix digestion. *Circ Res* 1994; **75:**181–9.
52. Saren P, Welgus HG, Kovanen PT. TNF-α and IL-1β selectively induce expression of 92-kDa gelatinase by human macrophages. *J Immunol* 1996; **157:**4159–65.
53. Galis Z, Sukhova G, Kranzhöfer R, Clark S, Libby P. Macrophage foam cells from experimental atheroma constitutively produce matrix-degrading proteinases. *Proc Natl Acad Sci USA* 1995; **92:**402–6.
54. Brown PD. Synthetic inhibitors of matrix metalloproteinases. In: *Matrix Metalloproteinases* (Parks WC, Mecham RP, eds), pp. 243–61. San Diego; Academic Press: 1998.
55. Kovanen PT. Role of mast cells in atherosclerosis. *Chem Immunol* 1995; **62:**132–70.
56. Wang Y, Kovanen PT. Heparin proteoglycans released from rat serosal mast cells inhibit proliferation of rat aortic smooth muscle cells in culture. *Circ Res* 1999; **84:**74–83.
57. Saarinen J, Kalkkinen N, Welgus HG, Kovanen PT. Activation of human interstitial procollagenase through direct cleavage of the Leu83–Thr84 bond by mast cell chymase. *J Biol Chem* 1994; **269:**18134–40.
58. Gruber BL, Marchese MJ, Suzuki K *et al.* Synovial procollagenase activation by human mast cell tryptase: dependence upon matrix metalloproteinase 3 activation. *J Clin Invest* 1989; **84:**1657–62.
59. Kaartinen M, Penttilä A, Kovanen PT. Mast cells in rupture-prone areas of human coronary atheromas produce and store TNF-α. *Circulation* 1996; **94:**2787–92.
60. Johnson JL, Jackson CL, Angelini GD, George SJ. Activation of matrix-degrading metalloproteinases by mast cell proteases in atherosclerotic plaques. *Arterioscler Thromb Vasc Biol* 1988; **18:**1707–15.
61. Lassila R, Lindstedt K, Kovanen PT. Native macromolecular heparin proteoglycans exocytosed from stimulated rat serosal mast cells strongly inhibit platelet–collagen interactions. *Arterioscler Thromb Vasc Biol* 1997; **17:**3578–87.
62. Pesonen E, Siitonen O. Acute myocardial infarction precipitated by infectious diseases. *Am Heart J* 1981; **101:**512–13.
63. Nieminen MS, Mattila K, Valtonen V. Infection and inflammation as a risk factor for myocardial infarction. *Eur Heart J* 1993; **14**(Suppl K):12–16.
64. Saikku P, Leinonen M, Mattila K *et al.* Serologic evidence of coronary artery disease and acute myocardial infarction. *Lancet* 1988; **2:**983–6.
65. Capron L. Chlamydia in coronary plaques: Hidden culprit or harmless hobo? *Nature Med* 1996; **2:**856–7.
66. Kol A, Sukhova GK, Lichtman AH, Libby P. Chlamydial heat shock protein 60 localizes in human atheroma and regulates macrophage tumor necrosis factor-α and matrix metalloproteinase expression. *Circulation* 1998; **98:**300–7.
67. Wick G, Schett G, Amberger A, Kleindienst R, Xu Q. Is atherosclerosis an immunologically mediated disease? *Immunol Today* 1995; **16:**27–33.
68. Mayr M, Metzler B, Kiechl S *et al.* Endothelial cytotoxity mediated by serum antibodies to heat shock proteins of *Escherichia coli* and *Chlamydia pneumoniae*. Immune reactions to heat shock proteins as a possible link between infection and atherosclerosis. *Circulation* 1999; **99:**1560–6.
69. Hajjar DP. Viral pathogenesis of atherosclerosis.

Am J Pathol 1991; **139:**1195–211.

70. Chiu B, Viira E, Tucker W, Fong IW. *Chlamydia pneumoniae*, cytomegalovirus, and herpes simplex virus in atherosclerosis of the carotid artery. *Circulation* 1997; **96:**2144–8.
71. Kovanen PT, Mänttäri M, Palosuo T, Manninen V, Aho K. Predictions of myocardial infarction in dyslipidemic men by elevated levels of immunoglobulin classes A, E, and G, but not M. *Arch Intern Med* 1998; **158:**1434–9.
72. Rus HG, Niculescu F, Constantinescu E, Cristea A, Vlaicu R. Immunoelectronmicroscopic localization of the terminal C5b–9 complement complex in human atherosclerotic fibrous plaque. *Atherosclerosis* 1986; **61:**35–42.
73. Libby P, Egan D, Skarlatos S. Roles of infectious agents in atherosclerosis and restenosis: an assessment of the evidence and need for future research. *Circulation* 1997; **96:**4095–103.
74. Jander S, Sitzer M, Schumann R *et al.* Inflammation in high-grade carotid stenosis: a possible role for macrophages and T cells in plaque destabilization. *Stroke* 1998; **29:**1625–30.
75. Dirksen MT, van der Wal AC, van den Berg FM, van der Loos CM, Becker AE. Distribution of inflammatory cells in atherosclerotic plaques relates to the direction of flow. *Circulation* 1998; **98:**2000–3.
76. Nagel T, Resnick N, Atkinson WJ, Dewey CF Jr, Gimbrone MA Jr. Shear stress selectively upregulates intercellular adhesion molecule-1 expression in cultured human vascular endothelial cells. *J Clin Invest* 1994; **94:**885–91.
77. Springer TA. Traffic signals on endothelium for lymphocyte recirculation and leukocyte emigration. *Annu Rev Physiol* 1995; **57:**827–72.
78. Endres M, Laufs U, Merz H, Kaps M. Focal expression of intercellular adhesion molecule-1 in the human carotid bifurcation. *Stroke* 1997; **28:**77–82.
79. DeGraba TJ, Siren AL, Penix L *et al*. Increased endothelial expression of intercellular adhesion molecule-1 in symptomatic versus asymptomatic human carotid atherosclerotic plaque. *Stroke* 1998; **29:**1405–10.
80. Walpola PL, Gotlieb AI, Cybulsky MI, Langille BL. Expression of ICAM-1 and VCAM-1 and monocyte adherence in arteries exposed to altered shear stress. *Arterioscler Thromb Vasc Biol* 1995; **15:**2–10.
81. Kling D, Fingerle J, Harlan JM, Lobb RR, Lang F. Mononuclear leukocytes invade rabbit arterial intima during thickening formation via CD18- and VLA-4-dependent mechanism and stimulate smooth muscle migration. *Circ Res* 1995; **77:**1121–8.
82. Kumar A, Hoover JL, Simmons CA, Lindner V, Shebuski RJ. Remodeling and neointimal formation in the carotid artery of normal and P-selectin-deficient mice. *Circulation* 1997; **96:**4333–42.
83. Yasukawa H, Imaizumi T, Matsuoka H, Nakashima A, Morimatsu M. Inhibition of intimal hyperplasia after balloon injury by antibodies to intercellular adhesion molecule-1 and lymphocyte function-associated antigen-1. *Circulation* 1997; **95:**1515–22.
84. Frijns CJ, Kappelle LJ, van Gijn J, Nieuwenhuis HK, Sixma JJ, Fijnheer R. Soluble adhesion molecules reflect endothelial cell activation in ischemic stroke and in carotid atherosclerosis. *Stroke* 1997; **28:**2214–18.
85. Hwang SJ, Ballantyne CM, Sharrett AR *et al.* Circulating adhesion molecules VCAM-1, ICAM-1, and E-selectin in carotid atherosclerosis and incident coronary heart disease cases: The Atherosclerosis Risk In Communities (ARIC) Study. *Circulation* 1997; **96:**4219–25
86. Ruggeri ZM. Mechanisms initiating thrombus formation. *Thromb Haemost* 1997; **78:**611–16.
87. Weiss H, Turitto VT, Baumgartner HR. Role of shear rate and platelets in promoting fibrin formation on rabbit subendothelium. *J Clin Invest* 1986; **78:**1072–8.
88. Lassila R, Badimon JJ, Vallabhajosula S, Badimon L. Dynamic monitoring of platelet deposition on severely damaged vessel wall during blood flow: effects of different stenoses on thrombus growth. *Arteriosclerosis* 1990; **10:**306–15.
89. The French Study of Aortic Plaques in Stroke Group. Atherosclerotic disease of the aortic arch as a risk factor for recurrent ischemic stroke. *N Engl J Med* 1996; **334:**1216–21.
90. Fuster V, Badimon L, Badimon JJ, Chesebro J. The pathogenesis of coronary artery disease and the acute coronary syndromes (part I). *N Engl J Med* 1992; **326:**245–50.
91. Sixma JJ, van Zanten GH, Saelman EUM *et al.* Platelet adhesion to collagen. *Thromb Haemost* 1995; **74:**454–9.
92. Siebler M, Sitzer M, Rose G, Bendfeldt D, Steinmetz H. Silent cerebral embolism caused by neurologically symptomatic high-grade carotid stenosis. *Brain* 1993;**116:**1005–15.
93. Moriwaki H, Matsumoto M, Handa N *et al.* Functional and anatomic evaluation of carotid

atherothrombosis. A combined study of Indium 111 platelet scintigraphy and B-mode ultrasonography. *Arterioscler Thromb Vasc Biol* 1995; **15:**2234–40.

94. Siebler M, Kleinschmidt A, Sitzer M, Steinmetz H, Freund H-J. Cerebral microembolism in symptomatic and asymptomatic high-grade internal carotid artery stenosis. *Neurology* 1994; **44:**615–18.
95. Sitzer M, Müller W, Siebler M *et al*. Plaque ulceration and lumen thrombus are the main source of cerebral microemboli in high-grade internal carotid artery stenosis. *Stroke* 1995; **26:**1231–33.
96. Coller BS. Blockade of platelet glycoprotein GIIb/IIIa receptors as an antithrombotic strategy. *Circulation* 1995; **92:**2373–80.
97. Bevers EM, Comfurius P, Zwaal RFA. Platelet procoagulant activity: physiological significance and mechanisms of exposure. *Blood Rev* 1991; **5:**146–56.
98. Mann K, Harker LA. Thrombosis and fibrinolysis. In: *Cardiovascular Thrombosis: Thrombocardiology and Thromboneurology* (Verstraete M, Fuster V, Topol EJ, eds), 2nd edn, pp. 1–22. Philadelphia; Lippincott-Raven Publishers: 1998.
99. Leung LLK, Gibbs GS. Modulation of thrombin's procoagulant and anticoagulant properties. *Thromb Haemost* 1997; **78:**577–80.
100. Rapaport SI, Rao LVM. The tissue factor pathway: how it has become a 'prima ballerina'. *Thromb Haemost* 1995; **74:**7–17.
101. Furie B, Furie BC. The molecular basis of platelet and endothelial cell interaction with neutrophils and monocytes: role of P-selectin and P-selectin ligand, PSGL-1. *Thromb Haemost* 1995; **74:**224–7.
102. Barkalow FJ, Goodman MJ, Gerritsen ME, Mayadas TN. Brain endothelium lack one of two pathways of P-selectin-mediated neutrophil adhesion. *Blood* 1996; **88:**4585–93.
103. Verstrate M. The fibrinolytic system: from Petri dishes to genetic engineering. *Thromb Haemost* 1995; **74:**25–35.
104. Siljander P, Carpén O, Lassila R. Platelet-derived microparticles associate with fibrin during thrombosis. *Blood* 1996; **87:**4651–63.
105. Ross R. Atherosclerosis – an inflammatory disease. *N Engl J Med* 1999; **340:**115–26.
106. Prospective Studies Collaboration. Cholesterol, diastolic blood pressure, and stroke: 13,000 strokes in 450,000 people in 45 prospective cohorts. *Lancet* 1995; **346:**1647–53.
107. Plehn JF, Davis BR, Sacks FM *et al*. Reduction of stroke incidence after myocardial infarction with pravastatin. The Cholesterol and Recurrent Events (CARE) Study. *Circulation* 1999; **99:**216–23.
108. Furberg CD. Natural statins and stroke risk. *Circulation* 1999; **99:**185–8.
109. Pasterkamp G, Schoneveld AH, van der Wal AC *et al*. Inflammation of the atherosclerotic cap and shoulder of the plaque is a common and locally observed feature in unruptured plaques of femoral and coronary arteries. *Arterioscler Thromb Vasc Biol* 1999; **19:**54–8.

15

Surgical and medical therapy in asymptomatic carotid lesions

Antonio Carolei and Carmine Marini

CONTENTS • **Introduction** • **Pathology** • **Diagnostic investigations** • **Surgical therapy** • **Angioplasty** • **Medical therapy**

INTRODUCTION

Carotid artery stenosis represents a major etiological determinant of focal cerebral ischemia that may remain undiagnosed until the occurrence of the first-ever stroke in most of the cases.[1] Asymptomatic carotid stenosis is commonly detected either incidentally or in the presence of a cervical bruit. A reduction in the vessel lumen diameter greater than 50% affects between 2 and 14% of the asymptomatic population over 65 years of age.[2–5] Prevalence rates range from 0.5% in individuals under 60 years of age to 10% in those over 80.[3,5]

Patients with asymptomatic carotid stenosis are at higher risk for ischemic stroke, myocardial infarction, and vascular death compared with those without carotid disease, even if the risk of stroke is lower than in patients with symptomatic stenosis.[6–13] Prognosis depends on lesion morphology and comorbidity. In patients with less than 50% carotid stenosis the risk of stroke is low while in the presence of a stenosis greater than 75% the overall annual risk of stroke ranges between 3 and 5%, the annual risk of ipsilateral stroke is 2.5%, while the annual risk of myocardial infarction is even greater (5–9%).[12–16] Rapid progression of the asymptomatic carotid lesion is associated with a risk of transient ischemic attack (TIA) and stroke as high as 18% while arterial occlusion is associated with a stroke risk of 20–30%.[15,17–20] Unstable or ulcerated plaques that carry the worse prognosis in symptomatic patients might also add to the risk of asymptomatic patients.[14,17,21–26] Morphological variations in the circle of Willis, as well as the presence of a concomitant severe stenosis or occlusion in the posterior circulation or in the contralateral carotid artery, also add to the stroke risk.[27–29] The presence of lesions on CT and MRI scans in 20% of the asymptomatic patients is associated with a worse outcome.[30] According to some predictive models, a combination of multiple recognized vascular risk factors and of signs or symptoms of cerebral, coronary, and peripheral vascular involvement increases by several times the risk for an individual patient.[31]

PATHOLOGY

Early carotid lesions occur most often in the posterolateral wall of the carotid bulb in the presence of high and low shear zones, and progress to stenosing plaques under the influence of known risk factors, such as hypertension, diabetes mellitus, cigarette smoking, and blood lipids.[32,33]

Carotid plaques in asymptomatic patients

are mostly fibrous and produce low grade stenosis while plaques in symptomatic patients are predominantly lipidic, with intraplaque hemorrhage, ulceration, and associated endoluminal thrombi.[21,23,24,34,35] The fibrous cap of the plaque, the cholesterol crystals of the core, and the breakdown products of hemorrhage all represent potential sources of emboli.[18]

Clinically silent cerebral infarctions, mostly in silent areas of the brain, are often associated with asymptomatic carotid stenosis.[24,30,36] Slow growing fibrous plaques in the presence of a good collateral circulation may remain asymptomatic even if they cause occlusion, while rapidly expanding plaques, because of intraplaque hemorrhage, are more likely to cause symptoms. Tandem intracranial lesions may contribute to the stroke risk by reducing the cerebral collateral reserve.[37,38]

DIAGNOSTIC INVESTIGATIONS

Investigations in patients with asymptomatic carotid stenosis largely depend on medical history and physical examination. Markers of atherothrombotic disease include: irregular pulse; hypertension; blood pressure differences between arms; funduscopic findings; abnormal heart sounds or murmurs; carotid, vertebral, subclavian, renal and iliofemoral bruits; and the absence of pulses. A cervical bruit, loudest in the middle and upper cervical region, is related to severe stenosis in up to 30% of the patients, while the absence of a bruit does not exclude a severe stenosis.[12,39]

Duplex ultrasonography, combining B-mode ultrasound and Doppler spectral analysis, has become the standard non-invasive test for the assessment of carotid lesions. B-mode ultrasound helps to detect early carotid disease and to define the density and composition of the carotid plaque, while spectral analysis is necessary to quantify various degrees of carotid stenosis.[31] Despite its high reliability, the accuracy of duplex scanning is operator-dependent.

In patients considered for carotid endarterectomy, angiography is recommended, being indicated for patients undergoing surgery, or when non-invasive tests have provided insufficient information for clinical management.[31] Magnetic resonance angiography (MRA) may help to define a carotid stenosis.[40] High resolution spiral CT scanning may also provide high quality imaging of the carotid arteries.

Brain CT may identify clinically silent cerebral infarctions, although MRI is more sensitive in detecting earlier and smaller areas of infarction.[41] Transcranial Doppler (TCD) may provide information regarding the adequacy of the intracranial circulation and help to predict clinical outcome.[24,42] Positron emission tomography and single photon emission computed tomography have improved our understanding of cerebral functioning, but they did not prove useful for patient management.[31]

Assessment of cardiac and renal function should be provided in all patients with carotid disease. Coexisting silent coronary artery disease contributes to the majority of the perioperative and most of the delayed mortality in patients undergoing carotid endarterectomy.[43,44] The presence of risk factors, such as age over 70 years, previous myocardial infarction, diabetes mellitus, angina, and congestive heart failure, help to identify patients in whom specific preoperative screening tests for coronary artery disease are required.[45] Tests may include 24 h Holter monitoring, treadmill testing, dipyridamole thallium scanning, and two-dimensional stress test using dipyridamole or dobutamine.[46–51] Patients with positive tests and those with evidence of coronary artery disease should be considered for coronary angiography.

SURGICAL THERAPY

Trials of surgical therapy

According to data from the National Hospital Discharge Survey,[52,53] the number of carotid endarterectomies performed in the United States stopped declining and increased again up to 91 000 in 1992, after the publication of two trials demonstrating a marked benefit of carotid endarterectomy in symptomatic patients with severe stenosis.[9,10,54–56] Unfortunately, data on carotid endarterectomies performed in patients with asymptomatic carotid stenosis are scanty. Recent reports estimated a proportion of carotid endarterectomies performed in the United States for asymptomatic stenosis ranging from 9 to 60%.[53,57–60] These estimates varied by surgeon, hospital, and geographical location and reflected the lack of specific guidelines.[53]

The first trial of carotid endarterectomy for asymptomatic carotid stenosis in patients with cervical bruits and abnormal ocular pneumoplethysmography was published in 1984.[61] Twenty-nine out of 57 eligible patients were randomized either to arteriography and surgery or to 650 mg aspirin twice daily. Eleven of the 15 patients in the surgical group (73%) and four of the 14 in the medical group (29%) had surgery. No perioperative strokes or deaths and no strokes during the follow-up were reported in either group. Three patients in the surgical and one in the medical group died during follow-up. The study was too small to draw any valid conclusions.[53]

The Carotid Artery Stenosis with Asymptomatic Narrowing: Operation Versus Aspirin (CASANOVA) trial was a randomized, multicenter study of patients with moderate asymptomatic stenosis (50–90% reduction in lumen diameter).[62] Rather than a trial of surgical vs. medical therapy, this study was a comparison between two different intervention policies, that is, immediate prophylactic surgery vs. selective delayed surgery for bilateral carotid lesions, progression of unilateral stenosis up to 90% or greater, progression of contralateral lesions up to 50% or greater, or development of symptoms.[62–64] All patients were treated with a combination of 330 mg aspirin and 75 mg dipyridamole three times daily. Of the 206 patients randomized to immediate surgery, 83% had at least one carotid endarterectomy, whereas of the 202 patients assigned to selective surgery, 20% had immediate carotid endarterectomy and 22% had carotid endarterectomy during the follow-up. No significant outcome differences were found between the treatment groups.[62] Stroke and death occurred as a complication of surgery in 3.0% of the patients, with an overall 1.2% perioperative mortality risk. The study was widely criticized because of its methodological failings and the insufficient statistical power to detect even large differences.[63,65]

The Mayo Asymptomatic Carotid Endarterectomy Trial randomized patients to either surgical treatment with carotid endarterectomy avoiding antiplatelet therapy, or to medical treatment with 80 mg aspirin daily.[66,67] The trial was terminated early, after only 71 patients had been randomized, because of a significantly higher number of TIAs and myocardial infarctions in the surgical than in the medical group that were attributed to lack of prophylactic antiplatelet therapy.[65,67]

The Veterans Affairs Cooperative Study was a randomized, controlled clinical trial performed in elderly, male veterans with asymptomatic stenosis (at least 50% reduction in lumen diameter) of the internal carotid artery.[16,68] Out of 1935 screened patients, 444 (23%) were randomly assigned to carotid endarterectomy plus optimal medical therapy or to medical therapy alone. In the surgical group, 195 patients had unilateral carotid endarterectomy, eight had staged bilateral procedures, and eight refused surgery after randomization. The recommended aspirin dose was 650 mg twice daily. Thirty-day perioperative mortality was 1.9% and the 30-day combined stroke and mortality rate was 4.3%. All perioperative deaths were attributed to cardiac causes, although one patient who died also had a stroke.[44] During a mean follow-up of 48 months, the combined incidence of ipsilateral stroke and TIA was 8% in the surgical group and 20.6% in the medical group, with an absolute risk reduction of 12.6% in the former group.[16] However, the inclusion of TIA as an end point was criticized as representing a possible source of observational bias and because the reduction of a non-disabling event does not justify perioperative morbidity and mortality as high as 4.3%.[65,69,70] Incidence of stroke and death was not different between the two treatment groups, within a sample size that was inadequate to provide a sufficient study power.

The Asymptomatic Carotid Atherosclerosis Study (ACAS) is the last published prospective multicenter, randomized trial of carotid endarterectomy in patients with asymptomatic carotid stenosis greater than 60%.[71,72] From among 42 000 patients screened, 1662 eligible patients (4%) were randomized to receive either medical treatment, consisting of risk factor control and 325 mg aspirin daily, or carotid endarterectomy plus medical treatment. Of the 828 patients included in the surgical group, 101 subsequently refused, whereas 45 patients of the 834 in the medical group had carotid endarterectomy. A procedure-related stroke developed in a small proportion (1.2%) of the 414 patients who underwent arteriography to verify the degree of stenosis and to exclude contraindications to endarterectomy, such as distal tandem lesions. During the perioperative period, 2.3% of the surgical patients had a stroke or died. The trial was stopped early after a statistically significant result was obtained in favor of surgery.[72] The cumulative 5-year risk of any perioperative stroke or death and of ipsilateral stroke during the follow-up was 11% for the medical group and 5.1% for the surgical group, with a 5.9% absolute risk reduction and a 53% relative risk reduction. As suggested, the incidence of cerebral infarction was reduced by carotid endarterectomy provided that stringent quality control measures were used to reduce surgical morbidity and mortality.[72] Despite the apparently straightforward methodology, the ACAS trial raised concerns about the choice and analysis of the primary endpoint (that was modified after the study started and the Veterans Affairs study was published), the early stopping of the trial, and the prominence given to relative risk reduction in the evaluation of the claimed overall benefit.[60,73,74] Indeed, the 5.9% absolute risk reduction within 5 years was small, whereas the immediate combined risk of arteriography and surgery reached 2.3%.[53]

Overview analysis

Considering that all the reported trials were flawed by insufficient study power, a meta-analysis was necessary in order to assess quantitatively the efficacy and safety of carotid endarterectomy in patients with asymptomatic stenosis.[75] Several searching strategies of all available sources were used to identify published and unpublished trials, in any language, that evaluated the efficacy of carotid endarterectomy in patients with asymptomatic carotid lesions. To be included in the meta-analysis: studies had to be randomized, controlled trials; they had to include patients with 50–99% asymptomatic carotid stenosis on ultrasonography or arteriography, either with no history of cerebrovascular disease or with previous strokes or TIAs in the vertebrobasilar circulation or in the contralateral carotid territory; and they had to compare medical treatment alone and endarterectomy with or without concomitant medical treatment.[75] Six randomized, controlled trials, including a study not fully published, were identified for potential inclusion (Table 15.1).[16,61,62,67,72,76] The CASANOVA study was excluded because its protocol precluded direct comparison of the results with the other studies.[62]

A total of 1215 patients were randomized to carotid endarterectomy and in 1225, carotid endarterectomy was withheld.[75] The follow-up varied from 2 to 5 years, with an overall mean of 3.1 years. Seventy-four per cent of patients were men and the mean age ranged from 64 to 67 years. Stenosis was initially assessed by Doppler ultrasonography in all trials but one, which combined oculoplethysmography and intra-arterial catheter angiography. Antiplatelet agents were advocated for both medically-treated patients and those assigned to carotid endarterectomy in three trials.[16,72,76] In the largest two, about one-third of the patients had symptoms or endarterectomy on the side contralateral to the qualifying asymptomatic carotid stenosis.[16,72]

The occurrence of the composite endpoint of perioperative stroke or death and ipsilateral stroke was 6.4% for the medically-treated patients and was reduced among patients allocated to carotid endarterectomy (odds ratio (OR) 0.62; 95% confidence interval (CI) 0.44–0.86) with no significant heterogeneity across the

Table 15.1 Characteristics of clinical trials of endarterectomy for asymptomatic carotid stenosis

Study	No. of patients	% of men	Mean age (years)	Mean follow-up (years)	Degree of stenosis (%)	Angiography (patients)	Aspirin (mg/day)	
							Surgical group	Medical group
Clagett *et al.*[60]	29	72	64	3	72	Surgical	None	1300
MACE[66]	71	58	NR	2	⩾50	Surgical	None	80
VA[15]	444	100	65	4	⩾50	All	1300	1300
ACAS[71]	1659	66	67	2.7	⩾60	Surgical	325	325
L'AURC[74]	237	73	64	5	⩾70	Surgical	1000	1000
CASANOVA[61]	410	73	55	3	⩾50 to ⩽90	All	975	975

Modified from Benavente *et al.*[75]
MACE = Mayo Asymptomatic Carotid Endarterectomy Trial; VA = Veterans Affairs Cooperative Study; ACAS = Asymptomatic Carotid Atherosclerosis Study; L'AURC = French L'AURC trial (unpublished); CASANOVA = Carotid Artery Stenosis with Asymptomatic Narrowing: Operation Versus Aspirin trial; NR = not reported.

Table 15.2 Effectiveness of endarterectomy for asymptomatic carotid stenosis

Study	*Surgical group %*	*Medical group %*	*Odds ratio*	*95% CI*
Ipsilateral stroke plus perioperative stroke or death				
Clagett *et al.*[60]	0	0	—	—
MACE[66]	8.33	0	—	—
VA[15]	7.58	10.30	0.71	0.37–1.38
ACAS[71]	4.00	6.24	0.63	0.40–0.98
L'AURC[74]	3.91	13.76	0.25	0.10–0.68
Total	4.40	6.40	0.62	0.44–0.86
All ipsilateral stroke (including perioperative)				
Clagett *et al.*[60]	0	0	—	—
MACE[66]	5.55	0	—	—
VA[15]	4.74	9.44	0.48	0.22–1.02
ACAS[71]	2.91	6.00	0.47	0.29–0.76
L'AURC[74]	3.13	13.76	0.20	0.07–0.57
Total	3.20	6.20	0.46	0.32–0.66
All stroke and perioperative stroke or death				
Clagett *et al.*[60]	0	0	—	—
MACE[66]	8.33	0	—	—
VA[15]	9.48	12.45	0.74	0.40–1.34
ACAS[71]	7.27	10.31	0.68	0.48–0.96
L'AURC[74]	6.25	14.68	0.39	0.16–0.92
Total	7.40	9.20	0.68	0.51–0.90

Modified from Benavente *et al.*[75]
MACE = Mayo Asymptomatic Carotid Endarterectomy Trial; VA = Veterans Affairs Cooperative Study; ACAS = Asymptomatic Carotid Atherosclerosis Study; L'AURC = French L'AURC trial (unpublished).

considered trials (Table 15.2, Fig. 15.1).[75] The absolute risk reduction after endarterectomy was about 2% over an average follow-up of 3.1 years. Consistent and significant risk reductions after carotid endarterectomy were also observed when considering ipsilateral stroke only (OR 0.46) or all strokes plus perioperative stroke or death (OR 0.68).[75]

Therefore, despite important differences among the studies, regarding the number of included patients and methodology, the results of this meta-analysis convincingly showed that carotid endarterectomy reduces the risk of stroke ipsilateral to the asymptomatic carotid stenosis. However, the magnitude of the benefit was not large. Assuming the 6.4% adjusted rate of perioperative stroke or death and of ipsilateral stroke in the non-surgical group, and the 2% absolute risk reduction by carotid endarterectomy, about 50 patients should be

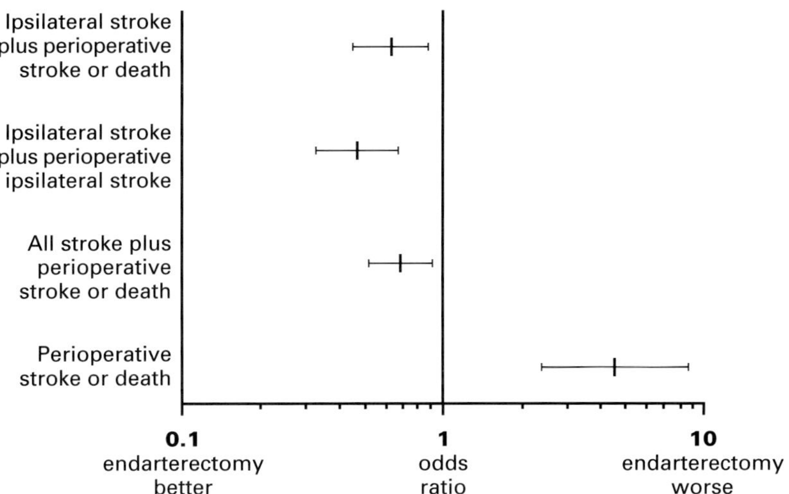

Figure 15.1 Effectiveness of carotid endarterectomy in asymptomatic patients on different outcomes

operated on to prevent a disabling or non-disabling stroke, or death, over an average 3.1 years of follow-up.[77] Based on these results, carotid endarterectomy should not be routinely recommended for unselected patients with asymptomatic carotid stenosis. On the other hand, if the risk of ipsilateral ischemic stroke associated with carotid stenosis persists in the unoperated patient for more than just 3 years, the benefit of endarterectomy may go on accruing for many years, reducing the number of patients who need to be treated to prevent one event. Moreover, it seems likely that specific subgroups of patients with asymptomatic carotid stenosis with a high incidence of ipsilateral stroke might substantially benefit from carotid endarterectomy.[78,79]

Safety requirements

Endarterectomy for asymptomatic carotid disease is a prophylactic operation. The potential risks of the operation are death and brain damage, the same events that the operation is designed to prevent. The efficacy of surgery may become apparent only if the operation can be performed with a very low risk. Death and stroke related to carotid endarterectomy are significantly lower in patients with asymptomatic than in patients with symptomatic carotid stenosis.[80] In fact, the positive results of endarterectomy in asymptomatic patients heavily depended on a very low combined perioperative stroke and mortality rate of 2.3%, achieved through surgeon selection and medical assistance during the perioperative period. However, community-based studies reported rates of perioperative stroke and death after endarterectomy in asymptomatic patients, ranging from 3.2 to 6.9%.[44,80–83] For these reasons, the marginal benefit shown by the procedure cannot be warranted in general practice.

Operations for asymptomatic carotid stenosis should be performed by surgeons of proven ability who must have completed a training program, must be familiar with methods for protecting cerebral circulation, vascular reconstruction and intraoperative assessment, and must be able to identify patients at higher risk. Since different surgical techniques are acceptable, individual surgeons should be encouraged to use those surgical techniques which provide the lowest morbidity and mortality and the best long-term results. The institutions in which carotid endarterectomy is performed should possess their own diagnostic facilities, and adequate emergency and perioperative nursing care.[31]

Few data are available on factors affecting the risk of endarterectomy outside the setting of a randomized, controlled trial.[31] Postoperative stroke and death were more frequent in women (5.3%) than in men (1.6%), in those aged 75 years or older (7.8%), and in those with a past history of congestive heart failure (8.6%). Other prognostic factors include coronary heart disease, presence of carotid plaque ulceration, mural thrombi or occlusion, diseases in the collateral circulation, recent infarcts in the brain, and severe uncontrolled hypertension.[31] Knowledge of these factors may help to assess the individual's postoperative risk better and therefore the anticipated benefit of surgery.[84]

Several measures have been suggested to ensure a high standard of surgical performance to all patients subjected to endarterectomy. The Ad hoc Committee of the American Heart Association[85] defined the upper limits for morbidity and mortality associated with carotid endarterectomy in patients with asymptomatic carotid stenosis. As suggested, the 30-day mortality rate from all causes should not exceed 2% and the combined stroke morbidity and mortality during or after carotid endarterectomy should be less than 3%.[85,86] The American Heart Association Consensus Conference[30] expanded these recommendations and suggested an auditing of the individual surgeons. Such an audit should include a registry of the results of all carotid endarterectomies together with all major complications and should establish the acceptable yearly surgical volume and perioperative morbidity and mortality.

In the ACAS trial, the criteria for auditing potential surgeons to be included into the study required the performance of at least 12 carotid endarterectomies per year and documentation of combined morbidity and mortality data referring to the last 50 consecutive carotid endarterectomies.[87] The success of the ACAS trial investigators in minimizing perioperative morbidity and mortality rates confirms the validity of the approach. Therefore, the widespread application of some quality controls may warrant the appropriate selection of surgeons who are justified to perform carotid endarterectomy in asymptomatic patients, while the failure of surgeons to meet minimum performance standards might raise concerns about informed consent and standard of care.[31,53]

Clinical indications

A very careful patient selection for low surgical risk allowed the inclusion of 4% of the screened patients in the ACAS trial.[72] This study included patients aged between 40 and 79 years; without previous cerebrovascular events in the carotid or vertebrobasilar arterial systems; without symptoms referable to the contralateral carotid territory within the previous 45 days; without contraindication to aspirin treatment; without disorders that could seriously complicate surgery; and without any condition likely to produce disability or death within 5 years.[72,88] Any extension of the indications of carotid endarterectomy beyond these eligibility requirements is inappropriate. In particular, if because of age and comorbidity, a patient is unlikely to survive long enough to reach the potential long-term benefits of surgical treatment, surgery should not be performed since such patients would only be exposed to a greater short-term risk. For women, available data do not support a favorable risk–benefit profile.

In patients with asymptomatic carotid artery stenosis, diagnostic work-up may identify plaque changes that may eventually predict symptoms, such as stenosis progression, particularly when it exceeds 80%, intraplaque hemorrhage, and the presence of a fresh thrombus.[89] All these observations may help to identify patients who should undergo carotid endarterectomy.

There is general consensus that population screening of truly asymptomatic patients is not worthwhile.[11,60,90,91] In fact, a screen-and-treat strategy requiring non-invasive tests on every healthy individual and carotid angiography on patients with a positive test, and finally performing endarterectomy on patients with internal carotid artery stenosis greater than 60%, would result in more ipsilateral strokes or deaths than the alternative strategy of not screening. The explanation relies on the low prevalence of a carotid stenosis greater than 60% in asymptomatic patients (5%), possible false-positive results of screening tests, and patient harm related to angiography.[92] Moreover, the majority of the adverse events using the screen-and-treat strategy would occur immediately, whereas adverse events using the alternative strategy may occur much more uniformly during the subsequent years.

When managing a patient with a positive screening test for severe asymptomatic carotid stenosis, one should consider the balance between the probability of being harmed rather than being helped by being referred for further tests or surgery, depending on the predictive power of the screening test, the risk of diagnostic and surgical procedures, and the potential benefit of surgery.[93] For a patient under 60 years of age with no additional risk factors, presenting to a clinic with a positive test, the probability of being a false-positive is about 88%, due to the 93% average specificity of screening tests and the low prevalence of asymptomatic carotid stenosis in the general population (approximately 1%).[93] Much higher prevalence of asymptomatic carotid stenosis ranging from 14 to 28% has been estimated in elderly patients who are current smokers, with hypertension, peripheral vascular disease, carotid bruit, or atrial fibrillation.[9,94] Only at a prevalence of over 20% were significant benefits reported.[93] However, even in these high prevalence groups, further screening and surgery would have limited public health impact, with at best 100 screened individuals needed to prevent one stroke.

Combined surgery

Elective coronary artery bypass grafting is performed in increasing proportions of elderly and high-risk patients in which the incidence of perioperative stroke morbidity is increased and preoperative screening programs often detect relevant asymptomatic carotid stenoses.[95] As a consequence, many surgeons consider patients with an asymptomatic carotid stenosis over 60% for simultaneous treatment of the concomitant disease. The analysis of large series suggests that the simultaneous treatment is safe and may be preferred to a staged approach.[96] Nevertheless, the performance of coronary artery bypass grafting and carotid endarterectomy in the same setting may increase the perioperative stroke risk. A randomized trial is necessary to address this issue better.

ANGIOPLASTY

Surgery for asymptomatic carotid stenosis has several disadvantages including anesthesia, 3–8-day hospitalization, risk of injury to cranial nerves, and the resulting scar.[97] Percutaneous transluminal angioplasty (PTA) avoids these disadvantages providing a potential alternative to surgery in asymptomatic patients. Furthermore, surgically inaccessible lesions and patients with contraindications to endarterectomy might be suitable candidates for PTA.[98]

A number of centers are treating carotid stenosis by PTA, while randomized, controlled trials are in progress in symptomatic patients.[98,99] Retrospective series suggest that the immediate risk of carotid PTA is similar to that of surgery, but the long-term efficacy of the procedure in dilating the carotid artery has not been fully established.[100] Balloon dilation in patients with severe carotid stenosis did not always result in full dilation of the artery and the probability of restenosis after the initial incomplete dilation is still uncertain. In the coronary circulation, stenting reduces the 6-month restenosis rate by 40%.[101] Although only one trial has shown sustained clinical benefit with stenting, carotid stenting has also been suggested as the treatment of choice for carotid stenosis.[102]

MEDICAL THERAPY

Antiplatelet agents, such as aspirin, should be considered in patients with asymptomatic carotid stenosis because of their significant effect in reducing the overall atherothrombotic risk.[103] Although a beneficial effect of aspirin has also been suggested in patients with asymptomatic high grade stenosis, prospective randomized confirmatory studies are not yet available.[104,105] A double-blind trial randomized 372 neurologically asymptomatic patients with carotid stenosis (reduction of lumen diameter of 50% or more on duplex ultrasonography) in at least one artery, to either 325 mg aspirin daily or placebo. After 2.3 years of follow-up, the annual rate of all ischemic events and death from any cause was 12.3% for the placebo group and 11.0% for the aspirin group. The adjusted hazard ratio was 0.99 (95% CI, 0.67–1.46), indicating a lack of benefit.[105] Treatment with ticlopidine has been shown to be beneficial in stroke prevention but is associated with some adverse events.[106]

Although data from clinical trials suggest that controlling blood lipids is effective in both primary and secondary prevention of myocardial infarction and death, there is no evidence that their control may favor regression of the carotid plaque.[107] Clopidogrel proved to be more effective than aspirin in the prevention of stroke, myocardial infarction and vascular death in patients with either stroke, acute myocardial infarction or peripheral arterial disease.[108] Although no data were reported on asymptomatic carotid stenosis, the high effectiveness found in the subgroup with peripheral arterial disease may also suggest a positive effect in patients with asymptomatic carotid stenosis.

The risk of stroke increases dramatically in asymptomatic patients after the development of initial symptoms, making it imperative that patients treated medically recognize and promptly report symptoms to their physician.[109] Since a TIA is painless and transitory, many patients may fail to report symptoms in time for clinical management. In one study,[31] despite patients receiving formal instruction and education and being highly trained in identifying TIA and stroke, 32.2% of patients experiencing a TIA and 44.9% of those experiencing a stroke referred to the study staff within 3 days of onset. Fast reporting was more frequent for TIA occurring early during follow-up and for stroke occurring after surgery. Therefore, frequent out-patient evaluation of high-risk patients and careful review of symptoms is necessary to determine when asymptomatic carotid stenosis has become symptomatic to provide appropriate therapy.

REFERENCES

1. Gelabert HA, Moore WS. Carotid endarterectomy: current status. *Curr Probl Surg* 1991; **28:**187–262.
2. Colgan MP, Strode GR, Sommer JD, Gibbs JL, Sumner DS. Prevalence of asymptomatic carotid disease: results of duplex scanning in 348 unselected volunteers. *J Vasc Surg* 1988; **8:**674–8.
3. Ricci S, Flamini OF, Celani MG, Marini M, Antonini D, Bartolini E. Prevalence of internal carotid artery stenosis in subjects older than 49 years: a population study. *Cerebrovasc Dis* 1991; **23:**1752–60.
4. O'Leary DH, Polak JF, Kronmal RA *et al.* Distribution and correlates of sonographically detected carotid artery disease in the Cardiovascular Health Study. *Stroke* 1992; **23:**1752–60.
5. Prati P, Vanuzzo D, Casaroli M *et al.* Prevalence and determinants of carotid atherosclerosis in a general population. *Stroke* 1992; **23:**1705–11.
6. Wolf PA, Kannel WB, Sorlie P, McNamara R. Asymptomatic carotid bruit and risk of stroke. The Framingham Study. *J Am Med Assoc* 1981; **245:**1442–5.
7. Meissner I, Wiebers DO, Whisnant JP, O'Fallon M. The natural history of asymptomatic carotid artery occlusive lesions. *J Am Med Assoc* 1987; **258:**2704–7.
8. Norris JW, Zhu CZ, Bornstein NM, Chambers BR. Vascular risk of asymptomatic carotid stenosis. *Stroke* 1991; **22:**1485–90.
9. North American Symptomatic Carotid Endarterectomy Trial Collaborators. Beneficial effect of carotid endarterectomy in symptomatic patients with high-grade carotid stenosis. *N Engl J Med* 1991; **325:**445–53.
10. The European Carotid Surgery Trialists' Collaborative Group. MRC European Carotid Surgery Trial: interim results for symptomatic patients with severe (70–99%) or with mild

(0–29%) carotid stenosis. *Lancet* 1991; **337:**1235–43.
11. European Carotid Surgery Trialists' Collaborative Group. Risk of stroke in the distribution of an asymptomatic carotid artery. *Lancet* 1995; **345:**209–12.
12. Chambers BR, Norris JW. Outcome in patients with asymptomatic neck cervical arterial bruits. *N Engl J Med* 1986; **315:**860–5.
13. Carolei A, Marini C, Nencini P *et al.* Prevalence and outcome of symptomatic carotid lesions in young adults. *Br Med J* 1995; **310:**1363–6.
14. Hennerici M, Hulsbomer HB, Hefter H, Lammerts D, Rautenberg W. Natural history of asymptomatic extracranial arterial disease. Results of a long-term prospective study. *Brain* 1987; **110:**177–91.
15. Norris JW, Zhu CZ. Stroke risk and critical carotid stenosis. *J Neurol Neurosurg Psychiat* 1990; **53:**235–7.
16. Hobson RW II, Weiss DG, Fields WS *et al.* Efficacy of carotid surgery for asymptomatic carotid stenosis. *N Engl J Med* 1993; **328:**221–7.
17. Moore DL, Miles RD, Goolev NA, Sumner DS. Noninvasive assessment of stroke risk in asymptomatic and nonhemispheric patients with suspected carotid disease. Five-year follow-up of 294 unoperated and 81 operated patients. *Ann Surg* 1985; **202:**491–504.
18. Mohr JP, Caplan LR, Melski J-W *et al.* The Harvard Cooperative Stroke Registry: a prospective registry. *Neurology* 1978; **28:**754–62.
19. Klop RB, Eikelboom BC, Taks AC. Screening of the internal carotid arteries in patients with peripheral vascular disease by colour-flow duplex scanning. *Eur J Vasc Surg* 1991; **5:**41–5.
20 Mackey AE, Abrahamowicz M, Langlois Y *et al.* Outcome of asymptomatic patients with carotid disease. *Neurology* 1997; **48:**896–903.
21. Langsfeld M, Gray-Weale AC, Lusby RJ. The role of plaque morphology and diameter reduction in the development of new symptoms in asymptomatic carotid arteries. *J Vasc Surg* 1989; **9:**548–57.
22. O'Hallerhan LW, Kennelly MM, McClurken M, Johnson JM. Natural history of asymptomatic carotid plaque. Five year follow-up study. *Am J Surg* 1987; **154:**659–62.
23. Lusby RJ, Ferrell LD, Ehrenfeld WE, Stoney RJ, Wylie EJ. Carotid plaque hemorrhage: its role in production of cerebral ischemia. *Arch Surg* 1982; **117:**1479–88.
24. Zukowski AJ, Nicolaides AN, Lewis RT *et al.* Incidence of CT scan cerebral infarction in relation to carotid plaque ulceration. *J Vasc Surg* 1984; **1:**782–6.
25. Imparato AM, Riles TS, Mintzer R, Baumann FG. The importance of hemorrhage in the relationship between gross morphologic characteristics and cerebral symptoms in 376 carotid artery plaques. *Ann Surg* 1983; **197:**195–203.
26. Hatsukami TS, Ferguson MS, Beach KW *et al.* Carotid plaque morphology and clinical events. *Stroke* 1997; **28:**95–100.
27. Ringelstein EB, Sievers C, Ecker S, Schneider PA, Otis SM. Noninvasive assessment of CO_2-induced cerebral vasomotor response in normal individuals and patients with internal carotid artery occlusions. *Stroke* 1988; **19:**963–9.
28. Reith W, Pfadenhauer K, Loeprecht H. Significance of transcranial Doppler CO_2 reactivity measurements for the diagnosis of hemodynamically relevant carotid obstructions. *Ann Vasc Surg* 1990; **4:**359–64.
29. Gur AY, Bova I, Bornstein NM. Is impaired cerebral vasomotor reactivity a predictive factor of stroke in asymptomatic patients? *Stroke* 1996; **27:**2188–90.
30. Norris JW, Zhu CZ. Silent stroke and carotid stenosis. *Stroke* 1992; **23:**483–5.
31. Consensus Group. Consensus statement on the management of patients with asymptomatic atherosclerotic carotid bifurcation lesions. *Intl Angiol* 1995; **14:**5–20.
32. Haust MD. The morphogenesis and fate of potential and early atherosclerotic lesions in man. *Human Pathol* 1971; **2:**1–29.
33. Zarins CK, Giddens DP, Glagov S. Atherosclerotic plaque distribution and flow velocity profiles in the carotid bifurcation. In: *Cerebrovascular Insufficiency* (Bergan JJ, Yao JST, eds.), p. 19. New York; Grune and Stratton: 1983.
34. Lusby RJ. Lesions, dynamics, and pathogenetic mechanisms responsible for ischemic events in the brain. In: *Surgery for Cerebrovascular Disease* (Moore WS, ed.), pp. 51–76. New York; Churchill Livingstone: 1987.
35. Grigg MJ, Papadakis K, Nicolaides AN *et al.* The significance of cerebral infarction and atrophy in patients with amaurosis fugax and transient ischaemic attack in relation to internal carotid stenosis: a preliminary report. *J Vasc Surg* 1988; **7:**215–22.
36. Herderschee D, Hijdra A, Algra A *et al.* Silent stroke in patients with transient ischemic attack

or minor ischemic stroke. The Dutch TIA Trial Study Group. *Stroke* 1992; **23:**1220–4.
37. Powers WJ. Cerebral haemodynamics in ischemic cerebrovascular disease. *Ann Neurol* 1991; **29:**231–40.
38. Schuler JJ, Flanigan DP, Lim LT, Kiefer T, Williams LR, Behrend AJ. The effect of carotid siphon stenosis on stroke rate, death, and relief of symptoms following elective carotid endarterectomy. *Surgery* 1982; **92:**1058–67.
39. Roederer GO, Langlois YE, Jager KA *et al.* The natural history of carotid arterial disease in asymptomatic patients with cervical bruits. *Stroke* 1984; **15:**605–13.
40. Welby GE, Sedwitz MM, Bergan JJ, Moreland SI, Bardin JA, Schmalback P. Cerebrovascular magnetic resonance angiography: a critical verification. *J Vasc Surg* 1992; **15:**238–9.
41. Kertesz A, Black SE, Nicholson L, Carr T. The sensitivity and specificity of MRI in stroke. *Neurology* 1987; **37:**1580–5.
42. Totaro R, Varroni A, Gizzi E, Marini C, Carolei A, Spartera C. Valutazione pre-, intra- e postoperatoria con Doppler transcranico di 85 pazienti sottoposti ad endarterectomia carotidea. *Clin Ter* 1998; **149:**267–70.
43. Riles TS, Kopelman I, Imparato AM. Myocardial infarction following carotid endarterectomy: a review of 683 operations. *Surgery* 1979; **85:**249–52.
44. Towne JB, Weiss DG, Hobson RW II. First phase report of cooperative Veterans Administration asymptomatic carotid stenosis study. Operative morbidity and mortality. *J Vasc Surg* 1990; **11:**252–9.
45. Eagle KA, Coley CM, Newell JB *et al.* Combining clinical and thallium data optimizes preoperative assessment of cardiac risk before major vascular surgery. *Ann Intern Med* 1998; **110:**859–66.
46. Coldschlager N, Selzer A, Cohn K. Treadmill stress tests as indicators of presence and severity of coronary artery disease. *Ann Intern Med* 1976; **85:**277–86.
47. Hendel RC, Cutler BS, Villegas BJ, Leppo JA. Dipyridamole-thallium imaging predicts both postoperative and late cardiac events in vascular patients [Abstract]. *Circulation* 1990; **82**(Suppl III):202.
48. Lette J, Waters D, Bernier H *et al.* Preoperative and long term cardiac risk assessment. Predictive value of 23 clinical descriptors, seven multivariate scoring systems, and quantitative dipyridamole imaging in 360 patients. *Ann Surg* 1992; **216:**192–204.
49. Mazika P, Nadazdin A, Oakley CM. Dobutamine stress echocardiography for detection and assessment of coronary artery disease. *J Am Coll Cardiol* 1992; **19:**1203–11.
50. Kennedy HC, Wiens RD. Ambulatory (Holter) electrocardiography and myocardial ischemia. *Am Heart J* 1989; **117:**164–8.
51. Landesberg G, Wolf Y, Schechter D *et al.* Preoperative thallium scanning, selective coronary revascularization, and long-term survival after carotid endarterectomy. *Stroke* 1998; **29:**2541–8.
52. Winslow CM, Solomon DH, Chassin MR, Kosecoff J, Merrick NJ, Brook RH. The appropriateness of carotid endarterectomy. *N Engl J Med* 1988; **318:**721–7.
53. Douglas J, Lanska DJ, Richard J, Kryscio RJ. Endarterectomy for asymptomatic internal carotid artery stenosis. *Neurology* 1997; **48:**1481–90.
54. North American Symptomatic Carotid Endarterectomy Trial (NASCET) Investigators. Clinical alert: benefit of carotid endarterectomy for patients with high-grade stenosis of internal carotid artery. *Stroke* 1991; **22:**816–7.
55. Mayberg MR, Wilson SE, Yatsu F *et al.* Carotid endarterectomy and prevention of cerebral ischemia in symptomatic carotid stenosis. *J Am Med Assoc* 1991; **266:**3289–94.
56. Tu JV, Hannan EL, Anderson GM *et al.* The fall and rise of carotid endarterectomy in the United States and Canada. *N Engl J Med* 1998; **339:**1441–7.
57. Maini BS, Mullins TF, Catlin J, O'Mara P. Carotid endarterectomy: a ten-year analysis of outcome and cost of treatment. *J Vasc Surg* 1990; **12:**732–40.
58. Wall CA, Long JB, Lampert NR, Clarke JC, Murray RE. Impact of changing attitudes in carotid surgery on community hospital practice. *Am J Surg* 1991; **162:**190–3.
59. Mattos MA, Modi JR, Mansour MA *et al.* Evolution of carotid endarterectomy in two community hospitals: Springfield revisited—seventeen years and 2243 operations later. *J Vasc Surg* 1995; **21:**719–28.
60. Barnett HJM, Eliasziw M, Meldrum HE, Taylor DW. Do the facts and figures warrant a 10-fold increase in the performance of carotid endarterectomy on asymptomatic patients? *Neurology* 1996; **46:**603–8.

61. Clagett GP, Youkey JR, Brigham RA *et al.* Asymptomatic cervical bruit and abnormal ocular pneumoplethysmography: a prospective study comparing two approaches to management. *Surgery* 1984; **96:**823–30.
62. CASANOVA Study Group. Carotid surgery versus medical therapy in asymptomatic carotid stenosis. *Stroke* 1991; **22:**1229–35.
63. Solis MM, Ranval TJ, Barone GW, Eidt JF, Barnes RW. The CASANOVA study: immediate surgery versus delayed surgery for moderate carotid artery stenosis? *Stroke* 1992; **23:**917.
64. Diener HC. The CASANOVA study: immediate surgery versus delayed surgery for moderate carotid artery stenosis? *Stroke* 1992; **23:**918.
65. Easton JD, Wilterdink JL. Carotid endarterectomy: trials and tribulations. *Ann Neurol* 1994; **35:**5–17.
66. Mayo Asymptomatic Carotid Endarterectomy Study Group. Effectiveness of carotid endarterectomy for asymptomatic carotid stenosis: design of a clinical trial. *Mayo Clin Proc* 1989; **64:**897–901.
67. Mayo Asymptomatic Carotid Endarterectomy Study Group. Results of a randomized controlled trial of carotid endarterectomy for asymptomatic carotid stenosis. *Mayo Clin Proc* 1992; **67:**513–8.
68. Role of carotid endarterectomy in asymptomatic carotid stenosis. A Veterans Administration cooperative study. *Stroke* 1986; **17:**534–9.
69. Warlow C. Endarterectomy for asymptomatic carotid stenosis? *Lancet* 1995; **345:**1254–5.
70. Barnett HJM, Haines SJ. Carotid endarterectomy for asymptomatic carotid stenosis. *N Engl J Med* 1993; **328:**276–9.
71. National Institute of Neurological Disorders and Stroke. Clinical advisory: carotid endarterectomy for patients with asymptomatic internal carotid artery stenosis. *Stroke* 1994; **25:**2523–4.
72. Executive Committee for the Asymptomatic Carotid Atherosclerosis Study. Endarterectomy for asymptomatic carotid artery stenosis. *J Am Med Assoc* 1995; **273:**1421–8.
73. Barnett HJM, Meldrum HE, Eliasziw M. The dilemma of surgical treatment for patients with asymptomatic carotid disease. *Ann Intern Med* 1995; **123:**723–5.
74. Barnett HJM, Meldrum HE. Update on carotid endarterectomy. *Curr Opin Cardiol* 1995; **10:**511–16.
75. Benavente O, Moher D, Pham B. Carotid endarterectomy for asymptomatic carotid stenosis: a meta-analysis. *Br Med J* 1998; **317:**1477–80.
76. Lagneau P. Stenoses carotidiennes asymptomatiques. *J Mal Vasc* 1993; **18:**209–12.
77. Warlow C. Carotid endarterectomy for asymptomatic carotid stenosis. *Br Med J* 1998; **317:**1468.
78. Robless P, Emson M, Thomas D, Mansfield A, Halliday A, on behalf of the Asymptomatic Carotid Surgery Trial collaborators. Are we detecting and operating on high risk patients in the Asymptomatic Carotid Surgery Trial? *Eur J Vasc Endovasc Surg* 1998; **16:**59–64.
79. Frey JL. Asymptomatic carotid stenosis: surgery's the answer, but that's not the question. *Ann Neurol* 1996; **39:**405–6.
80. Rothwell PM, Slattery J, Warlow CP. A systemic comparison of the risks of stroke and death due to carotid endarterectomy for symptomatic and asymptomatic stenosis. *Stroke* 1996; **27:**266–9.
81. Brott TG, Labutta RJ, Kempczinski RF. Changing patterns in the practice of carotid endarterectomy in a large metropolitan area. *J Am Med Assoc* 1986; **255:**2609–12.
82. Fode NC, Sundt TM Jr, Robertson JT, Peerless SJ, Shields CB. Multicenter retrospective review of results and complications of carotid endarterectomy in 1981. *Stroke* 1986; **17:**370–6.
83. Rubin JR, Pitluk HC, King TA *et al.* Carotid endarterectomy in a metropolitan community: the early results after 8535 operations. *J Vasc Surg* 1988; **7:**256–60.
84. Goldstein LB, Samsa GP, Matchar DG, Oddone EZ. Multicenter review of preoperative risk factors for endarterectomy for asymptomatic carotid artery stenosis. *Stroke* 1998; **29:**750–3.
85. Beebe HG, Clagett GP, De Weese JA *et al.* Assessing risk associated with carotid endarterectomy: a statement for health professionals by an Ad Hoc Committee on Carotid Surgery Standards of the Stroke Council, American Heart Association. *Stroke* 1989; **20:**314–5.
86. Moore WS, Mohr JP, Najafi H, Robertson JT, Stoney RJ, Toole JF. Carotid endarterectomy: practice guidelines: report of the Ad Hoc Committee to the Joint Council of the Society for Vascular Surgery and the North American Chapter of the International Society for Cardiovascular Surgery. *J Vasc Surg* 1992; **18:**469–79.

87. Moore WS, Vescera CL, Robertson JT, Baker WH, Howard VJ, Toole JF. Selection process for surgeons in the Asymptomatic Carotid Atherosclerosis Study. *Stroke* 1991; **22:**1353–7.
88. The Asymptomatic Carotid Atherosclerosis Study Group. Study design for randomized prospective trial of carotid endarterectomy for asymptomatic atherosclerosis. *Stroke* 1989; **20:**844–9.
89. Carr S, Farb A, Pearce WH, Virmani R, Yao JST. Atherosclerotic plaque rupture in symptomatic carotid artery stenosis. *J Vasc Surg* 1996; **23:**755–66.
90. Mayberg MR, Winn HR. Endarterectomy for asymptomatic carotid artery stenosis: resolving the controversy. *J Am Med Assoc* 1995; **273:**1459–61.
91. Perry JR, Szalai JP, Norris JW, for the Canadian Stroke Consortium. Consensus against both endarterectomy and routine screening for asymptomatic carotid artery stenosis. *Arch Neurol* 1997; **54:**25–8.
92. Oddone E, Waters K. Endarterectomy for asymptomatic carotid artery stenosis. *J Am Med Assoc* 1995; **274:**1506.
93. Whitty CJM, Sudlow CLM, Warlow CP. Investigating individual subjects and screening populations for asymptomatic carotid stenosis can be harmful. *J Neurol Neurosurg Psychiatry* 1998; **64:**619–23.
94. Alexandrova NA, Gibson WC, Norris JW, Maggisano R. Carotid artery stenosis in peripheral vascular disease. *J Vasc Surg* 1996; **23:**645–9.
95. Takach TJ, Reul GJ Jr, Cooley DA *et al.* Is an integrated approach warranted for concomitant carotid and coronary artery disease? *Ann Thorac Surg* 1997; **64:**16–22.
96. Dunn EJ. Concomitant cerebral and myocardial revascularization. *Surg Clin North Am* 1986; **66:** 385–95.
97. Crawley F, Clifton A, Markus H, Brown MM. Delayed improvement in carotid artery diameter after carotid angioplasty. *Stroke* 1997; **28:**574–9.
98. Robertson JT. Carotid endarterectomy: a saga of clinical science, personalities, and evolving technology. The Willis lecture. *Stroke* 1998; **29:**2345–441.
99. Sivaguru A, Venables GS, Beard JD, Gaines PA. European carotid angioplasty trial. *J Endovasc Surg* 1996; **3:**16–20.
100. Brown MM. Balloon angioplasty for cerebrovascular diseases. *Neurol Res* 1992; **4**(Suppl.): 159–73.
101. Serruys PW, De Jaegere P, Kiemeneij F *et al.* A comparison of balloon-expandable-stent implantation with balloon angioplasty in patients with coronary artery disease. *N Engl J Med* 1994; **331:**489–95.
102. Bergeron P, Chambran P, Hartung O, Bianca S. Cervical carotid artery stenosis: which technique, balloon angioplasty or surgery? *J Cardiovasc Surg* 1996; **37**(Suppl. 1):73–5.
103. Barnett HJM. Aspirin in stroke prevention: an overview. *Stroke* 1990; **21**(Suppl. IV):40–3.
104. Hobson RW, Krupski WC, Weiss DG. Influence of aspirin in the management of asymptomatic carotid stenosis. *J Vasc Surg* 1993; **18:**257–63.
105. Côté R, Battista RN, Abrahamowicz M *et al.* Lack of effect of aspirin in asymptomatic patients with carotid bruits and substantial carotid narrowing. *Ann Intern Med* 1995; **123:**649–55.
106. Hass WK, Easton JD, Adams HP Jr *et al.* A randomized trial comparing ticlopidine hydrochloride with aspirin for the prevention of stroke in high risk patients. *N Engl J Med* 1989; **321:**501–7.
107. Report of the National Cholesterol Education Program Expert Panel on Detection, Evaluation, and Treatment of High Blood Cholesterol in Adults. *Arch Intern Med* 1988; **148:**36–69.
108. CAPRIE Steering Committee. A randomized, blinded trial of clopidogrel versus aspirin in patients at risk of ischaemic events (CAPRIE). *Lancet* 1996; **348:**1329–38.
109. Castaldo JE, Nelson JJ, Reed JF III, Longenecker JE, Toole JF, for the Asymptomatic Carotid Atherosclerosis Study Investigators. The delay in reporting symptoms of carotid artery stenosis in an at-risk population. *Arch Neurol* 1997; **54:**1267–71.

16

Stenting and angioplasty for cerebrovascular disease

Randall T Higashida, Adel M Malek, Constantine C Phatouros, Todd E Lempert, Philip M Meyers, Christopher F Dowd and Van V Halbach

CONTENTS

INTRODUCTION

Stroke from atherosclerotic disease represents a major source of mortality in the Western hemisphere and is associated with an enormous medical and social cost. This is the result of more than 600 000 cases of new or recurrent strokes yearly,[1] of which up to 30% may be attributed to the atherosclerosis of the carotid bifurcation and proximal internal carotid artery.

Recent advances in neurointerventional catheter-based techniques, microballoon and stent design have occurred in the past 10 years which have enabled the treatment of complex vascular lesions, previously deemed unapproachable using catheter-based techniques.[2] The endovascular approach is providing greater therapeutic options for patients who pose a great surgical risk and who are symptomatic despite maximal medical therapy. Such lesions include severe atherosclerosis in patients with significant comorbidity, such as tandem intracranial stenosis, contralateral carotid occlusion and recurrent stenosis of vessels having previously undergone endarterectomy.

Percutaneous balloon angioplasty alone or when combined with stent placement (stent-assisted angioplasty) is also providing alternatives to the treatment of carotid dissection, intracranial atherosclerosis or recalcitrant acute thrombosis refractory to intraluminal thrombolysis, wide-necked aneurysms, and intracranial vasospasm resulting from subarachnoid hemorrhage.

We will review in this chapter the key topics relating to the technique of angioplasty and stent deployment and their current role in the management of cerebrovascular ischemic disease (Fig. 16.1, Tables 16.1 and 16.2).

ANGIOPLASTY OF THE EXTRACRANIAL VESSELS

Percutaneous balloon angioplasty is credited to Dotter and Judkins;[3] subsequent innovation led to the first report of angioplasty in the coronary artery 15 years later[4] with a subsequent revolution in coronary intervention. Percutaneous angioplasty of the extracranial carotid artery began initially with modest efforts tempered by fears of distal intracranial embolization from plaque rupture during angioplasty.[5] A review by Kachel summarizing the cumulative experience of angioplasty of the carotid, vertebral, subclavian, and innominate arteries reported until 1995, described 1971 cases with a technical success rate of 94.6%[6] (Table 16.3). The mortality varied by territory from 0 to 2.1% with overall morbidity of 0.9% and minor tech-

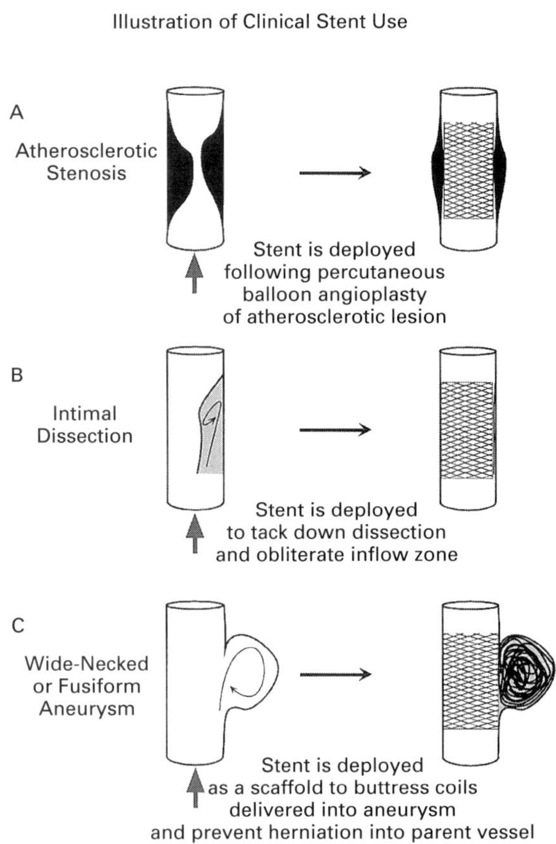

Figure 16.1 Illustration of typical vascular pathologies involving the cervical and intracranial arterial circulation to which stent deployment is playing an increasing role: (A) atherosclerotic stenosis, (B) intimal dissection (spontaneous, traumatic, or iatrogenic), and (C) stent-assisted coil embolization of wide-necked aneurysm or pseudoaneurysm.

nical complications of 0–6.3%. The author's experience included percutaneous angioplasty of 74 symptomatic carotid lesions with a technical success of 93%, a risk of major stroke of 1.4%, two minor complications for a risk of major stroke of 2.7% and no reported restenosis at 70 months follow-up. Higashida and Tsai reported angioplasty of 256 extracranial vessels with greater than 70% stenosis with one major stroke (0.4%), five transient ischemic events (2%), no mortality and 15 cases (6%) of restenosis at 6–12 months' follow-up.[7]

In the posterior circulation, Higashida reported percutaneous angioplasty in 42 patients of the vertebral artery (34 proximal, five distal, three basilar) with stroke in two cases and vessel rupture in one (7.1% permanent complications), two cases of spasm, and two cases of cerebral ischemia lasting less than 30 min (9.5% transient complications); clinical improvement was noted in 92.9% of patients at follow-up with three cases of restenosis (7.1%) of the proximal vertebral artery, two of which underwent successful repeat percutaneous angioplasty (Fig. 16.2).[8]

Measurements of middle cerebral artery velocity using transcranial Doppler insonation has also enabled the assessment of intracranial hemodynamics prior to and after angioplasty. Although restenosis is one of the reported concerns following angioplasty, there is evidence for a delayed and persistent improvement in cerebral reactivity and hemodynamics beyond the immediate post-angioplasty period to 1 and 6 months.[9] Indeed, quantitative angiographic measurement of stenotic lesions (mean of 87%) treated with percutaneous angioplasty showed an improvement from 47% immediately post-dilatation to 28% at 1 year follow-up, suggesting an active expansile structural remodeling process.[10]

Recent experience in the percutaneous angioplasty of the subclavian artery for aortoarteritis (32 vessels) and atherosclerosis (23 vessels) has been performed by Tyagi *et al.* with 92.8% success in stenotic lesions and 60% success in recanalizing totally occluded arteries.[11] The average stenosis decreased from 88.7% to 15.5% for atherosclerosis and from 89% to 8.3% for aortoarteritis following percutaneous angioplasty without neurological complications and with good long-term symptomatic relief (3–120 months).[11]

A prospective analytical study of 29 patients having undergone carotid angioplasty for severe symptomatic ipsilateral carotid stenosis by NASCET criteria, was recently reported by Schoser *et al.*[12] Neurological and ultrasonographic follow-up (mean 33 months) revealed

Table 16.1 Location of reported arterial and venous sites where a stent has been deployed either primarily or following percutaneous balloon angioplasty

Arterial		*Venous*
Anterior circulation	*Posterior circulation*	
Innominate artery	Subclavian artery	Internal jugular vein
Common carotid artery	Vertebral artery	Transverse sinus*
Carotid artery bifurcation	Origin stenosis	Occipital sinus*
Internal carotid	Cervical vertebral artery	
Cervical	Intracranial vertebral artery*	
Petrous*	Basilar artery*	
Cavernous*	Midbasilar trunk*	
Supraclinoid*		

*Intracranial location

Table 16.2 Various indications for which a stent has been deployed intravascularly

Arterial	*Venous*
Atherosclerotic stenosis (>70% NASCET criteria)	Maintenance of patency
Restenosis following carotid endarterectomy	Recanalization of occluded sinus
Tandem stenotic lesions	
Intimal dissection (spontaneous, iatrogenic, chronic)	
Pseudoaneurysm without coiling (spontaneous thrombosis)	
Scaffold for coiling of wide-necked intracerebral aneurysm	
Scaffold for coiling of pseudoaneurysm	

that 78% of patients suffered no further neurological sequelae, 10% suffered a single episode of ipsilateral transient ischemia or amaurosis fugax, and 7% suffered recurrent such episodes, with no patient suffering a stroke. Fifty per cent of treated vessels remained with normal ultrasound (<50% stenosis), 40% with mild stenosis (50–70%), and 10% with severe stenosis (>70%). These findings suggest that angioplasty alone is salutary and can have sustained benefit even to 6.5 years of follow-up[12] with an acceptable risk profile (Table 16.3).

Table 16.3 Summary of technical success, complications, and morbidity in reported studies in the literature

Author	*Number of patients*	*Technical success (%)*	*Major complications or stroke (%)*	*Minor complications or TIAs (%)*	*Mortality rate (%)*	*Restenosis rate (%)*
Angioplasty						
Kachel[6] (review)	1971	94.6	0.9	4.2	0	–
Kachel[6] (series)	74	93.2	1.4	1.4	0	0
Higashida[2]	325	100	2.4	5.5	0	7.4
Iyer[17]	100	97	7	3	3	1
Mathias[82]	79	100	0	2.5	0	0
Théron[35]	482	100	2	2	0.6	16
Stent-assisted angioplasty						
Diethrich[83]	110	99	6.4	4.5	1.8	4
Vitek[21]	404	98	0.7	5.8	1.9	0
GSCAS[15]	2048	98.6	1.32	3.1	1.37	4.8
Vozzi[84]	22	96	4	4	0	–
Henry[85]	163	99.4	1.8	3	0	2.3

GSCAS: Global status of carotid artery stent placement
TIA: Transient ischemic attack

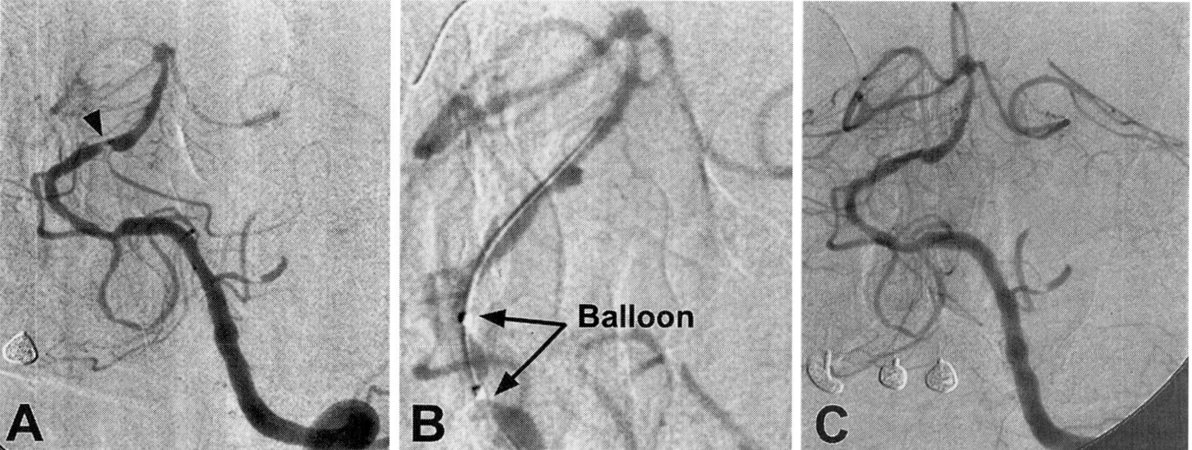

Figure 16.2 A 77-year-old man with hypertension presented with increased gait unsteadiness and multiple falls. Hypercholesterolemia was diagnosed with vertebrobasilar insufficiency and multiple drop attacks despite oral anticoagulant and platelet anti-aggregation therapy with warfarin and ticlopidine. (A) Digital subtraction angiography (DSA) of the left vertebral artery revealed a focal severe stenosis (arrowhead) of the proximal basilar artery. (B) A coaxial microcatheter/microguidewire system was used to cross the lesion and navigate an exchange guidewire into the right P1 segment of the posterior cerebral artery. A 2.5 mm diameter balloon (Charger, Cordis Endovascular; arrows) was guided coaxially over the exchange microguidewire and used to perform percutaneous angioplasty of the focal stenosis. (C) DSA following treatment confirms significant improvement in appearance and in flow rate. The patient tolerated the procedure well and has had improved symptoms.

ANGIOPLASTY AND STENTING OF THE EXTRACRANIAL CAROTID ARTERY

Current state

Trials of stent-assisted vs. simple percutaneous balloon angioplasty of the coronary circulation have consistently demonstrated a persistent benefit in event-free survival at 1 year and a lower rate of repeat angioplasty.[13,14] The increased acceptance and reliance on stent placement in the coronary and peripheral vascular interventions has led to a similar trend in the treatment of supra-aortic cervical vessels including the carotid,[15–17] subclavian,[11] and vertebral arteries (Fig. 16.3).[18]

Recently, Yadav *et al.* reported their experience with balloon angioplasty and stenting of carotid restenosis in a series of 22 patients having previously undergone carotid endarterectomy.[19] They were able to decrease the stenosis successfully by 79 ± 13% with a morbidity of 4% (a minor stroke in a single patient) and no restenosis (>50%) at 6 months' follow-up (Figs 16.4 and 16.5). Given the high risk of re-operation on previous endarterectomized lesions which have been reported to suffer operative complication rates of 10.5% (Tables 16.4 and 16.5),[20] balloon angioplasty and stenting is a promising approach (Table 16.3).

Vitek and Roubin reported having treated a total of 445 vessels in 404 patients using stent-assisted angioplasty using predilatation, placement of stent, followed by stent dilatation.[21] Patients were pretreated with aspirin and ticlopidine and were not maintained under intravenous anticoagulation

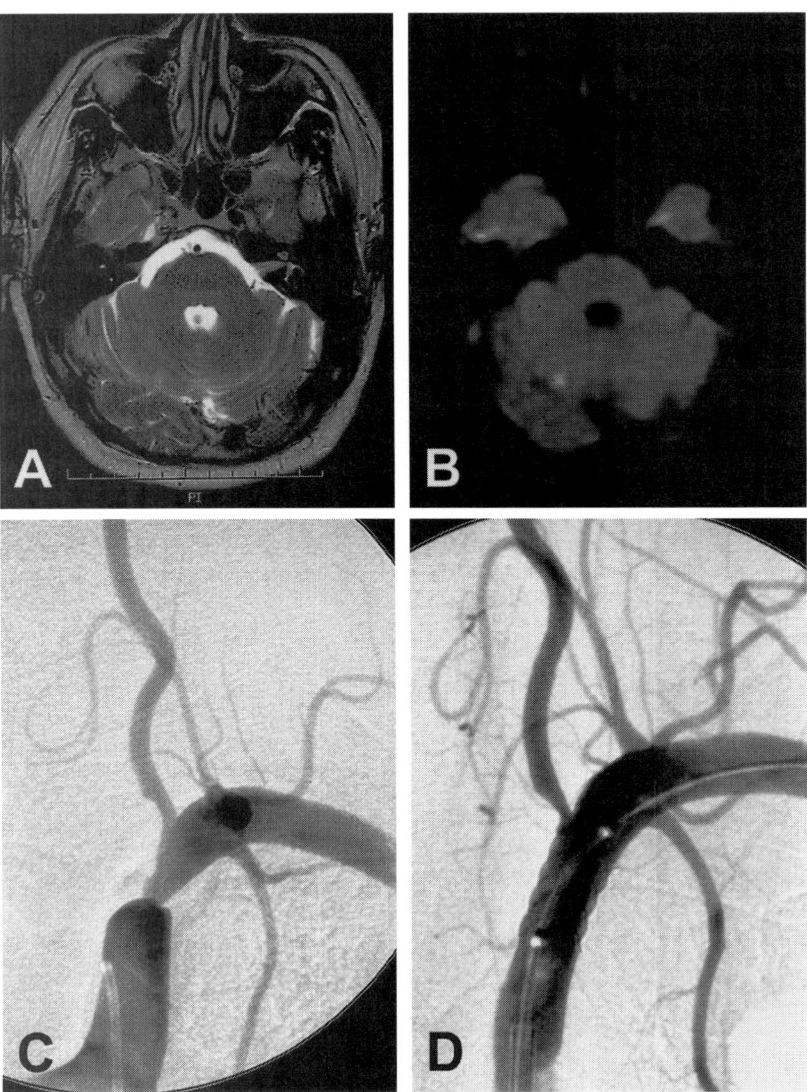

Figure 16.3 A 56-year-old man presented with symptoms of vertebrobasilar insufficiency and episodes of right ocular obscuration and underwent MR imaging revealing a focus of infarction in the right posterior fossa on T2-weighted MR (A) and perfusion weighted MR (B). (C) Digital subtracted angiography revealed an occluded right vertebral artery and a focal stenosis (70%) of the left subclavian artery proximal to the origin of the left vertebral artery with a subclavian steal syndrome. A Palmaz stent was mounted on a 10 × 20 mm balloon catheter (Optra, Cordis Endovascular) and used to perform primary angioplasty after crossing the lesion with a 0.035 inch exchange guidewire. Post-deployment DSA confirms excellent placement proximal to the origin of the left vertebral artery (D).

following the procedure, with same day and 23-h discharges when possible. They reported on the treatment of 40 patients with contralateral carotid occlusion and 70 patients with post-endarterectomy restenosis. Overall technical success was 98%, with a 30-day mortality/morbidity and death rate of 1.9% (0.7% neurological and 1.2% systemic), 0.7% risk of major stroke and 5.8% minor stroke (Table 16.3). The authors determined their annual risk of minor stroke and showed a steady decline from 7.2% in 1994–1995, to 4.4% and 2.2% in each successive year. The decrease in complication rate with experience illustrates the fact that stent-assisted angioplasty is still in its infancy; nonetheless, stent-assisted balloon angioplasty appears to have a short-term risk comparable to that reported for carotid endarterectomy. Six-month follow-up obtained in 80% of patients uncovered stenosis greater than 50% in 5% of

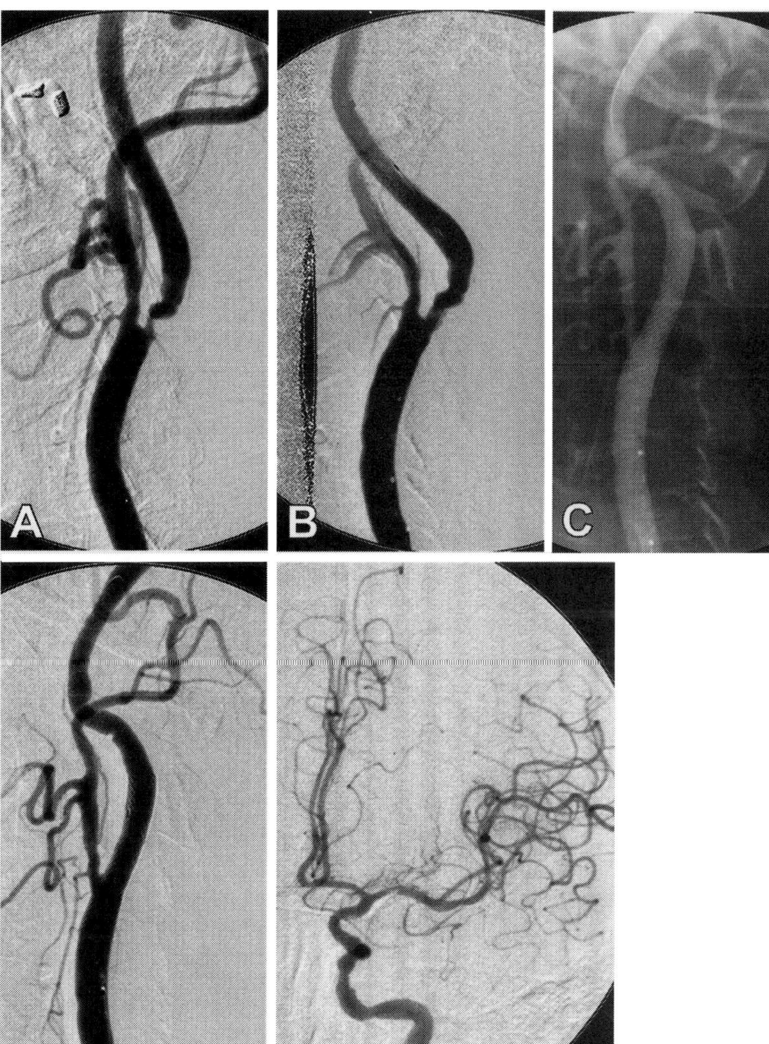

Figure 16.4 An 82-year-old right-handed man with coronary artery disease who suffered transient ischemic attacks involving his right hand and cognitive function. Magnetic resonance imaging and angiography (MRI/MRA) confirmed a focal high-grade stenosis. He was referred for carotid percutaneous angioplasty. (A) DSA of the left common carotid artery revealed a focal 85% stenosis near the origin of the left internal carotid artery. (B) DSA of the left common carotid artery after percutaneous angioplasty with a 4 × 18 mm balloon (Titan, Cordis Endovascular). (C) Unsubtracted angiography and (D) DSA of the left common carotid artery after deployment of a 8 × 20 mm WallStent and post-dilatation with a 6 × 20 mm balloon (Jupiter, Cordis Endovascular).

patients; 3.3% was the result of the collapse of the Palmaz balloon expandable stent[22] which was treated successfully in three patients (0.75%).

Vitek *et al.* reported clinical follow-up in 95% of patients with two neurological deaths and one major and three minor strokes, for a rate of freedom from any stroke of 92% and freedom from disabling stroke or death of 98%, both at 2 years.

Mathur *et al.* recently reported their analysis of multiple factors that portend a higher risk of complication in stent-assisted angioplasty of the carotid artery in 271 vessels of 231 patients.[23] Their patients constituted a high-risk subset suffering from coronary disease (71%), bilateral carotid disease (39%), and contralateral carotid occlusion (12%). The treated vessels had undergone previous endarterectomy (22%), contained

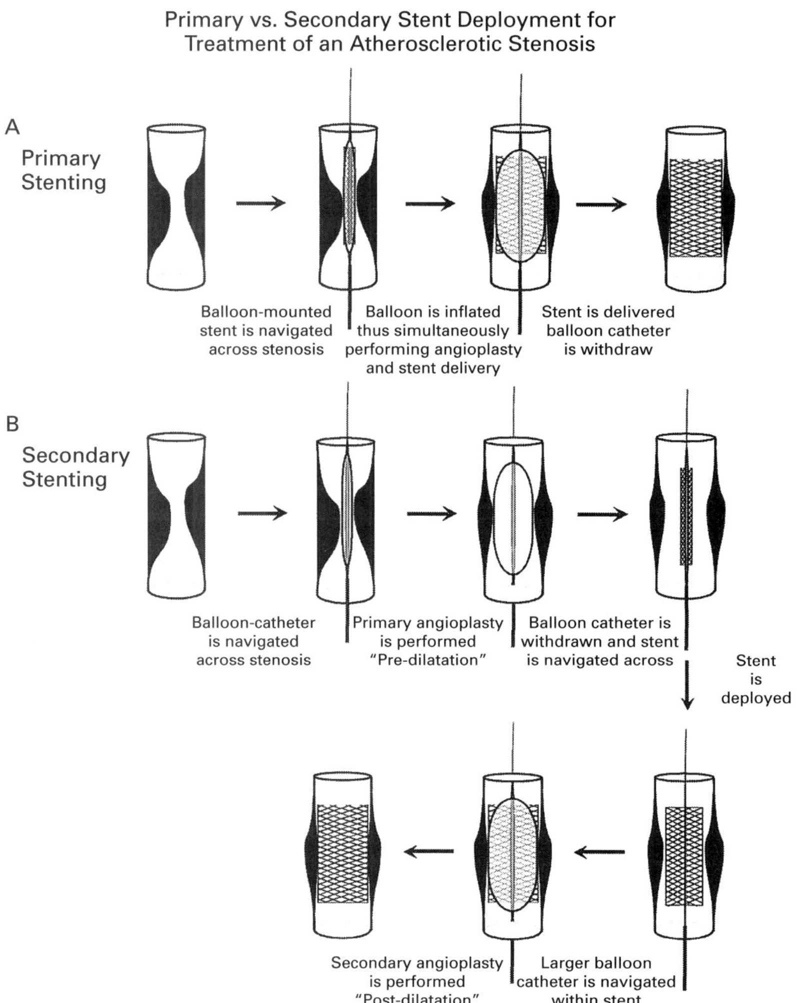

Figure 16.5 Illustration of the two methods of stent deployment for treatment of an atherosclerotic stenosis. (A) Primary stenting in which the lesion is crossed with a wire over which a balloon-mounted stent is navigated across the lesion; the balloon is inflated thus deploying the stent and performing angioplasty in one step. (B) Secondary stenting which may be required in more severe or highly tortuous anatomy, in which a smaller profile balloon is navigated across the lesion and inflated to predilate the lesion; the first balloon is then withdrawn and a stent is deployed (in this case a self-expanding one, although it could also be balloon-mounted), followed by advancement of another larger-caliber balloon through the deployed stent, and angioplasty of the stenosis through the stent. Highly irregular or complex lesions may necessitate the use of a microcatheter (2.3 Fr) and microwire (0.014 inch) combination to cross the lesion prior to removal of the microwire and advancement of a long exchange guidewire (300 cm long) through the microcatheter.

ulcerated plaques (24%), or were calcified lesions (32%). Only 14% of these patients would have been eligible to undergo endarterectomy by NASCET criteria: the rate of minor stroke was 6.2% and that of major stroke was 0.7% during the first 30 days after and including the procedure. Furthermore, the rate of any stroke for the NASCET eligible subset was 2.7% for the same time interval.

Multivariate analysis revealed advanced age and long or multiple stenoses to be independent predictors of procedure-related stroke in carotid stent-assisted angioplasty.[23] These rates compare favorably with the risk of procedural stroke or death from endarterectomy in NASCET[24] which was 5.8%, and in ACAS[25] which was 2.3%, especially considering these high-risk patients,[20] and rates of up to 18% in other high-risk subsets.[20,26] In addition, they also compare favorably to the retrospective analysis of 3111 carotid endarterectomies performed by Sundt *et al.* (Tables 16.4 and 16.5)[20,26] given that a large proportion of the patients undergoing stent-assisted angioplasty constitute Sundt class III and IV.[26]

Table 16.4 Sundt's classification system based on retrospective analysis of 3111 consecutive endarterectomy patients. (From Sundt *et al.*[26]).

Sundt's class	*Criteria for classification*	*Combined surgical morbidity/(mortality)*
Class I	Neurologically stable, no major medical/ angiographically defined risk, with unilateral/ bilateral ulcerative-stenotic disease	0.9%
Class II	Neurologically stable, no major medical risks, with or without angiographic risks	1.7%
Class III	Neurologically stable, major medical risks, with or without angiographic risks	3.7% (1.3%)
Class IV	Neurologically unstable, with or without medical/ angiographic risks	8.1% (2.9%)
Class V	Acute internal carotid artery occlusion, progressive neurological deficit within 6 h of exam	Not included in study
Class VI	Recurrent symptomatic carotid stenosis	Not included in study

Table 16.5 Sundt's definition of medical, neurological and angiographic risk (from Sundt *et al.*[26])

Risk	*Definition*
Medical	Coronary artery disease (angina, myocardial infarction <6 months, congestive heart failure), hypertension (>180/110 mmHg), severe peripheral vascular disease, chronic obstructive pulmonary disease, age > 70 years, severely obese
Neurological	Neurological deficit within 24 h, general cerebral ischemia, recent cerebrovascular accident (<7 days), frequent transient ischemic attacks
Angiographic	Contralateral internal carotid artery occlusion, siphon stenosis, plaque > 3 cm distally in internal carotid artery or >5 cm proximal in common carotid artery, bifurcation at C2 vertebra, short thick neck, and soft thrombus extending from an ulcerative lesion

Angioplasty-induced particulate embolization

Ultrasound has been shown to be sufficiently sensitive to detect stenosis when compared to angiography in a series of 170 stent placements in 119 patients.[27] Robbin *et al.* found that ultrasound did not fail to detect any significant stenosis and was promising in its ability to assess intra-stent intimal hyperplasia.[27]

Angioplasty of atherosclerotic lesions has been reported to induce the release of multiple emboli including atheroma, cholesterol crystals, thrombus, and platelet aggregates.[28–31] Markus *et al.* monitored embolic signals using transcranial Doppler insonation of the ipsilateral middle cerebral artery in 10 patients and detected emboli immediately after angioplasty in nine out of 10 patients, and in eight out of 10 after catheter withdrawal from the artery.[9] The frequency decreased to one out of five patients at 4 h, one out of six at 1 week, and one out of 10 at 1 month.[9]

Embolization of microparticles has also been demonstrated during open endarterectomy and has been shown to correlate with complex plaque morphology[32] and with clinical postoperative cerebral ischemia.[33] A direct contemporaneous analysis of 14 patients undergoing percutaneous angioplasty and 14 undergoing endarterectomy with shunt placement revealed that endarterectomy resulted in significantly greater total occlusion time (337 s vs. 26 s), but a lower count of microembolic signals (52 vs. 202 events) compared to angioplasty , although neither parameter was predictive of later neurological events.[30] It is unclear whether stent placement concomitant with angioplasty may help to decrease the microembolic shower by trapping them under the metal interstices or whether primary stenting would decrease emboli compared to secondary stenting (Fig. 16.5).

The problem of distal embolization during balloon dilatation of atherosclerotic stenoses has engendered interest in various methods of protection. Distal protection using a specially designed triple-coaxial catheter has been described by Théron *et al.*[34] Distal embolic complications were found in three of 38 patients undergoing angioplasty without (8%) and in none of 136 undergoing angioplasty (0%) with distal protection.[35] A number of commercial devices are currently under development to provide distal protection as a means of decreasing the thromboembolic burden associated with angioplasty.

Complications related to angioplasty and stenting

Although angioplasty and stent therapy have certain advantages when compared to the current standard of open surgery,[36] they are also characterized by a set of unique complications of which the operator must be acutely cognizant during both the procedure and the subsequent in-patient recovery.[37] These can be segregated according to Dorros[37] to be related to: arterial access, including hematoma, retroperitoneal hemorrhage, pseudoaneurysm, arteriovenous fistula, arterial thrombosis, groin infection; catheterization, including arterial dissection, embolism of air or thrombus, vessel perforation, tear or rupture; contrast media, including allergic reaction, hypotension, and acute renal failure; and stent placement, including pseudoaneurysm formation and stent infection and arteritis. A recent study reported that permanent neurological complications from diagnostic cerebral angiography was 0.8% in a consecutive series of 500 patients with no deaths.[38]

In a recent meta-analysis, angiography-associated risk of combined and transient neurological complications ranged from 0.8 to 3.0% for patients undergoing the procedure for subarachnoid hemorrhage or for transient ischemic attack/stroke, respectively. The rate of permanent neurological complication was found to be very low at 0.07% for patients presenting with subarachnoid hemorrhage.[39] An excellent account of the multitude of technical complications relating to carotid stent-assisted angioplasty has recently been published by Théron *et al.*[40] The authors eloquently described the type and mechanism of complications encountered, as well as precautionary measures needed for the avoidance of such pitfalls, such as: (1) distal embolism into the internal carotid artery; (2) reflux of thrombus into an ophthalmic artery with a variant origin of the meningolacrimal branch of the middle meningeal artery and into a right vertebral artery via the right subclavian, both encountered during the thrombus flushing phase of protected angioplasty;[35] (3) internal carotid artery thrombosis from insufficient anticoagulation of a complex plaque; (4) internal carotid artery occlusion following deployment of a stent into a false lumen resulting from intimal dissection; (5) vasospasm during protective balloon use; (6) persistent thromboembolic events resulting from the use of a low radial force variant of the WallStent leading to poor apposition of the stent mesh to the luminal lesion surface; and (7) carotid-cavernous fistula formation from inflation of the protective balloon after it had inadvertently migrated distally to the cavernous internal carotid artery as a result of over-aggressive flushing.

Future trends

These complications make it clear that stent-assisted balloon angioplasty of the carotid artery is a more technically complex procedure than it would initially seem, and is fraught with a number of dangerous pitfalls that belie its seductive label as 'minimally invasive'. The endovascular approach presents certain advantages compared to open surgical procedures in its ability to reach areas of the carotid and vertebral arteries which are not readily accessible by open techniques, such as the innominate artery, high cervical and petrous segments of the internal carotid artery.[2]

A recent comparison of carotid stent-assisted angioplasty (107 patients) and endarterectomy (166 patients) by Jordan *et al.*[41] reported an early minor stroke rate of 6.6% for the former and 0.6% for the latter, and a combined major stroke/death rate of 2.8% for the former and 4.2% for the latter: these findings suggest promising results for stent-assisted angioplasty at its current early stage[41] and bode well for its future given the recent report of improved annual risk profile with accumulated technical experience even in the absence of distal protection.[21]

On the other hand, an attempt at a randomized study in an institutional setting for 23 patients with symptomatic stenosis greater than 70% resulted in a prohibitively high risk among the stent-assisted angioplasty group prompting an early halt of the trial in favor of endarterectomy.[42] The stent-assisted angioplasty procedure was performed by a radiologist specialized in peripheral interventional procedures; it is unclear what led to the inordinately elevated rate of procedure-related stroke given the accumulating evidence from different centers pointing to significantly better results (Table 16.3).[15]

The consensus of experienced operators in the field suggests that extensive experience with carotid and cerebral angiography and with interventional procedures is one of the mandatory requisites for achieving a low technical complication rate.[15,40,43] In experienced hands, results from multiple centers (Table 16.3) suggest that carotid stent-assisted angioplasty is currently an acceptable alternative to carotid endarterectomy in select patient subsets which are known to constitute very high risk for surgical complication (Tables 16.4 and 16.5).[20,26]

Future developments in carotid-specific stent design, angioplasty catheters, and methods of distal protection, coupled with long-term clinical radiological follow-up will ultimately determine the role of stent-assisted angioplasty compared to surgical endarterectomy.[36,43] There is an ongoing randomized trial of carotid and vertebral stent-assisted angioplasty and open surgery (CAVATAS),[44,45] and future randomized prospective studies should shed light on the debate and provide the needed scientific data for appropriate decision-making in various patient subsets.

Protocol for carotid angioplasty and stenting at UCSF Medical Center

The patients undergoing balloon angioplasty and stent deployment at UCSF Medical Center mostly belong to Sundt's classes III–VI and include patients with atherosclerosis as well as dissection who have failed maximal medical therapy. In the carotid artery territory, are high-risk patients such as patients with multiple advanced medical problems, contralateral occluded carotid artery with no collateral flow, high cervical and petrous lesions or low common carotid lesions, which are not readily accessible by surgery. Lesions treated in the posterior circulation include subclavian stenosis, vertebral artery origin stenosis, extracranial and intracranial vertebral stenosis and dissection.[18,46]

Technique

The patient is first subjected to a complete and thorough angiographic evaluation, including selective catheterization when deemed safe, using a high-quality digital subtraction unit to determine the location of the lesion, the degree of stenosis, the adequacy of collateral blood supply to the affected territory, the presence of any anatomic variant or aberrant anomaly. Following the study or in certain cases following femoral access, the patient undergoes measurement of a baseline activated clotting time (ACT) and receives an initial weight-based (70 units/kg) intravenous bolus of heparin followed by a post-heparin ACT determination to achieve an ACT value equal to or greater than 2.5 times the baseline value (>250 s). The patient then receives either an hourly dose equal to half the initial bolus or is placed on a heparin drip of 15–20 U/kg/h. Patients are administered enteric-coated aspirin (325 mg daily) and either ticlopidine (Ticlid 250 mg twice a day) or clopidogrel (Plavix 75 mg daily) starting 1–2 days prior to the procedure. Following the procedure, the patient is kept on daily aspirin indefinitely and on ticlopidine or clopidogrel for 6 weeks. The role of glycoprotein IIb/IIIa inhibitors, which have been shown to decrease mortality and morbidity in a number of coronary stent studies,[47] remains to be defined in carotid and vertebral angioplasty and stenting.

During the procedure of cervical carotid angioplasty patients undergo placement of external cutaneous pacing leads and are constantly monitored by a transcutaneous pacer/defibrillator device in case of severe bradycardia or asystole from carotid body stimulation during angioplasty. In addition, patients are administered atropine 0.5–1 mg intravenously or an appropriate dose of glycopyrrolate prior to balloon dilatation of the carotid artery to blunt any parasympathetic discharge. The patients are maintained well hydrated during the procedure although this is tailored to the specific patient and their cardiac status.

The procedure consists of placing a 7-9 Fr sheath (Avanti, Cordis Endovascular) depending on the type of stent to be used (7 Fr for low-profile balloon-mounted coronary stent catheter such as the GFX (Arterial Vascular Engineering, Santa Rosa, CA, USA), GR-2 (Cook Cardiology, Bloomington, IN, USA) or Multi-Link (Guidant, Santa Clara, CA, USA) designs, or 8–9 Fr in the case of the Palmaz (Johnson and Johnson, New Brunswick, NJ, USA) or WallStent (Schneider, Plymouth, MN, USA) designs). In the case of a complex, severely stenosed lesion, or in a high-cervical or intracranial location, a 2.3 Fr microcatheter (Rapid Transit, Cordis Endovascular, Miami Lakes, FL, USA) is used coaxially over a 0.014 inch microguidewire (Transend 14, Scimed Inc., MN, USA). After crossing the lesion using the microcatheter with meticulous care, a 300 cm long 0.014 inch exchange microguidewire (Stabilizer, Cordis Endovascular) is passed through the microcatheter and placed in the cavernous segment of the internal carotid artery or in the posterior cerebral artery, and the microcatheter is then withdrawn. With the exchange guidewire in place, primary or secondary stent-assisted angioplasty is performed (Figs 16.4 and 16.5). In case of secondary stent placement, a low-profile angioplasty balloon catheter is used to cross and pre-dilate the lesion (Fig. 16.5). Once the stenosis has been decreased, the stent is deployed, and a high-pressure non-compliant angioplasty balloon is then used to post-dilate the stent in order to embed it firmly into the plaque. In the case of less complicated and more proximal lesions, a 0.035 guidewire may be used as an exchange guidewire to cross the lesion, bypassing the need for microcatheterization.

Stent designs

The current experience in our center with extracranial carotid atherosclerosis is similar to others[15] and involves the use of the Palmaz and WallStent stainless steel stents primarily, neither of which are specifically designed for use in the carotid artery. The Palmaz stent is balloon-mounted, provides greater radial force, has less metal surface area coverage with larger and fewer interstices and is non-compliant. The WallStent is a self-expandable design with significant lower radial force, and with a greater metal surface area coverage with finer and more numerous interstices.

A problem detected with the Palmaz non-compliant type of stent is that of external stent compression resulting in stenosis.[22] This has been treated by repeat angioplasty but appears to be a fundamental problem with non-compliant stents used in the cervical region. In the case of the WallStent, its compliant design and the consequently lower radial force can be a hindrance in severely calcified lesions. In such lesions, poor embedding of the stent into the vessel wall may lead to focal regions of flow stasis and predilection for thrombus formation.[40] Stent design is an active area with imminent new products some of which have been specifically designed for use in the carotid artery territory.

Intracranial angioplasty and stenting for treatment of atherosclerotic lesions

Percutaneous angioplasty of the intracranial vessels has been used by a number of groups in a preliminary fashion to treat intracranial atherosclerosis in patients who have previously failed maximal medical therapy. Terada reported treatment of 12 lesions with greater than 70% stenosis in patients with clinical symptoms consistent with transient ischemic attack (TIA) despite maximal medical therapy.[48] The angioplasty was performed in the distal vertebral and basilar arteries using a balloon with a 2.0–3.5 mm diameter inflated to 6 atmospheres. The overall stenosis decreased from 84 to 44%; eight patients had no complications, two suffered intimal dissection with subsequent small-size infarcts and two sustained thromboembolism with consequent TIA.[48] Long-term follow-up in 11 patients surviving beyond 6 months showed persistent freedom from symptoms in 10 patients and recurrent transient ischemia in one patient.

A recent development has been the treatment of intracranial atherosclerotic stenoses of the carotid and vertebral arteries with stent placement following, or concurrently with, angioplasty.[49] This treatment is reserved for lesions that are symptomatic despite maximum medical management including oral antiplatelet and anticoagulant treatment. In the carotid artery, stent placement has been performed or reported in the intracranial petrous,[50–52] cavernous, and proximal supraclinoid segment.[53] In the posterior circulation, stents have been deployed along the entire course of the extracranial vertebral artery, in the intracranial V4 segment and in the mid-segment of the basilar artery.[49,53] Compromise of median and paramedian perforator vessels by physical occlusion remains a limiting factor which may preclude the use of mid-basilar stent placement except as a last resort. Intimal dissection is not unexpected following plaque rupture by balloon angioplasty, and is anticipated to heal in the long-run. Stent placement can be used as a bailout measure for treatment of a flow-limiting angioplasty-induced intimal dissection. Intracranial stent-assisted angioplasty is felt to decrease the incidence of vessel recoil following conventional angioplasty.

We are currently treating focal high-grade intracranial atherosclerotic lesions using primary stent-assisted angioplasty with second-generation low-profile balloon-premounted coronary stents (GFX, GR-2, MultiLink). The significantly improved mechanical properties of this new generation of stent catheters has enabled the safe navigation of the vessels at the base of the skull, and in certain cases inside the intracranial circulation.[49] We have performed 12 such procedures in the intracranial vertebral and intracranial carotid artery (Fig. 16.6). Treatment of severe stenoses in the intracranial vessels entails a significantly greater risk of complications because of the delicate vascular structure and the near lack of media and muscular layers. Typical complications may include intimal dissection, vessel rupture, acute vessel thrombosis, and reperfusion injury.[54] We currently limit our treatment of intracranial atherosclerotic lesions to patients who have failed

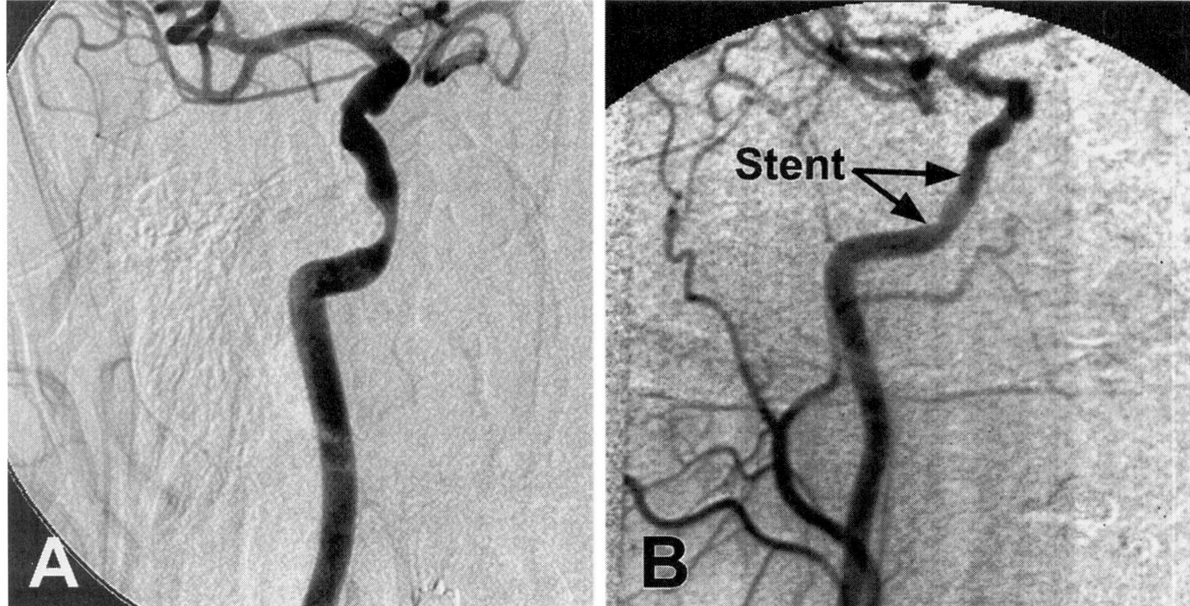

Figure 16.6 The patient described in the previous figure was noted to harbor a hemodynamically significant 70% stenosis in the right petrous portion of the internal carotid artery as evidenced by this right anterior oblique DSA of the right internal carotid artery injection. He underwent primary stent placement using a balloon-premounted stent measuring 3.5 × 12 mm (MultiLink, Cook) with excellent resolution of the stenosis as evidenced by follow-up DSA of the right common carotid artery on post-procedure day 20. The stent is sufficiently radio-opaque to be readily visualized through the petrous bone.

maximum medical therapy and are left with no options short of high-risk surgical bypass or revascularization procedures. As with all emerging indications, we advocate very close clinical and angiographic follow-up in order to outline the appropriate indications better and to define the drawbacks of this therapy in the future.

Intracranial angioplasty and stenting as an adjunct for thrombolysis of acute vessel occlusion

Angioplasty of the cerebral arteries for acute occlusion has been reported to be of benefit in the treatment of acute middle cerebral artery occlusion following a failed thrombolysis attempt.[55] The underlying mechanism remains unclear. It is possible that angioplasty may treat an underlying stenotic lesion. It is hypothesized that the increased flow resulting from the caliber improvement by the dilatation may increase the endogenous production of endothelial nitric oxide and prostacyclin, both of which have vasodilatory and platelet-inhibitory effects,[56,57] and increase the release and production of tissue-type plasminogen activator (tPA).[58] A host of endothelium-derived factors and cytokines have been shown to be regulated by prevailing flow and associated shear stress conditions.[59] The contribution of platelet aggregation to restenosis following successful thrombolysis has been recently confirmed by successful treatment of this condition using the glycoprotein IIb/IIIa inhibitor abciximab.[60]

We have recently reported a case of recalcitrant basilar thrombosis despite thrombolysis and angioplasty which responded to intracranial mid-basilar stent deployment (Fig. 16.7).[49]

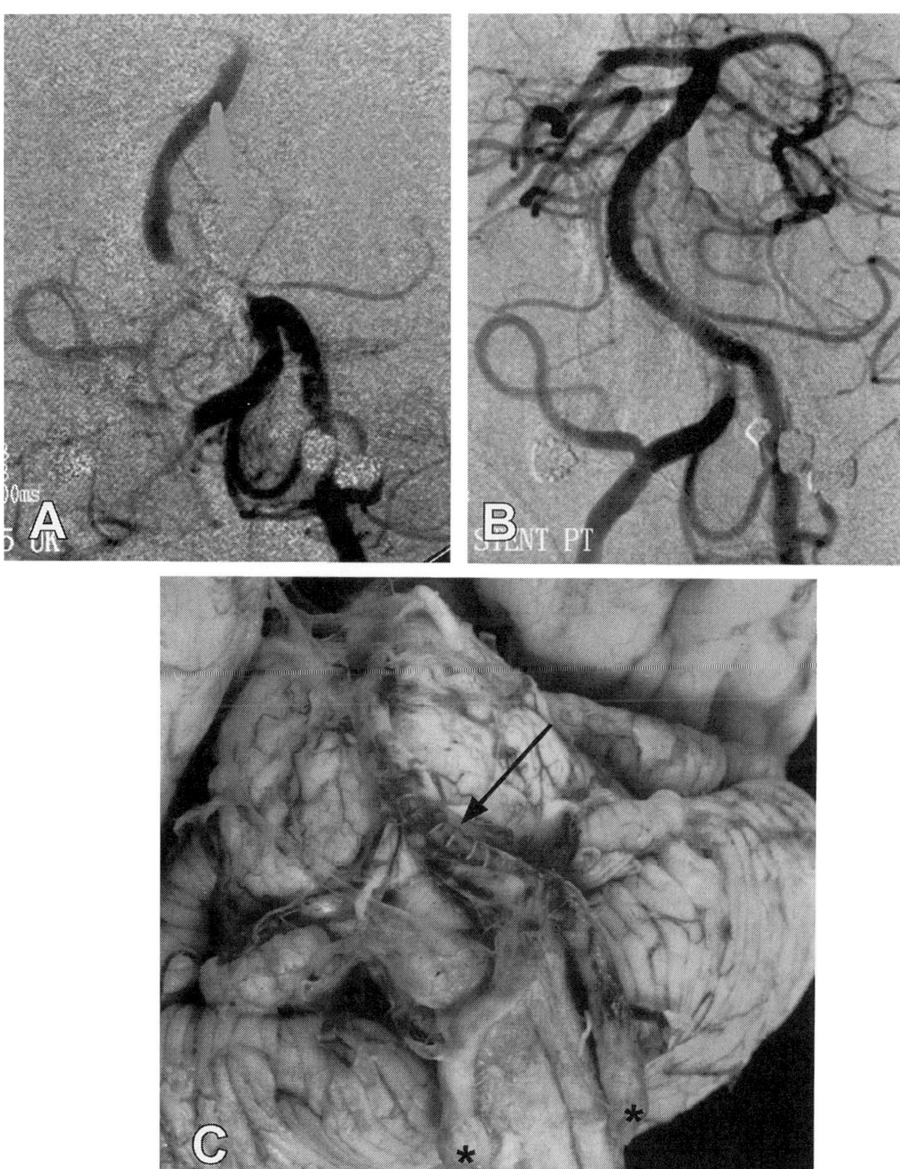

Figure 16.7 An 83-year-old man with a history of hypertension, hypercholesterolemia and coronary artery disease presented with a 6-day history of headaches and presyncope and intermittent locked-in state. He underwent digital subtraction angiography which confirmed acute thrombosis of the basilar artery, which was treated with intraluminal infusion of 750 000 units of urokinase. This resulted in transient patency of the basilar artery followed by recurrent rethrombosis (A). A balloon-premounted coronary stent with widely-spaced strut design (GR-2, Cook) was navigated into the basilar artery and deployed across the lesion (B). The patient improved neurologically, but succumbed later from a retroperitoneal hemorrhage following intravenous antifibrinolytic therapy for myocardial infarction on post-procedure day 10. Post-mortem image of the brainstem shows the bilateral intracranial vertebral arteries (highlighted by *) and the complex yellow atherosclerotic plaque. The stent and its struts can be easily identified through the translucent gossamer-like basilar arterial wall (arrow); this illustrates the delicate vascular structure with the thin media layer and lack of surrounding mesenchymal support such as may be present in the coronary circulation.

A similar benefit of angioplasty when combined with suboptimal thrombolysis was also demonstrated in three cases of intracranial vertebrobasilar occlusion,[61] and in four cases by Yokote *et al.*[62] A preliminary report recently confirmed the merit of a similar approach in 11 out of 68 patients who had failed thrombolysis using superselective intraluminal urokinase.[63]

Stent deployment for treatment of cerebral aneurysms and extracranial cervical pseudoaneurysms

Stents have become increasingly useful for the treatment of wide-necked intracranial aneurysms and extracranial pseudoaneurysms. A stent has been deployed in the basilar artery across the wide neck of a mid-basilar aneurysm to serve as an endovascular scaffold with subsequent placement of a microcatheter between the interstices of the stent.[64] Guglielmi detachable coils (GDC) were then deployed within the otherwise untreatable aneurysm because the stent precluded herniation of the coils within the parent vessel lumen.

Such stent-assisted coil embolization of aneurysms has since been reported for the treatment of carotid[65] and vertebral aneurysms[66,67] and has also been used successfully in the treatment of a petrous internal carotid dissecting pseudoaneurysm.[68] There have also been numerous reports on the effect of stent deployment on alteration of intra-aneurysmal hemodynamics with eventual thrombosis even in the absence of coil embolization.[69,70] Future advances in stent technology including a lower-profile design with greater flexibility and specifically tailored strut porosity for intracranial use is expected to expand the use of stents in the treatment of aneurysms.

Percutaneous balloon angioplasty for treatment of intracranial vasospasm

Cerebral vasospasm following subarachnoid hemorrhage is a leading source of delayed cerebral ischemia following intracranial aneurysmal rupture and is the single most important cause of death and disability for survivors.[71–73] Angioplasty of intracranial arteries for the treatment of vasospasm following subarachnoid hemorrhage is a useful technique for the treatment of cerebral hypoperfusion unresponsive to maximal hypertensive, hypervolemic and hemodilutional therapy (triple-H therapy).[74–76]

The angioplasty is performed while the patient is anticoagulated and utilizes a specifically designed low-profile compliant balloon mounted on an atraumatic flexible catheter. The balloon catheter is deployed via a guide catheter positioned in the extracranial internal carotid or vertebral artery. Upon deployment within the intracranial vessel to be treated, typically the intradural portion of supraclinoid internal carotid artery, the balloon is gently inflated under a digital roadmap technique with a dilute mixture of radio-opaque contrast material in short durations to enable intermittent cerebral perfusion. More distally, the M1 segment of the middle cerebral artery is the most commonly treated vessel. On rare occasions, and in particular when one of the anterior cerebral arteries is dominant, the A1 segment is amenable to angioplasty as well (Fig. 16.8).

A recent study by Elliott *et al.* indicated that there is a longer-lasting benefit with mechanical balloon angioplasty than with intraluminal infusion of papaverine.[74] Intracranial vasospasm was assessed by using transcranial Doppler (TCD) measurement pre- and post-treatment in 101 vessel segments treated with angioplasty alone and 24 vessel segments treated with superselective intraluminal infusion of papaverine alone. Papaverine-treated vessels showed an average decrease in TCD velocity of 20% on postprocedure day 1, which by postprocedure day 2 was no longer significantly different from pretreatment velocities. In contrast, vessels treated with angioplasty showed a 45% lower mean TCD velocity which remained sustained on postprocedure day 2. Eskridge *et al.* demonstrated a similar long-lasting effect by angiographic, clinical and TCD velocity criteria, with only one out of 170

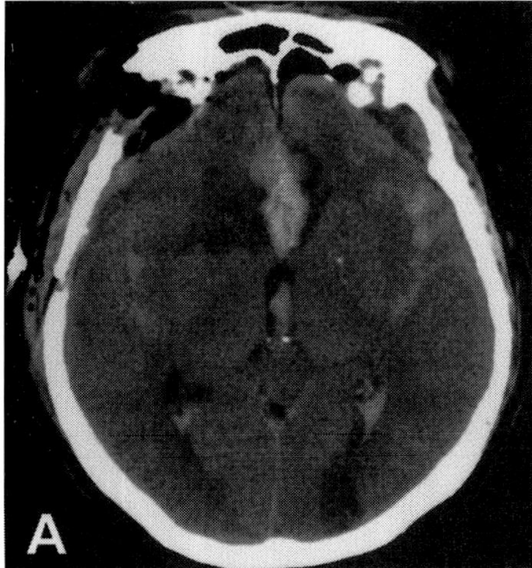

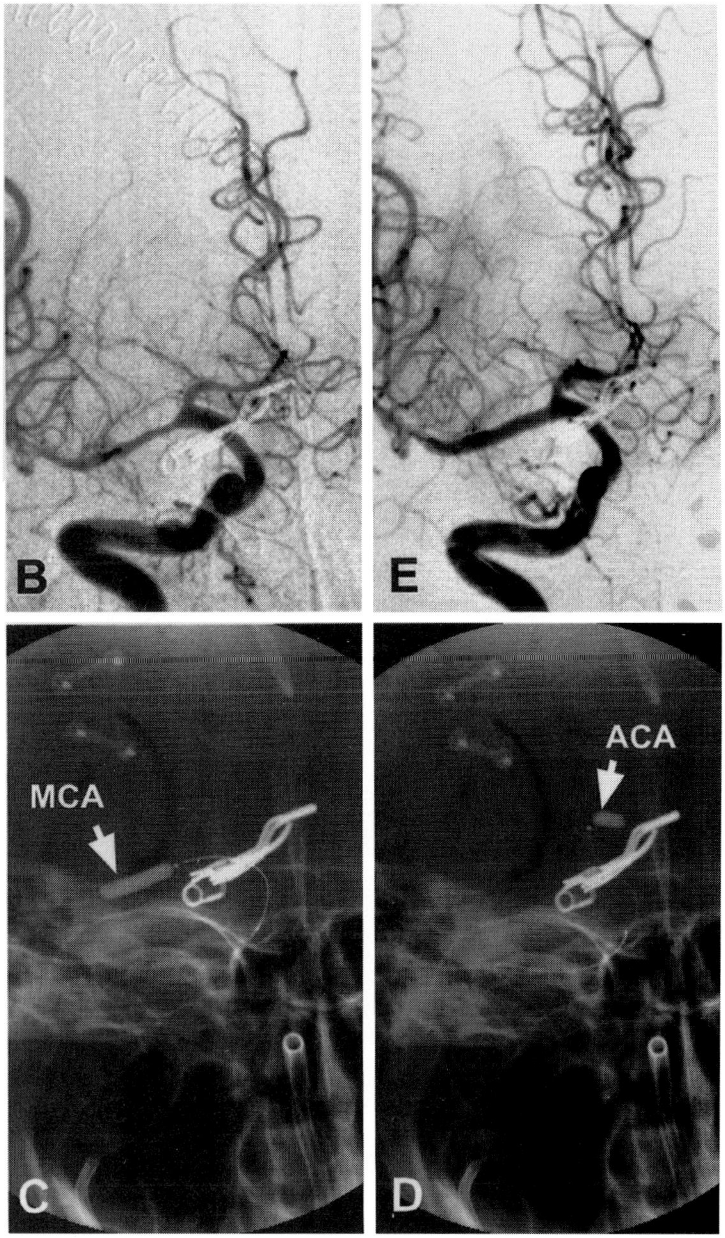

Figure 16.8 A 46-year-old man presented with a Hunt and Hess Grade I subarachnoid hemorrhage and underwent surgical clipping of an anterior communicating artery and a right posterior communicating artery aneurysm (computed tomography: A, postoperative). Postoperative transcranial Doppler insonation confirmed elevated middle cerebral and anterior cerebral velocities which were confirmed by DSA of the right internal carotid artery which showed severe vasospasm in the A1 and M1 segments of the anterior and middle cerebral arteries (B). Plain fluorography outlines the inflated compliant non-detachable balloon-microcatheter (NDSB 0.85, Target Therapeutics, Fremont, CA, USA) in the M1 stem of the middle cerebral artery (C) and the A1 stem of the dominant right anterior cerebral artery (D). Postangioplasty DSA of the right internal carotid artery confirms angiographic resolution of the vasospasm (E).

treated vessel segments requiring repeat angioplasty.[75]

Balloon-dilatation of intracranial vessel segments using a compliant microballoon catheter has established its efficacy and relative safety in the treatment of subarachnoid hemorrhage-related intracranial vasospasm which has failed maximum hypertensive, hypervolemic, and hemodilutional therapy.

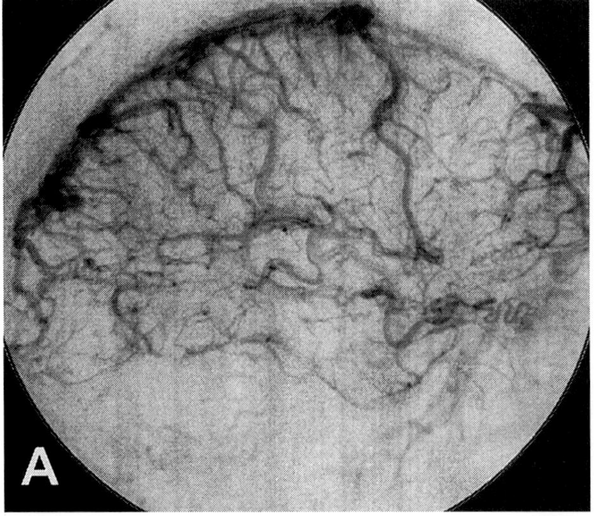

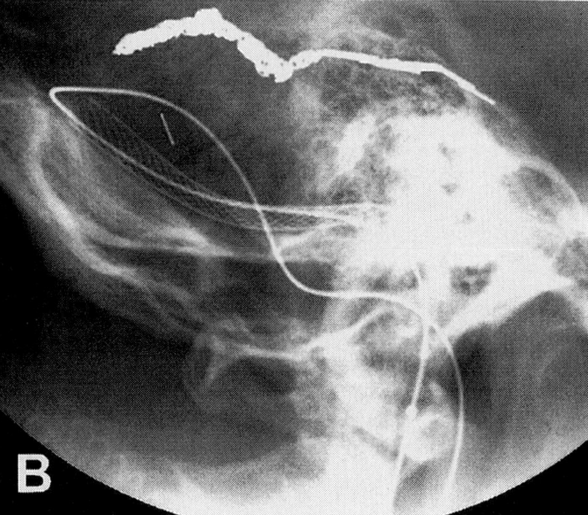

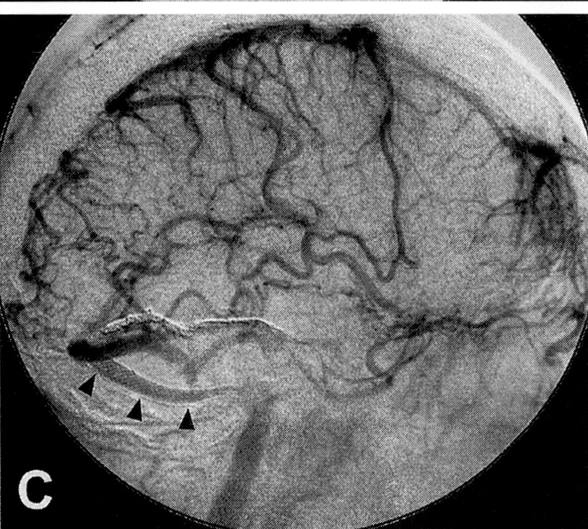

Figure 16.9 A 13-year-old boy with a history of chronic venous sinus thrombosis of the superior sagittal, straight, bilateral transverse, and occipital sinuses (venous phase DSA of the left internal carotid artery; A) presented with increasing headache, aphasia, right hemiparesis and engorged scalp veins consistent with intracranial venous hypertension despite oral warfarin and aspirin therapy. He underwent successful recanalization of the occipital sinus which underwent venous sinus percutaneous angioplasty, followed by deployment of a self-expanding 8 × 40 mm WallStent (Schneider, Plymouth, MN, USA; B). Late venous-phase DSA of the left internal carotid artery confirmed patency of the stent with the occipital sinus now as the only patent venous sinus outflow pathway (arrowheads; C). The patient remained neurologically stable at 1 year of follow-up with a documented persistently patent stent at 3 months postprocedure.

Angioplasty and stenting for treatment of intracranial venous hypertension

Venous hypertensive disease can result from either stenosis or thrombosis of the dural sinuses of the internal jugular vein. Angioplasty of the transverse sinus has been reported to decrease intracranial venous draining pressure.[77] Based on experience in peripheral interventional procedures, stents have a higher risk of thrombosis when placed in the venous than in the arterial circulation. This higher thrombotic[78] tendency in the venous system may be the result of the lower flow velocity and lower shear stress for the same reasons described previously. Stent placement in the venous circulation has mainly consisted of treatment of stenosis in dialysis fistula, axillary-subclavian thrombosis and fresh venous thrombus.[79] We have successfully deployed a stent following recanalization of an occipital sinus in a patient suffering from pan-sinus cerebral thrombosis with excellent patency at 3 months' angiographic follow-up (Fig. 16.9).[80] A stent has similarly been deployed in the left internal jugular vein of a patient with post-traumatic bilateral internal jugular vein thrombosis; this procedure resulted in a measured decrease in both intracranial pressure and sigmoid sinus with resumption of venous drainage and maintained patency at 6 months.

Although venous-side stenting for intracranial hypertension has provided clinical relief in a number of reported cases, it remains a procedure of last resort at the present time, also requiring oral anticoagulation with coumadin to decrease the likelihood of re-thrombosis.[81] Accumulation of future clinical experience and follow-up will help to define the guidelines and limitations of such therapy.

CONCLUSION

Advances in endovascular techniques are making it possible to treat increasingly complex vascular lesions involving both the extracranial and intracranial arterial and venous aspects of the cerebrovascular vasculature in an effort to combat ischemia and thwart cerebral infarction. Angioplasty and stenting in the extracranial carotid artery is becoming a viable alternative to surgical carotid endarterectomy in certain subsets of very high-risk patients. Long-term clinical and angiographic follow-up as well as randomized prospective trials will help to determine the role of percutaneous angioplasty with stenting in the treatment of carotid stenosis. The role of angioplasty has become more clearly established in the treatment of intracranial vasospasm from subarachnoid hemorrhage. Further experience will help to determine the role of percutaneous angioplasty and stent deployment in the treatment of lesions that have no current low-risk surgical alternative, such as intracranial atherosclerosis, cerebral venous hypertension, and carotid and vertebral dissection.

REFERENCES

1. American Heart Association. *1999 Heart and Stroke Statistical Update*. Dallas, Texas; American Heart Association: 1999.
2. Higashida RT, Tsai FY, Halbach VV *et al*. Transluminal angioplasty, thrombolysis, and stenting for extracranial and intracranial vascular disease. *J Interven Cardiol* 1996; **9**:245–55.
3. Dotter CT, Judkins MP. Transluminal treatment of arteriosclerotic obstruction: description of a new technique and a preliminary report of its application. *Circulation* 1964; **30**:654–70.
4. Gruntzig A. Transluminal dilatation of coronary-artery stenosis [letter]. *Lancet* 1978; **i**:263.
5. Kerber CW, Cromwell LD, Loehden OL. Catheter dilatation of proximal carotid stenosis during distal bifurcation endarterectomy. *Am J Neuroradiol* 1980; **1**:348–9.
6. Kachel R. Results of balloon angioplasty in the carotid arteries. *J Endovasc Surg* 1996; **3**:22–30.
7. Higashida RT, Tsai FY, Halbach VV *et al*. Cerebral percutaneous transluminal angioplasty. *Heart Dis Stroke* 1993; **2**:497–502.
8. Higashida RT, Tsai FY, Halbach VV *et al*. Transluminal angioplasty for atherosclerotic disease of the vertebral and basilar arteries. *J Neurosurg* 1993; **78**:192–8.
9. Markus HS, Clifton A, Buckenham T *et al*. Carotid angioplasty. Detection of embolic signals during and after the procedure. *Stroke* 1994; **25**:2403–6.
10. Crawley F, Clifton A, Markus H *et al*. Delayed improvement in carotid artery diameter after carotid angioplasty. *Stroke* 1997; **28**:574–9.
11. Tyagi S, Verma PK, Gambhir DS *et al*. Early and long-term results of subclavian angioplasty in aortoarteritis (Takayasu disease): comparison with atherosclerosis. *Cardiovasc Intervent Radiol* 1998; **21**:219–24.
12. Schoser BG, Becker VU, Eckert B *et al*. Clinical and ultrasonic long-term results of percutaneous transluminal carotid angioplasty. A prospective follow-up of 30 carotid angioplasties. *Cerebrovasc Dis* 1998; **8**:38–41.
13. Macaya C, Serruys PW, Ruygrok P *et al*. Continued benefit of coronary stenting versus balloon angioplasty: one-year clinical follow-up of Benestent trial. Benestent Study Group. *J Am Coll Cardiol* 1996; **27**:255–61.
14. Serruys PW, van Hout B, Bonnier H *et al*. Randomised comparison of implantation of heparin-coated stents with balloon angioplasty

in selected patients with coronary artery disease (Benestent II). *Lancet* 1998; **352:**673–81.

15. Wholey MH, Wholey M, Bergeron P *et al.* Current global status of carotid artery stent placement. *Cathet Cardiovasc Diagn* 1998; **44:**1–6.
16. Yadav JS, Roubin GS, Iyer S *et al.* Elective stenting of the extracranial carotid arteries. *Circulation* 1997; **95:**376–81.
17. Iyer SS, Roubin GS, Yadav S *et al.* Elective carotid stenting. *J Endovasc Surg* 1996; **3:**42–62.
18. Storey GS, Marks MP, Dake M *et al.* Vertebral artery stenting following percutaneous transluminal angioplasty. Technical note. *J Neurosurg* 1996; **84:**883–7.
19. Yadav JS, Roubin GS, King P *et al.* Angioplasty and stenting for restenosis after carotid endarterectomy. Initial experience. *Stroke* 1996; **27:**2075–9.
20. Piepgras DG, Sundt TM Jr, Marsh WR *et al.* Recurrent carotid stenosis. Results and complications of 57 operations. *Ann Surg* 1986; **203:**205–13.
21. Vitek J, Roubin G, Iyer S. *Immediate and Late Outcome of Carotid Angioplasty With Stenting.* Joint Section Meeting, AANS/CNS/ASITN, Nashville 1999.
22. Mathur A, Dorros G, Iyer SS *et al.* Palmaz stent compression in patients following carotid artery stenting. *Cathet Cardiovasc Diagn* 1997; **41:**137–40.
23. Mathur A, Roubin GS, Iyer SS *et al.* Predictors of stroke complicating carotid artery stenting. *Circulation* 1998; **97:**1239–45.
24. North American Symptomatic Carotid Endarterectomy Trial Collaborators. Beneficial effect of carotid endarterectomy in symptomatic patients with high-grade carotid stenosis. *N Engl J Med* 1991; **325:**445–53.
25. Executive Committee for the Asymptomatic Carotid Atherosclerosis Study. Endarterectomy for asymptomatic carotid artery stenosis. *J Am Med Assoc* 1995; **273:**1421–8.
26. Sundt TMJ, Meyer FB, Piepgras DG *et al.* Risk factors and operative results. In: Sundt's Occlusive Cerebrovascular Disease (Meyer FB, ed.), 2nd edn, pp. 241–7. Philadelphia, PA; W.B. Saunders: 1994.
27. Robbin ML, Lockhart ME, Weber TM *et al.* Carotid artery stents: early and intermediate follow-up with Doppler US. *Radiology* 1997; **205:**749–56.
28. Théron J. Cerebral protection during carotid angioplasty [letter; comment]. *J Endovasc Surg* 1996; **3:**484–6.
29. Muller M, Behnke S, Walter P *et al.* Microembolic signals and intraoperative stroke in carotid endarterectomy. *Acta Neurol Scand* 1998; **97:**110–17.
30. Crawley F, Clifton A, Buckenham T *et al.* Comparison of hemodynamic cerebral ischemia and microembolic signals detected during carotid endarterectomy and carotid angioplasty. *Stroke* 1997; **28:**2460–4.
31. Bladin CF, Bingham L, Grigg L *et al.* Transcranial Doppler detection of microemboli during percutaneous transluminal coronary angioplasty. *Stroke* 1998; **29:**2367–70.
32. Gaunt ME, Brown L, Hartshorne T *et al.* Unstable carotid plaques: preoperative identification and association with intraoperative embolisation detected by transcranial Doppler. *Eur J Vasc Endovasc Surg* 1996; **11:**78–82.
33. Levi CR, O'Malley HM, Fell G *et al.* Transcranial Doppler detected cerebral microembolism following carotid endarterectomy. High microembolic signal loads predict postoperative cerebral ischaemia. *Brain* 1997; **120:**621–9.
34. Théron J, Courtheoux P, Alachkar F *et al.* New triple coaxial catheter system for carotid angioplasty with cerebral protection. *Am J Neuroradiol* 1990; **11:**869–77.
35. Théron JG, Payelle GG, Coskun O *et al.* Carotid artery stenosis: treatment with protected balloon angioplasty and stent placement. *Radiology* 1996; **201:**627–36.
36. Zarins CK. Carotid endarterectomy: the gold standard. *J Endovasc Surg* 1996; **3:**10–15.
37. Dorros G. Complications associated with extracranial carotid artery interventions. *J Endovasc Surg* 1996; **3:**166–70.
38. Komiyama M, Yamanaka K, Nishikawa M *et al.* Prospective analysis of complications of catheter cerebral angiography in the digital subtraction angiography and magnetic resonance era. *Neurol Med Chir* 1998; **38:**534–40.
39. Cloft HJ, Joseph GJ, Dion JE. Risk of cerebral angiography in patients with subarachnoid hemorrhage, cerebral aneurysm, and arteriovenous malformation: a meta-analysis. *Stroke* 1999; **30:**317–20.
40. Théron J, Guimaraens L, Oguzman C *et al.* Complications of carotid angioplasty and stenting. *Neurosurg Focus* 1998; **5:**4.
41. Jordan WD Jr, Voellinger DC, Fisher WS *et al.* A comparison of carotid angioplasty with stenting versus endarterectomy with regional anesthesia. *J Vasc Surg* 1998; **28:**397–402.

42. Naylor AR, Bolia A, Abbott RJ *et al*. Randomized study of carotid angioplasty and stenting versus carotid endarterectomy: a stopped trial. *J Vasc Surg* 1998; **28:**326–34.
43. Dorros G. Carotid arterial obliterative disease: should endovascular revascularization (stent supported angioplasty) today supplant carotid endarterectomy? *J Interven Cardiol* 1996; **9:**193–6.
44. Sivaguru A, Venables GS, Beard JD *et al*. European carotid angioplasty trial [see comments]. *J Endovasc Surg* 1996; **3:**16–20.
45. Naylor AR, London NJ, Bell PR. Carotid and Vertebral Artery Transluminal Angioplasty Study [letter; comment]. *Lancet* 1997; **349:**1324–5.
46. Feldman RL, Rubin JJ, Kuykendall RC. Use of coronary Palmaz–Schatz stent in the percutaneous treatment of vertebral artery stenoses. *Cathet Cardiovasc Diagn* 1996; **38:**312–15.
47. Tcheng JE. Glycoprotein IIb/IIIa receptor inhibitors: putting the EPIC, IMPACT II, RESTORE, and EPILOG trials into perspective. *Am J Cardiol* 1996; **78:**35–40.
48. Terada T, Higashida RT, Halbach VV *et al*. Transluminal angioplasty for arteriosclerotic disease of the distal vertebral and basilar arteries. *J Neurol Neurosurg Psychiatr* 1996; **60:**377–81.
49. Phatouros CC, Higashida RT, Malek AM *et al*. Endovascular stenting of an acutely thrombosed basilar artery: technical case report and review of the literature. *Neurosurgery* 1999; **44:**667–73.
50. Dorros G, Cohn JM, Palmer LE. Stent deployment resolves a petrous carotid artery angioplasty dissection. *Am J Neuroradiol* 1998; **19:**392–4.
51. Feldman RL, Trigg L, Gaudier J *et al*. Use of coronary Palmaz–Schatz stent in the percutaneous treatment of an intracranial carotid artery stenosis. *Cathet Cardiovasc Diagn* 1996; **38:**316–19.
52. Mencken GS, Wholey MH, Eles GR. Use of coronary artery stents in the treatment of internal carotid artery stenosis at the base of the skull. *Cathet Cardiovasc Diagn* 1998; **45:**434–8.
53. Bernard JD, Vang MC, Williams JS. Intracranial primary stent-assisted angioplasty: a case series. Joint Section Meeting, AANS/CNS/ASITN, Nashville: 1999.
54. Schoser BG, Heesen C, Eckert B *et al*. Cerebral hyperperfusion injury after percutaneous transluminal angioplasty of extracranial arteries. *J Neurol* 1997; **244:**101–4.
55. Ueda T, Sakaki S, Nochide I *et al*. Angioplasty after intra-arterial thrombolysis for acute occlusion of intracranial arteries. *Stroke* 1998; **29:**2568–74.
56. Berthiaume F, Frangos JA. Flow-induced prostacyclin production is mediated by a pertussis toxin-sensitive G protein. *FEBS Lett* 1992; **308:**277–9.
57. Tsao PS, Lewis NP, Alpert S *et al*. Exposure to shear stress alters endothelial adhesiveness. Role of nitric oxide. *Circulation* 1995; **92:**3513–19.
58. Diamond SL, Eskin SG, McIntire LV. Fluid flow stimulates tissue plasminogen activator secretion by cultured human endothelial cells. *Science* 1989; **243:**1483–5.
59. Malek AM, Izumo S. Molecular aspects of signal transduction of shear stress in the endothelial cell [editorial]. *J Hypertens* 1994; **12:**989–99.
60. Wallace RC, Furlan AJ, Moliterno DJ *et al*. Basilar artery rethrombosis: successful treatment with platelet glycoprotein IIB/IIIA receptor inhibitor. *Am J Neuroradiol* 1997; **18:**1257–60.
61. Nakayama T, Tanaka K, Kaneko M *et al*. Thrombolysis and angioplasty for acute occlusion of intracranial vertebrobasilar arteries. Report of three cases. *J Neurosurg* 1998; **88:**919–22.
62. Yokote H, Terada T, Ryujin K *et al*. Percutaneous transluminal angioplasty for intracranial arteriosclerotic lesions. *Neuroradiology* 1998; **40:**590–6.
63. Budzik R, Farkas J, Schwamm LH *et al*. Intra-arterial balloon assisted thrombolysis for acute stroke. Joint Section Meeting, AANS/CNS/ASITN, Nashville 1999.
64. Higashida RT, Smith W, Gress D *et al*. Intravascular stent and endovascular coil placement for a ruptured fusiform aneurysm of the basilar artery. Case report and review of the literature. *J Neurosurg* 1997; **87:**944–9.
65. Perez-Cruet MJ, Patwardhan RV, Mawad ME *et al*. Treatment of dissecting pseudoaneurysm of the cervical internal carotid artery using a wall stent and detachable coils: case report. *Neurosurgery* 1997; **40:**622–6.
66. Sekhon LH, Morgan MK, Sorby W *et al*. Combined endovascular stent implantation and endosaccular coil placement for the treatment of a wide-necked vertebral artery aneurysm: technical case report. *Neurosurgery* 1998; **43:**380–4.
67. Lylyk P, Ceratto R, Hurvitz D *et al*. Treatment of a vertebral dissecting aneurysm with stents and coils: technical case report. *Neurosurgery* 1998; **43:**385–8.
68. Mericle RA, Lanzino G, Wakhloo AK *et al*. Stenting and secondary coiling of intracranial internal carotid artery aneurysm: technical case

report. *Neurosurgery* 1998; **43:**1229–34.

69. Lieber BB, Stancampiano AP, Wakhloo AK. Alteration of hemodynamics in aneurysm models by stenting: influence of stent porosity. *Ann Biomed Eng* 1997; **25:**460–9.
70. Wakhloo AK, Lanzino G, Lieber BB *et al.* Stents for intracranial aneurysms: the beginning of a new endovascular era? *Neurosurgery* 1998; **43:**377–9.
71. Awad IA, Carter LP, Spetzler RF *et al.* Clinical vasospasm after subarachnoid hemorrhage: response to hypervolemic hemodilution and arterial hypertension. *Stroke* 1987; **18:**365–72.
72. Origitano TC, Wascher TM, Reichman OH *et al.* Sustained increased cerebral blood flow with prophylactic hypertensive hypervolemic hemodilution ('triple-H' therapy) after subarachnoid hemorrhage. *Neurosurgery* 1990; **27:**729–40.
73. Higashida RT, Halbach VV, Cahan LD *et al.* Transluminal angioplasty for treatment of intracranial arterial vasospasm. *J Neurosurg* 1989; **71:**648–53.
74. Elliott JP, Newell DW, Lam DJ *et al.* Comparison of balloon angioplasty and papaverine infusion for the treatment of vasospasm following aneurysmal subarachnoid hemorrhage. *J Neurosurg* 1998; **88:**277–84.
75. Eskridge JM, McAuliffe W, Song JK *et al.* Balloon angioplasty for the treatment of vasospasm: results of first 50 cases. *Neurosurgery* 1998; **42:**510–17.
76. Higashida RT, Halbach VV, Dowd CF *et al.* Intravascular balloon dilatation therapy for intracranial arterial vasospasm: patient selection, technique, and clinical results. *Neurosurg Rev* 1992; **15:**89–95.
77. Marks MP, Dake MD, Steinberg GK *et al.* Stent placement for arterial and venous cerebrovascular disease: preliminary experience. *Radiology* 1994; **191:**441–6.
78. Malek AM, Izumo S. Control of endothelial cell gene expression by flow. *J Biomech* 1995; **28:**1515–28.
79. Rutherford RB. Primary subclavian-axillary vein thrombosis: the relative roles of thrombolysis, percutaneous angioplasty, stents, and surgery. *Semin Vasc Surg* 1998; **11:**91–5.
80. Malek AM, Higashida RT, Balousek PA *et al.* Endovascular recanalization with balloon angioplasty and stenting of an occluded occipital sinus for treatment of intracranial venous hypertension: technical case report. *Neurosurgery* 1999; in press.
81. Duke BJ, Ryu RK, Brega KE *et al.* Traumatic bilateral jugular vein thrombosis: case report and review of the literature. *Neurosurgery* 1997; **41:**680–3.
82. Mathias K. Stent placement in supra-aortic artery disease. In: *Stents. State of the Art and Future Developments* (Lieberman DD, ed.), pp. 87–92. Morin Heights, Canada; Polyscience Publication: 1995.
83. Diethrich EB, Ndiaye M, Reid DB. Stenting in the carotid artery: initial experience in 110 patients. *J Endovasc Surg* 1996; **3:**42–62.
84. Vozzi CR, Rodriguez AO, Paolantonio D *et al.* Extracranial carotid angioplasty and stenting. Initial results and short-term follow-up. *Tex Heart Inst J* 1997; **24:**167–72.
85. Henry M, Amor M, Masson I *et al.* Angioplasty and stenting of the extracranial carotid arteries. *J Endovasc Surg* 1998; **5:**293–304.

17

Migrainous stroke: diagnosis and treatment

Marie-Germaine Bousser

INTRODUCTION

The relationship between migraine and stroke has long been thought to be rather simple: migraine was viewed as a purely vasospastic disorder with arterial constriction and decreased cerebral blood flow during the aura and dilatation during the headache. Sometimes the vasoconstriction was so severe that blood flow decreased below the threshold of ischemia thus inducing a stroke, designated as 'migrainous infarct'.

Apart from this rare arterial complication, there seemed to be little in common between migraine and stroke. Migraine is an essentially benign whole life condition, usually starting before the age of 40 and affecting 12% of the population with a 3:1 female preponderance. It is characterized by recurrent attacks of severe headache with nausea and vomiting which are sometimes preceded by transient neurological disturbances. Stroke is a dramatic acute event occurring at a mean age of 70 and affecting two subjects per thousand per year with a 2:1 male preponderance. It is characterized by a more or less extensive focal deficit of sudden onset leading to death in up to 20% of cases and to sequelae in nearly half the survivors.

Recent studies have emphasized the diversity of migraine, the heterogeneity of stroke and the complexity of their relationship.[1–5] Despite recent advances in identifying the role of neuronal factors in migraine besides that of vascular factors (e.g., cortical spreading depression, trigeminovascular system, calcium channel gene), this condition remains an enigma and it is still not established which of the neuronal or of the vascular factors occur first. We do not even know whether migraine is a single entity, a syndrome, or a combination of various disorders. As regards stroke, it includes intracerebral hemorrhages (20%) and ischemic infarctions (80%). Among infarctions (ischemic strokes), there is a tremendous etiological heterogeneity, the three main varieties being atherosclerosis (30%), small artery diseases (20%), and cardiac emboli (20%). Some 100 other causes have been identified but, despite extensive investigations, the cause of stroke remains undetermined in up to 40% of cases, particularly in the young. Given the diversity and heterogeneity which characterize these two conditions, it is not surprising that their relationship is far more complex than the mere ischemic consequence of an unusually pronounced vasoconstriction. As we will see, migraine is now viewed more as a risk factor for stroke than as a cause, and when migraine and stroke coexist, particularly in young subjects, the possibility of a common underlying disorder should always be considered.

DIAGNOSIS OF MIGRAINOUS STROKE

The classical description

Although a few cases of intracerebral hemorrhage have been reported in migrainous patients,[6] there is no good evidence of a link between migraine and hemorrhagic stroke. By contrast, there is a huge amount of literature devoted to migrainous infarcts with numerous data on their incidence, anatomical features, clinical presentation, neuroimaging characteristics and pathophysiology.

In hospital-based studies of stroke in the young, migraine has been said to be the cause of stroke in up to 27% of cases[2,5] and several hundreds of 'migrainous stroke' or 'migrainous infarcts' case reports have been published. In the Oxfordshire community stroke project, it was found that seven (3%) of 244 first cerebral infarctions were due to 'migrainous infarcts', corresponding to an incidence of 3.36 per 100 000 per year and to an absolute number of 1700 new cases of migrainous infarcts each year in the UK.[7] Such figures obviously raise concern as to the usually held view that migraine is a benign condition. It is, however, of interest to note that among the seven strokes attributed to migraine, only two had a CT scan confirmation of infarct, only one underwent cerebral angiography, only one had echocardiography, three were hypertensive and one had severe widespread atheroma. It is thus highly debatable to consider these seven cases as 'migrainous infarcts' and to use them to calculate incidence rates.

Several cases of fatal stroke in migraine have been reported since that of Féré in 1883[8–14] Without going into the details of the pathological findings, it is remarkable that there was no single consistent pattern of infarcts which were either large or small, single or multiple, cortical or subcortical, carotid or basilar. There was no consistent pattern either of arterial changes; thrombosis, embolism, spasm, dissection and normal arteries have all been reported in these lethal cases of migraine.[2,5]

Such inconsistency applies equally to the clinical and neuroimaging presentations of these migrainous infarcts, which can affect any large arterial territory (although mostly the posterior cerebral artery territory), or present as single or multiple small deep infarcts or even purely affect the eye, encompassing all varieties of retinal infarcts and ischemic optical neuropathies.[2–5] Cerebral angiography is usually normal but various vascular abnormalities have been reported which can again affect large or small arteries: thrombotic or embolic occlusion, localized or diffuse spasm, local or proximal dissection, simple dilatation or aneurysms, early venous drainage.[2–5]

Given this wide variety of infarcts and arterial changes, it is not surprising that no single mechanism can account for every case.[5] The prevailing idea has long been that a primarily vascular mechanism is implicated, such as spasm sometimes visualized at angiography,[15,16] vessel wall hyperplasia as in the lethal case reported by Neligan,[11] embolism as suggested in a number of cases of sudden onset in the absence of arterial wall disease,[17] or local arterial dissection.[9] More recently, the oligemia of the neuronal spreading depression has been suspected to play a role but it has long been known from cerebral blood flow (CBF) studies[18,19] and more recently from positron emission tomography (PET)[20] and magnetic resonance imaging (MRI) studies[21,22] that the decrease in CBF during the aura does not usually reach the level of ischemia as illustrated by a normal diffusion-weighted MRI despite reduced perfusion.[22]

This rapid review of what has been reported as 'migrainous infarcts' shows that a variety of situations has been mixed up, such as any stroke occurring in a migrainous patient; stroke with migrainous features in non-migrainous patients; sometimes any stroke with headache; or even no stroke but a long-lasting deficit in migraine with aura. Such a situation was obviously due to a total lack of consistency not only in the definition of migrainous infarcts but also in the definition of migraine and sometimes of stroke itself. The classification proposed in 1988 by the International Headache Society (IHS) has clarified this issue in suggesting a restricted definition of migrainous infarcts.[23]

The IHS definition

The IHS definition of migrainous infarction includes four major criteria.

1. The patient previously had a migraine with aura.
2. The present attack is typical of previous attacks, which means that the symptoms of the infarct are, at least partly, those of the aura.
3. Neurological deficits are not completely reversible within 7 days and/or neuroimaging demonstrates ischemic infarction in the relevant area.
4. Other causes of infarction are ruled out by appropriate investigations.

This definition is a major improvement, although the 7-days rule is debatable since it leads to the inclusion of cases with long-lasting deficits but without any cerebral infarction (see below). However, the crucial issue concerns the need for appropriate investigations in order to rule out other causes of cerebral infarction: which investigations should be performed and when?

We performed an extensive review of over 200 cases of migrainous infarcts reported before 1988 and we used IHS criteria, requiring at least transthoracic echocardiography and cerebral angiography (any variety) as the minimal 'appropriate investigations'. The number of migrainous infarcts was dramatically reduced to 40.[2] Interestingly in a review of the literature from 1977 to 1997, Moskowitz also found 44 cases, although with slightly different criteria.[24] this number would obviously further decrease if blood tests such as antiphospholipid antibodies (APL) or homocysteinemia were required as 'appropriate investigations'. Furthermore, the absence of other causes at the time of the infarct does not necessarily imply that migraine is the cause since, first, among ischemic stroke in the young, about half occur without detectable undisputable cause, and second, it is sometimes years later that another potential cause can be detected. This was the case in a number of our patients who satisfied all IHS criteria for migrainous infarcts at the time of their stroke, including the absence of other causes at an extensive etiological work-up. One patient, who had a typical posterior cerebral artery (PCA) migrainous infarct with an arterial occlusion, was found 2 years later to have an aneurysm at the site of occlusion.[25] Another that we reported as 'a migrainous cerebral infarction studied by PET'[26] was found to have an atrial septal aneurysm years later when transesophageal echocardiography became available.[27] A third patient was a 20-year-old woman who also had a typical migrainous PCA infarct, but for an isolated positive venereal disease research laboratory (VDRL) test (this was years before APL syndrome was reported). Ten years later she had a miscarriage and a deep vein thrombosis which led to the discovery of a primary APL syndrome.

Migrainous infarcts: do they exist?

From what we have seen so far, the very existence of migrainous infarcts could be questioned. Yet there are documented cases satisfying IHS criteria and occurring in the absence of other causes, even after a long follow-up. One of the most illustrative cases is one of the oldest:[28] it is that of the pathologist Frank Mallory who, at the age of 47, suffered one of his typical attacks of migraine with a scintillating scotoma in the left visual field. Instead of totally recovering as usual, he was left with an upper left quadrant defect. He died 30 years later and, at autopsy his co-worker Polyak found an old small infarct confined to the right lower calcarine lip, in the absence of arterial disease or any other cause.

Thus, migrainous infarcts exist but they are extremely rare and, at present, vastly overdiagnosed.[1–5,24] Until we have specific diagnostic tools for migraine, it is good clinical practice to use restrictive criteria in order not to overlook other potentially treatable causes. The symptoms should:

1. be a documented infarct, and not just a long-lasting deficit;
2. occur during an attack of migraine with aura;

3. be in a subject with a history of migraine with aura;
4. be characterized clinically by the persistence of all or some of the symptoms of the aura;
5. be in the absence of other causes after extensive and repeated etiological investigations including at least ultrasound studies, angiography (magnetic resonance angiography, MRA, or conventional), transesophageal echocardiography (TEE) and APL.

Migrainous infarcts so defined frequently involve the PCA territory (because visual auras are the most frequent) and they are likely to be due to an unusually severe hypoperfusion during the aura, the precise mechanism of which remains unknown.

Migraine as a risk factor for stroke

The issue of migraine as a risk factor for stroke has been addressed in two cohorts[29,30] and seven case–control studies.[31–37] In the Physicians Health Study[29] and in the NHANES study,[30] the risk of ischemic stroke was slightly more than doubled in migrainous subjects, but these two studies suffer a major shortcoming as regards their diagnosis. The seven case–control studies are summarized in Table 17.1. The most consistent finding is that migraine is a risk factor for ischemic stroke in young women, with a relative risk (RR) of approximately 3.[33–37] The risk is higher in migraine with aura (RR 6)[34] and is markedly increased by smoking (RR 10)[34] and by oral contraceptives (RR 14). These risk factors seem to have more than a multiplicative effect since the odds ratio for ischemic stroke in young female migrainous patients who take oral contraceptives and who smoke reaches 34.4 (3.27–361).[37] Even with such an increased relative risk, the absolute risk of stroke remains low in young women but it is far from negligible and it requires practical preventive measures (see treatment).

In the most recent case–control study devoted to migraine and stroke in young women,[37] it has been stressed that 'up to 40% of strokes in migrainous women seem to develop directly out of a migraine attack—a so called migrainous stroke'. This statement is based on the fact that 67–73% of strokes occurring in women with a prior history of migraine were preceded by headache and other features of migraine within the 3 previous days compared with 24–31% of those occurring in controls. This argument is insufficient since first, the risk of other varieties of headache is increased in migrainous subjects, second, as admitted by the authors, their data are not precise enough to verify that the neurological deficit is identical to the aura symptoms, and third, it is not indicated which investigations were performed to rule out other causes of ischemic stroke. There is thus again a confusion between migraine as a risk factor for cerebral infarction (which is now a well established fact in young women) and migraine as a cause of cerebral infarction—so called 'migrainous infarction' which remains extremely rare.

By contrast to what is observed in young women, there is no good evidence so far that migraine is a risk factor in older age groups. This is further illustrated by recent data from the Framingham cohort-based study on 2100 subjects examined during 1971–1989. Visual migrainous auras were present in 1.23% and started at a mean age of 56.2 ± 18.7 years. This group had no increased risk of stroke (11.5%) compared with subjects without aura (13%) and in subjects with transient ischemic attacks (33%).[38]

The mechanism by which migraine increases the risk of ischemic stroke in young women remains unknown. In most cases other established or debated risk factors for ischemic stroke are involved, such as hypertension, smoking, oral contraceptives, mitral valve prolapse,[5] patent foramen ovale,[39] hereditary thrombophilia[40] or increased platelet aggregation.[41] It thus seems that an accumulation of risk factors puts migrainous women at risk for stroke but the exact immediate mechanism remains unknown.

One possible link between migraine and cerebral infarction is the occurrence of a dissection of cervical arteries. In a number of cases of so called 'migrainous infarcts', a carotid narrowing was seen at angiography which was interpreted as spasm but was strikingly similar

Table 17.1 Recent case–control studies on the association between migraine and stroke in young women

Authors	*Patients*	*Diagnosis of migraine*	*Risk of stroke in migraine patients*
Tzourio *et al.*[33]	212 patients aged 15–80 years with ischemic stroke 212 hospitalized controls matched for sex, age, and history of hypertension	Direct interview by neurologists, IHS criteria	OR = 4.3 (1.2, 16.3) in women < 45 years
Tzourio *et al.*[34]	72 females aged 15–44 years hospitalized for an ischemic stroke 173 hospitalized controls matched for age	Direct interview by neurologists, IHS criteria	OR = 3.0 (1.5, 5.8) MWA OR = 6.2 (2.1, 18.0) MA
Lidegaard[35]	692 females aged 15–44 years with ischemic stroke registered on a national registry 1584 controls matched for age	Questionnaire	OR = 2.8 ($P < 0.001$)
Carolei *et al.*[36]	308 patients aged 15–44 years hospitalized for transient ischemic attack or stroke 591 hospitalized controls matched for age and sex	Direct interview by neurologists, IHS criteria	OR = 3.7 (1.5, 9) in women < 35 years OR 8.6 (1, 75) MA
Chang *et al.*[32]	291 females aged 20–44 years with stroke 736 age- and hospital-matched controls	Questionnaire Modified IHS criteria	OR = 3.5 (1.3, 9.6) OR = 2.9 (0.6, 13.5) MWA OR = 3.8 (1.2, 11.5) MA

IHS indicates International Headache Society. OR; odds ratio. MWA; migraine without aura. MA; migraine with aura.

to the characteristic 'string sign' of carotid dissections.[42,43] Furthermore, migraine was found in a case–control study to be a risk factor for dissections.[44] There is thus an intriguing association between migraine and dissections which needs to be studied further.

DIFFERENTIAL DIAGNOSIS

Prolonged migrainous deficits without infarcts

Migrainous infarcts should be differentiated from very long-lasting deficits that can occur after a migrainous attack without CT scan or MRI evidence of infarcts and which recover completely. This has been particularly well documented in familial hemiplegic migraine (FHM), an autosomal dominant variety of migraine with aura in which hemiplegia, often associated with aphasia, hemianopia,[45–47] drowsiness and sometimes coma, can last up to several weeks and then resolve without sequelae. During these severe attacks which mimic a massive middle cerebral artery infarction, there is a major swelling of the hemisphere and severe electroencephalogram (EEG) disturbances.[48,49] In one case studied by PET, there was a diffuse metabolic depression with a relative increase in CBF, a major decrease in oxygen extraction fraction and a moderate decrease in the cerebral metabolic rate of oxygen ($CMRO_2$).[49] Such a pattern is not that of an infarct and it is a unique example of severe neuronal dysfunction with a preserved $CMRO_2$.

These cases demonstrate that very long-lasting deficits can occur in migraine without cerebral infarction and that the time limit of 7 days suggested by the IHS classification[23] is far too short. Whether these long-lasting deficits are specifically related to the involvement of the calcium-channel gene CACNL 1 A4 implicated in 50% of FHM families or to other genes remains to be determined.[50–52]

Ischemia-induced migraine

The idea that stroke can induce migraine has been vigorously defended by Olesen *et al.*[53] who suggested that 'ischaemia-induced (symptomatic) migraine attacks may be more frequent than migraine-induced ischaemic insults'. To make the point, they described a few cases of ischemic stroke causing single or recurrent attacks of migraine with aura and a few other cases of severe carotid stenosis or occlusion with decreased CBF causing a flurry of attacks of migraine with aura. Interestingly, two of the cases had carotid dissection which is, as seen above, a great mimic of so called migrainous infarction.[43,54] The possible triggering of an attack of migraine with aura by focal ischemia is further supported by animal studies showing that cerebral ischemia can induce cortical spreading depression. There is thus good evidence that attacks of symptomatic migraine can be triggered by focal ischemia but there are no data so far to demonstrate that migraine as a disease can be the consequence of cerebral ischemia.

Migraine and stroke sharing a common cause

There are a number of conditions, local or general, which can cause stroke and are also associated with high frequency of migraine.

Among local causes, the most classical one is arteriovenous malformations (AVM) which have long been thought to be a cause of migraine (symptomatic migraine).[55,56] The situation is not so clear because of the lack of large-scale, well conducted case–control studies and also because of the unpredictable effect of the AVM treatment. There are well documented cases of migraine attacks satisfying all IHS criteria which stopped after AVM removal but there are equally well documented cases of attacks persisting unchanged after surgery.[57] A strong argument in favor of a causal relationship is the overwhelming correlation between the side of the aura or headache and the side of the AVM. In his review of the literature, Haas found that only one patient out of 15 experienced his aura ipsilateral to the malformation and one out of 11 had unilateral headache contralateral to the AVM. There is thus a strong suggestion that AVM can trigger attacks of migraine particularly with aura. By contrast, the relation of migraine to saccular aneurysm remains poorly substantiated, provided that thunderclap headache[58] and sentinel headache[59] are not mistaken for migraine. A number of other local conditions can manifest themselves as stroke and/or as more or less typical migraine attacks: leptomeningeal angiomatosis of the Sturge–Weber type,[60–62] lymphocytic meningitis which always raises the question of migraine attacks with pleiocytosis,[46] and some rare cases of cerebral venous thrombosis.[63]

Many general conditions are also characterized by both migraine attacks (most commonly with aura), and ischemic strokes: thrombocythemia,[64] thrombocytopenia,[65] leukemia,[66] systemic lupus erythematosus,[67] antiphospholipid antibody syndrome,[68,69] hereditary hemorrhagic telangiectasia[70] and mitochondrial cytopathies.[71–75] Stroke and migraine are major features of MELAS syndrome, which is associated with the 3243 point mitochondrial DNA mutation in the tRNA leu (UUR) gene. The frequency of migraine attacks in this condition has led to the hypothesis that mitochondrial mutations could play a role in migraine with aura and in 'migrainous stroke', but the 3243 mutation was not detected in two groups of subjects suffering a migraine with aura.[73,75] However, more work is needed on this topic because other mutations not yet detected on this huge gene could play a role in both migraine and ischemic stroke.

A most remarkable example of a condition which can cause migraine and stroke is CADASIL (Cerebral Autosomal Dominant Arteriopathy with Subcortical Infarcts and Leukoencephalopathy). CADASIL is the acronym that we suggested in 1993 to designate an autosomal dominant small artery disease of the brain characterized clinically by recurrent small deep infarcts, subcortical dementia, mood disturbances and migraine with aura.[76–79] When it is present, migraine is usually the first symptom of the disease, appearing at a mean age of 30, some 15 years before the first ischemic stroke. Symptoms of migraine correspond clinically to those defined as migraine with aura by the IHS, with an unusual frequency of attacks with prolonged aura and of attacks of acute onset aura without headache that are sometimes indistinguishable from transient ischemic attacks.[76,79] However, MRI in CADASIL is always abnormal, showing striking white matter abnormalities in T2WI and, later in the disease, small subcortical areas of hyposignal on T1WI suggestive of small deep infarcts. These abnormalities should not be interpreted just as white matter changes related to migraine which have been reported to be particularly frequent in migraine with aura.[80,82] The finding of white matter abnormalities in subjects who suffer migraine with aura and have a family history of stroke or dementia is suggestive of CADASIL. In some families, however, the migraine phenotype may be preponderant leading to greater diagnostic difficulties.[83,84]

The CASASIL gene has now been identified as Notch 3 and the mutations are remarkably stereotyped (mis-sense mutations leading to an unpaired number of cysteine residues) and clustered within the epidermal-growth-factor (EGF)-like repeats in the extracellular domain of exons 3 and 4. This allows a diagnostic test that detects the pathogenic mutation in about 75% of subjects with a clinical and MRI pattern suggestive of CADASIL.[86] This disease, which affects small cerebral and leptomeningeal arteries, is a fascinating model to speculate about the relationships between migraine with aura and ischemic stroke. It is unlikely that migraine is the consequence of ischemia since, first, infarcts are subcortical whereas the visual aura points typically to the occipital lobe, and second, infarcts occur some 15–20 years after the onset of migraine. Migraine and ischemic stroke might both be due to the arteriopathy itself through the activation of the smooth muscle cells responsible for migraine at an early stage, and their destruction with thickening of the arterial wall responsible for stroke at a later stage. A third hypothesis would be that the arteriopathy would cause the ischemic strokes but that migraine could be directly due to Notch 3 alterations which might modulate the calcium-channel gene involved in migraine. This is totally speculative but the understanding of the exact role of Notch 3 mutations might be crucial for the elucidation of the pathogenesis of migraine with aura and of the migraine–stroke connection.

TREATMENT

Prevention

Since migraine is a risk factor for stroke in young women, young female migrainous patients should be considered as a good target group for stroke prevention.[87]

This means that other potential risk factors should be taken into consideration as well as potential protective factors. Making sure that the blood pressure is normal and that there are no other diseases (e.g., hyperlipemia, diabetes, familial thrombophilia) that might increase the risk of stroke is the obvious first step. When present, which is rare in young female migrainous patients, these conditions should be appropriately treated.

The major question relates to oral contraceptives and smoking which, when combined, dramatically increase the risk of ischemic stroke in young female migrainous patients.[88] This has led some specialists to firmly contraindicate oral contraceptives to all young migrainous patients. We believe that a less rigid position can be taken, first because of the obvious benefits of oral contraceptives for many young women, and second, because of the low absolute risk of stroke, provided that migrainous women who take the pill do not smoke. Smoking, more than oral contraceptives, is what should be discouraged since it is the single most important modifiable risk factor for stroke in the young and since more and more women smoke and at an ever younger age. If oral contraceptives are used, low-estrogen content pills or even progestin pills alone should be advised, particularly in women who suffer migraine with aura. There has been much debate about the use of daily aspirin for stroke prevention.[87] We do not favor the systematic use of aspirin because of its risk for gastric ulcers and bleeding and because of its absence of efficacy in primary stroke prevention[89] (in contrast to secondary stroke prevention). We only recommend aspirin in the very rare cases of migraine with aura who have very frequent attacks, more because of its preventive effect on migraine itself[90] than for stroke prevention.

Not only should risk factors be appropriately managed but protective measures should be encouraged such as having a regular physical activity, which has been shown in a number of studies to decrease the risk of stroke effectively.[91] For the prevention of true migrainous infarcts (an infarct due to severe ischemia during a migraine attack in the absence of other causes), it would seem appropriate to use prophylactic migraine drugs[88] but this is very debatable since drugs, such as beta blockers[92] and methysergide, have been held responsible for some migrainous infarcts. At present, there are no data to suggest that migraine prophylaxis decreases the risk of migrainous infarcts.

As regards the acute treatment of migraine attacks, there is a case, particularly in migraine with aura, for trying analgesics and non-steroidal anti-inflammatory drugs first, before turning to ergot-derivatives and triptans, which are ineffective when taken during the aura and should only be used during the headache phase of migraine.

Acute treatment

There is no specific treatment of migrainous infarcts. The treatment, as well as the investigation, should be as for any cerebral infarct in the young, according to its severity and presumed mechanism. After the infarct, the usual measures of secondary stroke prevention should be taken: suppression of oral contraceptives and of smoking, daily use of antiplatelet drugs such as aspirin[89] or clopidogrel,[93] regular check-up of blood pressure, glycemia and cardiac status.

The treatment of migraine after a cerebral infarct definitely excludes the use of ergot derivatives and triptans. Preventive treatment is usually unnecessary because of the prophylactic effect of aspirin on migraine.

CONCLUSIONS

Migrainous infarcts (i.e., infarcts due to a severe migraine attack with aura in the absence of other causes) are extremely rare and should be diagnosed only by exclusion. Their etiological work-up and treatment should be identical to those of stroke occurring in non-migrainous patients. The debate over the risk of angiography which was not found to be increased in migrainous patients[94] except in FHM,[79] is now closed with the widespread use of ultrasound and MRA. Many conditions can mimic migrainous infarcts such as prolonged aura symptoms, or ischemia-induced migraine attacks, and many conditions can induce both ischemic stroke and migraine attacks, such as AVM, mitochondrial cytopathies, and CADASIL. Finally, migraine, particularly with aura, is an established risk factor for ischemic stroke in young women, through an unknown mechanism. Young migrainous women thus constitute a good target group for stroke prevention, and should be strongly advised not to smoke.

REFERENCES

1. Bousser MG, Baron JC, Chiras J. Ischemic strokes and migraine. *Neuroradiology* 1985; **27**:583–7.
2. Iglesias S, Bousser MG. Migraine et infarctus cerebral. *Circ Métab Cerv* 1990; **7**:237–49.
3. Welch KMA, Levine SR. Migraine-related stroke in the context of the International Headache Society. Classification of head pain. *Arch Neurol* 1990; **47**:458–62.
4. Welch KMA. Relationship of stroke and migraine. *Neurology* 1994; **44**(Suppl 7):33–6.
5. Welch KMA, Tatemichi TK, Mohr JP. Migraine and stroke. In: *Stroke, Pathophysiology, Diagnosis and Management* (Barnett HJM, Mohr JP, Stein BM, Yatsu FM, eds), 3rd edn, pp. 845–67. Philadelphia; Churchill Livingstone: 1998.
6. Cole AJ, Aube M. Migraine with vasospasm and delayed intra cerebral hemorrhage. *Arch Neurol* 1990; **47**:53–6.
7. Henrich JB, Sandercock PAG, Warlow CP, Jones LN. Stroke and migraine in the Oxfordshire community stroke project. *J Neurol* 1986; **233**:257–62.
8. Féré Ch. Note sur un cas de migraine ophthalmique à accès répétés et suivis de mort. *Rev Méd* 1883; **3**:194–201.
9. Sinclair W. Dissecting aneurysm of the middle cerebral artery associated with the migraine syndrome. *Am J Pathol* 1953; **29**:1083–90.
10. Guest IA, Woolf AL. Fatal infarction of the brain in migraine. *Br Med J* 1964; **18**:267–336.
11. Neligan P, Harriman DG, Pierce J. Respiratory arrest in familial hemiplegic migraine. *Br Med J* 1977; **11**:732–4.
12. Selby G, Fryer JA. Fatal migraine. *Clin Exp Neurol* 1984; **20**:85–92.
13. Lindboe CF, Dahl T, Rostad B. Fatal stroke in migraine: a case report with autopsy findings. *Cephalalgia* 1989; **9**:277–80.
14. Buckle RM, Du Boulay G, Smith B. Death due to cerebral vasospasm. *J Neurol Neurosurg Psychiat* 1964; **27**:440–4.
15. Dukes HT, Vieth RG. Cerebral arteriography during migraine prodrome and headache. *Neurology* 1964; **14**:636–9.
16. Solomon S, Lipton RB, Harris PY. Arterial stenosis in migraine: spasm or arteriopathy? *Headache* 1990; **30**:51–61.
17. Rascol A, Cambier J, Guiraud B, Manelfe C, David J, Clanet M. Accidents ischémiques cérébraux au cours des crises migraineuses. A propos des migraines compliquées. *Rev Neurol* 1979; **135**:867–84.
18. Olesen J, Larsen B, Lauritzen M. Focal hyperemia followed by spreading oligemia and impaired activation of rCBF in classic migraine. *Ann Neurol* 1981; **9**:344–52.
19. Lauritzen M, Olsen TS, Lassen NA, Paulson OB. Changes in regional cerebral blood flow during the course of classic migraine attacks. *Ann Neurol* 1983; **13**:633–41.
20. Woods RP, Iacoboni M, Mazziotta JC. Bilateral spreading cerebral hypoperfusion during spontaneous migraine headache. *New Engl J Med* 1994; **331**:1689–92.
21. Welch KMA, Cao Y, Aurora S, Wiggins G, Vikingstad EM. MRI of the occipital cortex, red nucleus and substantia nigra during visual aura of migraine. *Neurology* 1998; **51**:1465–9.
22. Cutrer FM, Sorensen AG, Weisskoff RM *et al.* Perfusion-weighted imaging defects during spontaneous migrainous aura. *Ann Neurol* 1998; **43**:25–31.
23. Headache Classification Committee of the International Headache Society. Classification and diagnostic criteria for headache disorders, cranial neuralgias, and facial pain. *Cephalalgia*

1988; **8**(Suppl 7):1–97.
24. Moskowitz M. Migraine and stroke. A review of cerebral blood flow. *Cephalalgia* 1998; **18**(Suppl 22):22–5.
25. Mas JL, Baron JC, Bousser MG, Chiras J. Stroke, migraine and intracranial aneurysm: a case report. *Stroke* 1986; **17:**1019–21.
26. Bousser MG, Baron JC, Iba-Zizen MT, Comar D, Cabanis E, Castaigne P. Migrainous cerebral infarction: a tomographic study of cerebral blood flow and oxygen extraction fraction with the 015 inhalation technique. *Stroke* 1980; **11:**145–8.
27. Tourbah A, Mas JL, Baron JC, Bousser MG. Complicated migraine, migrainous infarction . . . or what? *Headache* 1988; **28:**689.
28. Polyak S. *The Vertebrate Visual System*, pp. 735–47. Chicago; University of Chicago Press: 1957.
29. Buring JE, Hebert P, Romero J *et al.* Migraine and subsequent risk of stroke in the Physicians Health Study. *Arch Neurol* 1995; **52:**129–34.
30. Merikangas KR, Fenton B, Cheng SH, Stolar MJ, Risch N. Association between migraine and stroke in a large scale epidemiological study of the United States. *Arch Neurol* 1997; **54:**362–8.
31. Collaborative Group for the Study of Stroke in Young Women. Oral contraceptives and stroke in young women. Associated risk factors. *J Am Med Assoc* 1975; **231:**718–22.
32. Henrich JB, Horwitz RJ. A controlled study of ischaemic stroke risk in migraine patients. *J Clin Epidemiol* 1989; **42:**773–80.
33. Tzourio C, Iglesias S, Hubert JB *et al.* Migraine and risk of ischemic stroke. *Br Med J* 1993; **308:**289–92.
34. Tzourio C, Tehindrazanarivelo A, Iglesias S *et al.* Case–control study of migraine and risk of ischaemic stroke in young women. *Br Med J* 1995; **310:**830–3.
35. Lidegaard Ö. Oral contraceptives, pregnancy and the risk of cerebral thromboembolism: the influence of diabetes, hypertension, migraine and previous thrombotic disease. *Br J Obstet Gynecol* 1995; **102:**153–9.
36. Carolei A, Marini C, De Matteis G and the Italian National Research Council Study Group in Stroke in the Young. History of migraine and risk of cerebral ischaemia in young adults. *Lancet* 1996; **347:**1503–6.
37. Chang CL, Donaghy M, Poulter N and WHO collaborative study of cardiovascular disease and steroid hormone contraception. *Br Med J* 1999; **318:**13–8.
38. Wijman CAC, Wolf PA, Kase CS, Kelly-Hayes M, Beiser AS. Migrainous visual accompaniments are not rare in late life. The Framingham Study. *Stroke* 1998; **29:**1539–43.
39. Del Sette M, Angeli S, Leandri M *et al.* Migraine with aura and right-to-left shunt on transcranial Döppler: a case–control study. *Cerebrovasc Dis* 1998; **8:**327–30.
40. D'Amico D, Moschiano F, Leone M *et al.* Genetic abnormalities of the protein C system: shared risk factors in young adults with migraine with aura and with ischemic stroke? *Cephalalgia* 1998; **18:**618–21.
41. Couch JR, Hassanein RS. Platelet aggregability in migraine. *Neurology* 1977; **27:**843–8.
42. Bousser MG, Baron JC, Mas JL. More on: unusual angiographic appearance during an attack of hemiplegic migraine. *Headache* 1986; **26:**487.
43. Shuaib A. Stroke from other etiologies masquerading as migraine-stroke. *Stroke* 1991; **22:**1068–74.
44. D'Anglejan-Chatillon J, Ribeiro V, Mas JL, Youl BD, Bousser MG. Migraine—a risk factor for dissection of cervical arteries. *Headache* 1989; **29:**560–1.
45. Whitty CWM. Familial hemiplegic migraine. *J Neurol Nuerosurg Psychiatr* 1953; **16:**172–7.
46. Fitzsimons RB, Wolfenden WH. Migraine coma. Meningitic migraine with cerebral oedema associated with a new form of autosomal dominant cerebellar ataxia. *Brain* 1985; **108:**555–77.
47. Münte TF, Müller-Vahl H. Familial migraine coma: a case study. *J Neurol* 1990; **237:**59–61.
48. Harrison MJG. Hemiplegic migraine. *J Neurol Neurosurg Psychiatr* 1981; **44:**652–3.
49. Baron JC, Serdaru M, Lebrun-Gandrie P, Bousser MG, Cabanis E, Lhermitte F. Débit sanguin cérébral et consommation d'oxygène locale au cours d'une migraine hémiplégique prolongnée. In: *Migraine et céphalées*, pp. 33–43, GREC. Colloque de Marseille; Sandoz Editions France: 1983.
50. Joutel A, Bousser MG, Biousse V *et al.* A gene for familial hemiplegic migraine maps to chromosome 19. *Nature Genet* 1993; **5:**40–5.
51. Ophoff RA, van Eijk R, Sandkuijl LA *et al.* Genetic heterogeneity of familial hemiplegic migraine. *Genomics* 1994; **22:**21–6.
52. Ducros A, Joutel A, Vahedi K *et al.* Mapping of a second locus for familial hemiplegic migraine to 1q21-q23 and evidence of further heterogeneity. *Ann Neurol* 1997; **42:**885–90.

53. Olesen J, Friberg L, Olsen TS *et al.* Ischaemia-induced (symptomatic) migraine attacks may be more frequent than migraine-induced ischaemic insults. *Brain* 1993; **116:**187–202.
54. Biousse V, d'Anglejan-Chatillon J, Massiou H, Bousser MG. Head pain in non-traumatic carotid artery dissection: a series of 65 patients. *Cephalalgia* 1994; **14:**33–6.
55. Waltimo O, Hokkanen E, Pirskanen R. Intracranial arteriovenous malformations and headache. *Headache* 1975; **15:**133–5.
56. Bruyn GW. Intracranial arteriovenous malformation and migraine. *Cephalalgia* 1984; **4:**191–207.
57. Haas DC. Arteriovenous malformations and migraine: case reports and an analysis of the relationship. *Headache* 1991; **31:**509–13.
58. Day JW, Raskin NH. Thunderclap headache: symptom of unruptured cerebral aneurysm. *Lancet* 1986; **ii:**1247–8.
59. Ostergaard JR. Headache as a warning symptom of unpending aneurysmal subarachnoid haemorrhage. *Cephalalgia* 1991; **11:**53–5.
60. Cambon H, Truelle JL, Baron JC, Chiras J, Tran-Dinh S, Chatel M. Ischemie chronique focale et migraine accompagnée: forme atypique d'une angiomatose de Sturge-Weber. *Rev Neurol* 1987; **143:**588–94.
61. Chabriat H, Pappata S, Traykov L, Kurtz A, Bousser MG. Angiomatose de Sturge-Weber responsable d'une hémiplégie sans infarctus cerébral en fin de grossesse. *Rev Neurol* 1996; **152:**536–41.
62. Klapper J. Headache in Sturge–Weber syndrome. *Headache* 1994; **34:**521–2.
63. Newman DS, Levine SR, Curtis VL, Welch KMA. Migraine-like visual phenomena associated with cerebral venous thrombosis. *Headache* 1989; **29:**82–5.
64. Bousser MG, Conard J, Lecrubier C, Bousser J. Migraine ou accidents ischémiques transitoires au cours d'une thrombocytémie essentielle? Action de la Ticlopidine. *Ann Med Int* 1980; **1312:**87–90.
65. Damasio H, Beck D. Migraine, thrombocytopenia and serotonin metabolism. *Lancet* 1978; **ii:**240–1.
66. Geller EB, Wen PY. Migraine with aura as the presentation of leukemia. *Headache* 1995; **35:**560–2.
67. Isenberg DA, Meyrick-Thomas, Snaith ML, McKeran RO, Royston JP. A study of migraine in systemic lupus erythematosus. *Ann Rheum Dis* 1982; **41:**30–2.
68. Tietjen GE. Migraine and antiphospholipid antibodies. *Cephalalgia* 1992; **12:**69–74.
69. Levine SR, Deegan MJ, Futrell N, Welch KMA. Cerebrovascular and neurologic diseases associated with antiphospholipid antibodies: 48 cases. *Neurology* 1990; **40:**1181–9.
70. Steele JG, Nath PU, Burn J, Porteus MEM. An association between migrainous aura and hereditary haemorrhagic telangiectasia. *Headache* 1993; **33:**145–8.
71. Pavlakis SG, Phillips PC, Di Mauro S, De Vivo DC, Rowland P. Mitochondrial myopathy, encephalopathy, lactic acidosis and stroke-like episodes: a distinct clinical syndrome. *Ann Neurol* 1984; **16:**481–8.
72. Andermann F, Lugaresi E, Dvorkin GS, Montagna P. Malignant migraine: the syndrome of prolonged classical migraine, epilepsia partialis continua, and repeated strokes: a clinically characteristic disorder probably due to mitochondrial encephalopathy. *Funct Neurol* 1986; **1:**481–6.
73. Klopstock A, May P, Siebel E, Papagiannuli E, Diezner NC, Heichmann H. Mitochondrial DNA in migraine with aura. *Neurology* 1996; **46:**1735–8.
74. Koo B, Becker L, Chuang S *et al.* Mitochondrial encephalomyopathy, lactic acidosis, stroke-like episodes (MELAS): clinical, radiological, pathological, and genetic observations. *Ann Neurol* 1993; **34:**25–32.
75. Ojaimi J, Katsabanis S, Bower S, Quigley A, Byrne E. Mitochondrial DNA in stroke and migraine with aura. *Cerebrovasc Dis* 1998; **8:**102–6.
76. Tournier-Lasserve E, Iba-Zizen MT, Romero N, Bousser MG. Autosomal dominant syndrome with stroke-like episodes and leukoencephalopathy. *Stroke* 1991; **22:**1297–302.
77. Tournier-Lasserve E, Joutel A, Melki J *et al.* Cerebral autosomal dominant arteriopathy with subcortical infarcts and leukoencephalopathy maps on chromosome 19q12. *Nature Genet* 1993; **3:**256–9.
78. Baudrimont M, Dubas F, Joutel A, Tournier-Lasserve E, Bousser MG. Autosomal dominant leukoencephalopathy and subcortical ischemic stroke. A clinicopathological study. *Stroke* 1993; **24:**122–5.
79. Chabriat H, Vahedi K, Iba-Zizen MT *et al.* Clinical spectrum of CADASIL: a study of 7 families. *Lancet* 1995; **346:**934–9.
80. Igarashi H, Sakai F, Kan S, Okada J, Tazaki Y. Magnetic resonance imaging of the brain in patients with migraine. *Cephalalgia* 1991; **11:**69–74.

81. Fazekas F, Koch M, Schmidt R *et al.* The prevalence of cerebral damage varies with migraine type: a MRI study. *Headache* 1992; **32:**287–91.
82. Pavese N, Canapicchi R, Nuti A *et al.* White matter MRI hyperintensities in 129 consecutive migraine patients. *Cephalalgia* 1994; **14:**342–5.
83. Chabriat H, Tournier-Lasserve E, Vahedi K *et al.* Autosomal dominant migraine with MRI white-matter abnormalities mapping to the CADASIL locus. *Neurology* 1995; **45:**1086–91.
84. Verin M, Rolland Y, Landgraf F *et al.* New phenotype of the cerebral autosomal dominant arteriopathy mapped to chromosome 19: migraine as the prominent clinical feature. *J Neurol Neurosurg Psychiatry* 1995; **59:**579–85.
85. Joutel A, Corpechot C, Ducros A *et al.* Notch 3 mutations in CADASIL, a hereditary adult-onset condition causing stroke and dementia. *Nature* 1996; **383:**707–10.
86. Joutel A, Vahedi K, Corpechot C *et al.* Strong clustering and stereotyped nature of Notch 3 mutations in CADASIL patients. *Lancet* 1997; **350:**1511–5.
87. Olesen J, Welch KMA, Carolei A, Easton JD. Treatment to prevent migraine-related stroke. *Cerebrovasc Dis* 1993; **3:**244–7.
88. Bousser MG. Migraine, female hormones and stroke. *Cephalalgia* 1999; **19:**75–9.
89. Antiplatelet Trialists' Collaboration. Collaborative overview of randomized trials of antiplatelet therapy. I: Prevention of death, myocardial infarction and stroke by prolonged antiplatelet therapy in various categories of patients. *Br Med J* 1994; **308:**81–106.
90. Buring JE, Peto R, Hennekens CH. Low-dose aspirin for migraine prophylaxis. *J Am Med Assoc* 1990; **264:**1711–3.
91. Shinton R, Sagar G. Lifelong exercise and stroke. *Br Med J* 1993; **307:**231–4.
92. Bardwell A, Trott JA. Stroke in migraine as a consequence of propranolol. *Headache* 1987; **27:**381–3.
93. The CAPRIE Steering Committee. A randomised, blinded trial of clopidogrel versus aspirin in patients at risk of ischaemic events (CAPRIE). *Lancet* 1996; **348:**1329–39.
94. Shuaib A, Hachinski V. Migraine and the risks from angiography. *Arch Neurol* 1988; **45:**911–2.

18

Vascular dementia: diagnosis, risk factors, prevention

Timo Erkinjuntti and Ingmar Skoog

CONTENTS • **Introduction** • **Clinical features** • **Criteria for vascular dementia** • **Risk factors** • **Prevention and treatment of vascular dementia**

INTRODUCTION

Dementia is a syndrome characterized by a decline in memory and other intellectual functions.[1] The concept of dementia does not imply prognosis, i.e., the course may be progressive, static, fluctuating or even reversible. The disturbance should, however, be a decline from a previously higher level and give rise to difficulties in activities of daily living. Vascular dementia (VaD) is a syndrome due to cerebrovascular disorders (CVD), but not only the traditional multi-infarct dementia.[2–4] This category does not include cases with vascular risk factors, but does include those without structural vascular changes in the brain.[5,6] Different types of cerebrovascular disorders have been related to VaD syndrome (Table 18.1).[4,7–9] Several vascular disorders, and often also coexisting neurodegenerative changes, can be present in the same patient, which may confound both the clinical picture and the study of the etiopathogenesis.

Table 18.1 Cerebrovascular disorders related to vascular dementia

Large artery disease
Artery-to-artery embolism
Occlusion of an extra- or intracranial artery
Cardiac embolic events
Small vessel disease
Lacunar infarcts
Ischemic white matter lesions
Hemodynamic mechanisms
Specific arteriopathies
Hemorrhages
Intracranial hemorrhage
Subarachnoidal hemorrhage
Hematological factors
Venous diseases
Hereditary entities

The pathophysiology of VaD includes: complex interactions between vascular etiologies (cerebrovascular disorders and vascular risk-factors); vascular (e.g. infarcts, white matter lesions) or degenerative (e.g. Alzheimer pathology, atrophy) changes in the brain; and host factors (age, education) leading to cognitive impairment.[6,10–13] The individual roles these factors play in causation have not been identified in detail, and it is not clear which of these mechanisms differentiate patients with VaD from non-demented patients with cerebrovascular disorders.[2,3,10,11,13,14]

Different types of ischemic lesions in the brain have been related to VaD (Table

Table 18.2 Brain changes in vascular dementia

Static lesions
Arterial territorial infarct
Distal field (watershed) infarct
Lacunar infarct
Ischemic white matter lesions
Incomplete ischemic injury
Atrophy
Functional ischemic changes
Focal (around the ischemic lesion)
Remote (disconnection, diaschisis)

18.2).[7,8,10,11] Incomplete ischemic injuries include laminar necrosis, focal gliosis, granular atrophy and incomplete white matter infarction.[15,16] Both focal (around the ischemic lesion) and remote (disconnection, diaschisis) functional ischemic changes may be involved, and the volume of functionally inactive tissue often exceeds that of the focal ischemic lesion itself.[17]

The mechanism by which vascular lesions in the brain cause cognitive impairment is not fully understood and may differ between different cases. For decades it has been debated whether type, extent, side, site and number of vascular lesions in the brain, as well as the tempo by which they evolve, is the key element in the pathogenesis of VaD.[7,10–12] It has been argued that VaD is related to the volume of brain infarcts (size reaching a critical threshold), the number of infarcts (additive, synergistic), the site of infarcts (bilateral, strategic cortical or sub-cortical sites), the ischemic white matter lesions (extent, site, type, density), other ischemic factors (incomplete ischemic injury, delayed neuronal death, functional changes), atrophic changes (origin, location, extent), and finally to the additive effects of other pathologies (Alzheimer's disease, Lewy body dementia, frontal lobe dementias).[7,10–12]

Vascular causes of cognitive impairment are common and may be prevented or even treated. Therefore, early detection and accurate diagnosis of VaD is desirable.[18]

MAIN SUBTYPES OF VASCULAR DEMENTIA

Multi-infarct dementia or cortical VaD, the small vessel dementia or the subcortical VaD and the strategic infarct dementia are the most frequently cited subtypes, but frequencies reported vary between studies (Table 18.3).[8,19,20]

Cortical VaD

Cortical VaD relates to ischemic stroke due to large vessel disease, cardiac embolic events and hypoperfusion. It presents predominantly with cortical and cortico–subcortical arterial territorial and distal field (watershed) infarcts. Typical clinical features are lateralized sensorimotor changes and abrupt onset of cognitive impairment and aphasia.[19] In addition, a combination of different cortical neuropsychological symptoms may be present.[21]

Subcortical VaD

Subcortical VaD, or small vessel dementia, incorporates 'the lacunar state', 'Binswanger's disease', and 'ischemic white matter dementia'. It relates to small vessel disease and hypoperfusion and presents predominantly with lacunar infarcts, focal and diffuse ischemic white matter lesions, and incomplete ischemic injury in subcortical areas of the brain.[19,21,22] Clinically, small vessel dementia is characterized by the symptoms of pure motor or sensory hemiparesis, bulbar signs and dysarthria in combination with symptoms of subcortical dementia such as psychomotor retardation, emotional lability or bluntness, and executive dysfunction.[21–24] Brain imaging shows extensive white matter lesions and lacunar infarcts in subcortical areas.

Strategic infarct dementia

Focal, often small, ischemic lesions involving specific sites critical for higher cognitive func-

Table 18.3 Vascular mechanisms and changes in the brain related to main subtypes of vascular dementia

Vascular mechanisms	*Changes in the brain*
Cortical vascular dementia or multi-infarct dementia	
Large vessel disease	Arterial territorial infarct
Cardiac embolic events	Distal field (watershed) infarct
Hypoperfusion	
Subcortical vascular dementia or small vessel dementia	
Small vessel disease	Lacunar infarct
Hypoperfusion	Focal and diffuse white matter lesions
	Incomplete ischemic injury
Strategic infarct dementia	
Large vessel disease	Arterial territorial infarct
Cardiac embolic events	Distal field (watershed) infarct
Small vessel disease	Lacunar infarct
Hypoperfusion	Focal and diffuse white matter lesions

tions may also be classified as causes of VaD. The angular gyrus and hippocampus are examples of cortical sites, whereas the thalamus, cyrus cinguli, fornix, basal forebrain, caudate, globus pallidus and genu of the anterior capsule are examples of subcortical sites.[2,7,10]

CLINICAL FEATURES

Cognitive symptoms

The cognitive symptoms of VaD differ depending on the type and location of the lesions. Cortical VaD often presents with a combination of different cortical neuropsychological symptoms, such as aphasia, apraxia, agnosia and visuospatial difficulties,[21] while the memory dysfunction may be less severe, at least in mild cases. Subcortical VaD is characterized by mild memory deficits (which are helped by cues), a dysexecutive syndrome, and slowed information processing. Compared to what is seen in Alzheimer's disease, the memory deficit in VaD is often less severe, and may not dominate in early cases. It is characterized by impaired recall, relative intact recognition and better benefit from cues.[25] The dysexecutive syndrome of VaD relates to lesions affecting the prefrontal subcortical circuit including the prefrontal cortex, caudate, pallidum, thalamus, and the thalamocortical circuit (capsular genu, anterior capsule, anterior centrum semiovale, and anterior corona radiata).[26] Symptoms include impairment in goal formulation, initiation, planning, organizing, sequencing, executing, set-shifting and set-maintenance, as well as disturbances in abstract thinking.[20,21,25] It has been suggested that the distribution of cognitive deficits in VaD show a more patchy distribution and a different pattern of evolution than is seen in primary degenerative dementias, such as Alzheimer's disease.

Neurological symptoms

Clinical neurological symptoms include mild motor or sensory deficits, decreased co-ordination, brisk tendon reflexes, Babinski's sign, visual field deficits, bulbar signs including dysarthria and dysphagia, extrapyramidal signs (mainly rigidity and akinesia), gait disorder (hemiplegic, apraxic–ataxic or small-stepped), unsteadiness and unprovoked falls, as well as urinary frequency and urgency.[19,22–24,27] It is often believed that the diagnosis of VaD is uncertain or unlikely in the absence of focal neurological signs, other than cognitive disturbance.[27] However, in a significant minority of cases the dementia may have a gradual onset with a slowly progressive course without major focal signs or symptoms.[4,28]

The typical clinical neurological findings in cortical VaD are lateralized sensimotor changes and abrupt onset of cognitive impairment and aphasia, and in subcortical VaD, they are pure motor hemiparesis, bulbar signs and dysarthria.[19]

Behavioral and psychological symptoms

Behavioral and psychological symptoms of vascular dementia include depression, anxiety, emotional lability and incontinence.[27] Depression, abulia, emotional incontinence, inertia and emotional bluntness and psychomotor retardation are especially frequent in subcortical VaD.[20,21] Furthermore, insight and personality are often relatively intact in mild and moderate cases of VaD.

Brain imaging

The typical findings on computed tomography (CT) and magnetic resonance imaging (MRI) are cortical or subcortical infarcts and the presence of diffuse subcortical white matter lesions. Several authors have suggested that bilateral ischemic lesions are of particular diagnostic importance.[2,10,11,13] It has further been suggested that the location of the infarct is of diagnostic importance. Some authors emphasize deep infarcts in the frontal and limbic areas, others emphasize cortical infarcts especially in the temporal and parietal areas. There are also controversies whether the number and volume of the infarcts, as well as the extent and location of atrophy, should be considered in the diagnostic evaluation. The diffuse and extensive white matter lesions have been suggested as important factors leading to functional disconnection of cortical brain areas.

The following conclusions on brain imaging in VaD may be drawn.

1. Not a single feature, but a combination of infarct features, extent and type of ischemic white matter lesions, degree and site of atrophy, and host factors are correlates of VaD.
2. Infarct features favoring VaD include: bilaterality, multiplicity (>2), location in the dominant hemisphere and in the limbic structures (fronto–limbic or prefrontal–subcortical and medial–limbic or medial–hippocampal circuits).
3. White matter lesion features favoring VaD are extensive white matter lesions (extending in periventricular white matter, and confluent to extending in the deep white matter) on CT or proton/T1-weighted MRI.
4. It is doubtful that only a single small lesion could support imaging evidence for a diagnosis of VaD.
5. Absence of cerebrovascular lesions on CT or MRI argue against a diagnosis of VaD.

The diagnosis of VaD is believed to be uncertain or unlikely in cases with an early memory deficit and a slow progressive course of cognitive deficits in the absence of corresponding focal lesions on brain imaging.[27] However, in a significant minority of cases, VaD may have a gradual onset with a slowly progressive course,[28] and focal signs or infarcts on brain imaging (especially when CT has been used) may be absent.[4,19] Furthermore, Alzheimer's disease and VaD are often present simultaneously. Thus, it is often difficult to differentiate VaD from Alzheimer's disease. To make it even more complicated, it has recently been found that the presence of mild cerebrovascular disease may be an important determinant as to whether individuals with Alzheimer lesions in their brains will express a dementia syndrome.[29]

Ischemic scores

Ischemic scores, such as the Hachinski Ischemic Score,[30] include cardinal features of VaD. In a recent neuropathological series, stepwise deterioration (odds ratio 6.0), fluctuating course (OR 7.6), history of hypertension (OR 4.3), history of stroke (OR 4.3) and focal neurological symptoms (OR 4.4) differentiated patients with definite VaD from those with definite Alzheimer's disease.[31] Nocturnal confusion and depression were not discriminatory features. However, the ischemic score could not differentiate pure VaD from Alzheimer's disease with concomitant cerebrovascular disease.

CRITERIA FOR VASCULAR DEMENTIA

The most widely used criteria for VaD are the Diagnostic and Statistical Manual of Mental Disorders (DSM-III-R and DSM-IV),[32,33] the International Classification of Disease (ICD-10),[34] the State of California Alzheimer's Disease Diagnostic and Treatment Centers (ADDTC),[35] and the National Institute of Neurological Disorders and Stroke and the Association Internationale pour la Recherche et l'Enseignement en Neurosciences (NINDS-AIREN).[27]

The two cardinal elements implemented in the clinical criteria for VaD are the definition of the cognitive symptoms of dementia,[36] and the definition of the vascular cause of the dementia.[37–39] All the clinical criteria used are consensus criteria, which are neither derived from prospective community-based studies on vascular factors affecting cognition, nor based on detailed natural histories.[27,35,39–41] All the cited criteria are based on the ischemic infarct concept and designed to have high specificity, although they have been poorly implemented and validated.[40,41] Furthermore, the dementia concept is based on the clinical symptoms seen in Alzheimer's disease, and requires the presence of memory impairment. The distribution and evolution of cognitive symptoms may be different in VaD,[18] and memory problems may be less severe in the early stages. Thus, current criteria for dementia may underestimate the frequency of VaD.

The most critical consequences in the variable definitions of the cognitive symptoms[36,42] and the vascular cause[37,43] are that the different criteria give different frequencies of VaD, they identify different groups of subjects, and identify different types and distribution of brain lesions.

DSM-IV criteria

The DSM-IV[33] definition for VaD requires the presence of dementia and focal neurological signs and symptoms (e.g. exaggeration of deep tendon reflexes, extensor plantar response, pseudobulbar palsy, gait abnormalities and weakness of an extremity) or laboratory evidence of cerebrovascular disease (e.g. multiple infarctions involving cortex and underlying white matter that are judged to be etiologically related to the disturbance). The course of the disorder is not specified, no details are given on how to judge whether cerebrovascular disease and dementia are related, and no details regarding brain imaging requirements are provided. The DSM-IV definition for VaD is reasonably broad and lacks detailed clinical and radiological guidelines. The dementia definition is identical to that for Alzheimer's disease.

ICD-10 criteria

The general ICD-10 criteria[34] for VaD require the presence of dementia, uneven distribution of deficits in higher cognitive functions, clinical evidence of focal brain damage (manifested as unilateral spastic weakness of the limbs, unilaterally increased tendon reflexes, extensor plantar response or pseudobulbar palsy), and evidence from the history, examination, or tests of a significant cerebrovascular disease, which may reasonably be judged to be etiologically related to the dementia. As in DSM-IV, the course of the disorder is not specified, no details are given on how to judge whether cerebrovascular disease and dementia are related,

Table 18.4 The NINDS-AIREN criteria for probable vascular dementia

I. The criteria for the clinical diagnosis of probable vascular dementia include *all* of the following.
   1. *Dementia*
   2. *Cerebrovascular disease*, defined by the presence of focal signs on neurological examination, such as hemiparesis, lower facial weakness, Babinski sign, sensory deficit, hemianopsia, dysarthria, etc. consistent with stroke (with or without history of stroke), and evidence of relevant CVD by brain imaging (CT or MRI) including multiple large-vessel strokes or a single strategically placed infarct (angular gyrus, thalamus, basal forebrain, PCA or ACA territories), as well as multiple basal ganglia and white matter lacunes or extensive periventricular white matter lesions, or combinations thereof.
   3. *A relationship between the above two disorders*, manifested or inferred by the presence of one or more of the following:
      a. onset of dementia within 3 months following a recognized stroke;
      b. abrupt deterioration in cognitive functions; or fluctuating, stepwise progression of cognitive deficits.

II. Clinical features consistent with the diagnosis of probable vascular dementia include the following.
   1. Early presence of a gait disturbance (small-step gait or marche a petits-pas, magnetic, apraxic–ataxic or Parkinsonian gait).
   2. History of unsteadiness and frequent, unprovoked falls.
   3. Early urinary frequency, urgency, and other urinary symptoms not explained by urological disease.
   4. Personality and mood changes, abulia, depression, emotional incontinence, other subcortical deficits including psychomotor retardation and abnormal executive function.

III. Features that make the diagnosis of vascular dementia uncertain or unlikely include the following.
   1. Early onset of memory deficit and progressive worsening of memory and other cognitive functions such as language (transcortical sensory aphasia), motor skills (apraxia), and perception (agnosia), in the absence of corresponding focal lesions on brain imaging.
   2. Absence of focal neurological signs, other than cognitive disturbance.
   3. Absence of cerebrovascular lesions on brain CT or MRI.

and no details regarding brain imaging requirements are provided. The dementia definition is similar to that for Alzheimer's disease, although uneven distribution of deficits is also required. The ICD-10 criteria also specify altogether six subtypes of VaD. The ICD-10 criteria for VaD have been shown to be highly selective and only a subset of those fulfilling the general criteria for ICD-10 VaD can be classified into defined subtypes.[37,38]

ADDTC criteria

The ADDTC criteria for ischemic vascular dementia (IVD)[35] require the presence of dementia, evidence of two or more ischemic strokes by history, neurological signs, and/or neuroimaging studies (CT or T1-weighted MRI) or in cases with a single stroke a clearly documented temporal relationship to the onset of dementia, and evidence of at least one infarct outside the cerebellum by CT or T1-weighted MRI. Ischemic white matter changes on CT or MRI do not qualify as brain-imaging evidence of probable IVD, but may support a diagnosis of possible IVD. A list of features supporting the diagnosis, as well as features casting doubt on a diagnosis of probable IVD are included in the criteria.

NINDS-AIREN criteria

The NINDS-AIREN research criteria for probable VaD[27] include the presence of dementia, cerebrovascular disease defined as focal signs consistent with stroke and relevant cerebrovascular disease by brain imaging (defined as multiple large-vessel infarcts, single strategically placed infarct, multiple lacunes in basal ganglia or white matter, and extensive periventricular white matter lesions), and evidence for a relationship between cerebrovascular disease and dementia (defined as onset of dementia within 3 months following stroke or abrupt deterioration in cognitive functions or a fluctuating stepwise progression) (Table 18.4). The criteria include a list of features consistent with the diagnosis, as well as a list of features that make the diagnosis uncertain or unlikely. It has to be noted that the criteria for probable VaD require both focal signs consistent with stroke, and brain imaging evidence of cerebrovascular disease, which is a rather strict definition. The criteria for possible VaD only require the presence of dementia and stroke for a diagnosis in the absence of a relationship between these (defined as dementia onset more than 3 months following stroke or subtle onset or variable course), which on the other hand is a broad definition. The selection of 3 months as the critical time limit for a diagnosis of probable VaD is not supported by empirical evidence, and may be difficult to apply in population studies.

The NINDS-AIREN criteria recognize heterogeneity[44] of the syndrome and variability of the clinical course in VaD, they highlight detection of ischemic lesions and a relationship between lesion and cognition, as well as stroke and dementia onset. The inter-rater reliability of the NINDS-AIREN criteria has been shown to be moderate to substantial (kappa 0.46–0.72).[45]

Comparison of the clinical criteria

The current criteria for VaD are not interchangeable; they identify different numbers and clusters of patients labeled as VaD. The DSM-IV criteria are less restrictive compared to the ICD-10, the ADDTC and the NINDS-AIREN criteria for probable VaD.[39,46]

The NINDS-AIREN criteria are currently most widely used in clinical drug trials on VaD and in epidemiological studies (even if no brain imaging has been performed), despite their limitations. In a neuropathological series, sensitivity of the NINDS-AIREN criteria was 58% and specificity 80%.[47] The criteria successfully excluded Alzheimer's disease in 91% of cases, and the proportion of combined cases misclassified as probable VaD was 29%.[47] Compared to the ADDTC criteria the NINDS-AIREN criteria were more specific and they excluded combined cases better (54% vs. 29%).[47]

RISK FACTORS

Risk factors of VaD (Table 18.5) have mainly been studied in relation to cortical VaD and can be divided into vascular factors (e.g. arterial hypertension, atrial fibrillation, myocardial infarction, coronary heart disease, diabetes, generalized atherosclerosis, lipid abnormalities, smoking), demographic factors (e.g. age, education), genetic factors (e.g. family history, individual genetic features), and stroke-related factors (e.g. type of cerebrovascular disease, site and size of stroke).[48,49] Hypertension is the main risk factor for subcortical VaD.[50] Hypoxic ischemic events (cardiac arrhythmias, congestive heart failure, myocardial infarction, seizures, pneumonia) may be an important risk factor for incident dementia in patients with stroke.[51]

PREVENTION AND TREATMENT OF VASCULAR DEMENTIA

Primary prevention

The aim of primary prevention is to preserve health by removing the precipitating causes

Table 18.5 Risk factors related to vascular dementia

- Vascular factors
  - Arterial hypertension
  - Atrial fibrillation
  - Cardiac abnormalities
    - Myocardial infarction
    - Coronary heart disease
  - Hypoxic ischemic events
  - Diabetes
  - Generalized atherosclerosis
  - Lipid abnormalities
  - Smoking
- Demographic factors
  - Advanced age
  - Low education
- Genetic factors
  - Family history
  - Individual genetic features
- Stroke related factors
  - Type of cerebrovascular disease
  - Site and size of stroke

and determinants of the disease, before the pathological process of the disease has started. In epidemiological terms, the aim of primary prevention is to reduce the incidence of disease by eliminating the causes or main risk factors.[52,53] Thus in relation to vascular dementia, primary prevention programs should be targeted at the risk factors for the underlying vascular disorder, or the factors that lead to cognitive impairment, or to promotion of potential protective factors (Table 18.6). In general, prevention programs can only be directed towards common disorders. Thus, in relation to VaD, risk factors related to vascular causes of cognitive impairment that could be eliminated, include those related to stroke and ischemic white matter lesions, and to cognitive impairment in general or to Alzheimer's disease.[6] The factors that may be amenable to prevention programs include arterial hypertension, atrial fibrillation, myocardial infarction, coronary heart disease, diabetes, generalized atherosclerosis, lipid abnormalities and smoking. Putative protective factors are estrogen,[54] anti-inflammatory agents and antioxidants which have been suggested to be protective for both vascular disorders and dementia in general.

Knowledge of the effects of primary prevention on these risk factors in relation to dementia or cognitive impairment is still scanty.[5,6] The Medical Research Council's treatment trial of hypertension in older adults did not show an effect on subsequent cognitive function.[55] The recent finding from the Syst-Eur trial[56] that treatment of isolated systolic hypertension with the long-acting calcium channel blocker nitrendipine reduces the incidence of dementia by 50%, further emphasizes vascular risk factors as possible targets for prevention. Positive effects in primary prevention of stroke support the idea that action on vascular risk factors could reduce the frequency of VaD.

Secondary prevention

The aim of secondary prevention is to prevent the disease from progressing into a more serious outcome by means of early detection followed by definite treatment.[53] Several criteria must be fulfilled before a secondary prevention program can start.[57,58] These can be divided into criteria relating to the disease, the screening, the treatment and the evaluation. In relation to VaD, the preventive approaches may be divided into those that are directed towards the vascular lesions and those directed specifically towards the cognitive deficits. Those against the vascular component include: (1) early diagnosis and treatment of acute stroke in order to limit the extent of ischemic brain changes and to promote recovery; (2) prevention of stroke recurrence; and (3) intensifying treatment of risk factors. Selection of treatment is guided by the etiology of cerebrovascular disorders, such as large artery disease (e.g. aspirin, dipyridamole, carotid endarterectomy), cardiac embolic events

Table 18.6 Prevention and treatment of vascular dementia

Type of therapy	*Main target*	*Degree of cognitive impairment*	*Action*
Prevention			
Primary	Brain at risk of CVD and any cognitive impairment	Normal	Treatment of and action on risk factors Promotion of protective factors
Secondary	CVD brain at risk of VCI and VaD	Normal Mild diffuse in several domains Significant in one domain	Diagnosis of the type of CVD Acute intervention on ischemic brain changes Treatment according to CVD type Intensifying treatment of risk factors
Treatment			
Slowing progression	Risk of progression of VCI and VaD	Significant in several domains Dementia	Intensifying primary and secondary prevention Targeted medications to: –increase cerebral blood flow –support neuronal metabolism –modify neurotransmission –neuroprotection
Secondary factors	Risk of intensifying VCI and VaD		Treatment of secondary factors affecting the cognition
AD strategies			AD treatments to prevent, slow progression and treat symptoms of impairment of cognition and behavior

CVD, cerebrovascular disease; VCI, vascular cognitive impairment; VaD, vascular dementia; AD, Alzheimer's disease.

(e.g. anticoagulation, aspirin), small-vessel disease (e.g. antiplatelet therapy), and hemodynamic mechanisms (e.g. control of hypotension and cardiac arrhythmias).[9,41,59] Hypoxic ischemic events (cardiac arrhythmias, congestive heart failure, myocardial infarction, seizures, pneumonia) are important risk factors for incident dementia in patients with stroke and should be taken into account in the secondary prevention of VaD.[51] Furthermore, aggressive treatment of hypertension may prevent further strokes, and thus the development of VaD in non-demented patients with stroke.

Detailed knowledge of the effects of secondary prevention directed towards the vascular component of VaD is still scanty. In a small series of patients with established VaD, control of high arterial blood pressure,[60] cessation of smoking[60] and use of aspirin[61] improved or stabilized cognition. It has been suggested that a lowering of plasma viscosity could also have an effect in VaD.[62] Effects of vitamins to reduce plasma homocysteine levels await randomized controlled trials.[63] Furthermore, absence of progressive cognitive decline in patients receiving placebo in symptomatic treatment trials of VaD may also reflect an effect of intensified risk factor control.[64]

Tertiary prevention

Tertiary prevention includes symptomatic treatment. A number of drugs have been studied for the symptomatic treatment of VaD including cerebro- and vasoactive drugs, inotropic drugs and some calcium antagonists, but these studies have largely shown negative results.[65] The studies have mostly included small numbers, short treatment periods, variations in diagnostic criteria and tools, often included mixed populations, and have had variations in the application of clinical endpoints. Recently nimodipine,[66] memantine,[67] and propentofylline[64] have raised expectations in the symptomatic treatment of VaD. A number of phase III double-blind, randomized, placebo-controlled trials in patients with VaD using these compounds are in progress, but the results have not been published yet (see Erkinjuntti[68] for review). It is possible that the symptomatic treatment with acetylcholinesterase inhibitors (such as tacrine, donepezil and rivastigmine), which are approved throughout the world for the treatment of Alzheimer's disease, may also prove to be effective on the cognitive symptoms of VaD.

REFERENCES

1. Skoog I, Blennow K, Marcusson J, Birren JE (eds.). *Encyclopedia of Gerontology*, pp. 383–404. San Diego; Academic Press Inc: 1996.
2. Erkinjuntti T, Hachinski VC. Rethinking vascular dementia. *Cerebrovasc Dis* 1993; **3:**3–23.
3. Chui HC. Rethinking vascular dementia: moving from myth to mechanism. In: *The Dementias* (Chui HC, Growdon JH, Rossor MN, eds), pp. 377–401. Boston; Butterworth-Heinemann: 1998.
4. Skoog I. Blood pressure and dementia. In: *Handbook of Hypertension* (Skoog I, Hansson L, Birkenhäger WH, eds), Vol. 18, pp. 303–31. Amsterdam; Elsevier Science: 1997.
5. Skoog I. The relationship between blood pressure and dementia: a review. *Biomed Pharmacother* 1997; **51:**367–75.
6. Skoog I. Status of risk factors for vascular dementia. *Neuroepidemiology* 1998; **17:**2–9.
7. Erkinjuntti T. Clinicopathological study of vascular dementia. In: *Vascular Dementia. Current Concepts* (Erkinjuntti T, Prohovnik I, Wade J *et al.*, eds), pp. 73–112. Chichester; John Wiley & Sons: 1996.
8. Brun A. Pathology and pathophysiology of cerebrovascular dementia: pure subgroups of obstructive and hypoperfusive etiology. *Dementia* 1994; **5:**145–7.
9. Amar K, Wilcock G. Vascular dementia. *Br Med J* 1996; **312:**227–31.
10. Tatemichi TK. How acute brain failure becomes chronic. A view of the mechanisms and syndromes of dementia related to stroke. *Neurology* 1990; **40:**1652–9.
11. Chui HC. Dementia: a review emphasizing clinicopathologic correlation and brain–behavior relationships. *Arch Neurol* 1989; **46:**806–14.
12. Desmond DW. Vascular dementia: a construct in evolution. *Cerebrovasc Brain Metabol Rev* 1996; **8:**296–325.

13. Pasquier F, Leys D. Why are stroke patients prone to develop dementia? *J Neurol* 1997; **244:**135–42.
14. Pantoni L, Garcia JH. The significance of cerebral white matter abnormalities 100 years after Binswanger's report. A review. *Stroke* 1995; **26:**1293–301.
15. Pantoni L, Garcia JH. Pathogenesis of leukoaraiosis: a review. *Stroke* 1997; **28:**652–9.
16. Englund E, Brun A, Alling C. White matter changes in dementia of Alzheimer's type. Biochemical and neuropathological correlates. *Brain* 1988; **111:**1425–39.
17. Mielke R, Herholz K, Grond M, Kessler J, Heiss WD. Severity of vascular dementia is related to volume of metabolically impaired tissue. *Arch Neurol* 1992; **49:**909–13.
18. Bowler JV, Hachinski V. Vascular cognitive impairment: a new approach to vascular dementia. *Baillieres Clin Neurol* 1995; **4:**357–76.
19. Erkinjuntti T. Types of multi-infarct dementia. *Acta Neurol Scand* 1987; **75:**391–9.
20. Cummings JL. Vascular subcortical dementias: clinical aspects. *Dementia* 1994; **5:**177–80.
21. Mahler ME, Cummings JL. The behavioural neurology of multi-infarct dementia. *Alzheimer Dis Assoc Disord* 1991; **5:**122–30.
22. Roman GC. Senile dementia of the Binswanger type. A vascular form of dementia in the elderly. *J Am Med Assoc* 1987; **258:**1782–8.
23. Babikian V, Ropper AH. Binswanger's disease: a review. *Stroke* 1987; **18:**2–12.
24. Ishii N, Nishihara Y, Imamura T. Why do frontal lobe symptoms predominate in vascular dementia with lacunes? *Neurology* 1986; **36:**340–5.
25. Desmond DW, Erkinjuntti T, Sano M *et al.* The cognitive syndrome of vascular dementia: implications for clinical trials. *Alzheimer Dis Assoc Disord* 1999; (in press).
26. Cummings JL. Fronto-subcortical circuits and human behavior. *Arch Neurol* 1993; **50:**873–80.
27. Roman GC, Tatemichi TK, Erkinjuntti T *et al.* Vascular Dementia: Diagnostic Criteria for Research Studies report of the NINDS-AIREN International Work Group. *Neurology* 1993; **43:**250–60.
28. Fischer P, Gatterer G, Marterer A, Simanyi M, Danielczyk W. Course characteristics in the differentiation of dementia of the Alzheimer type and multi-infarct dementia. *Acta Psychiatr Scand* 1990; **81:**551–3.
29. Snowdon DA, Greiner LH, Mortimer JA, Riley KP, Greiner PA, Markesbery WR. Brain infarction and the clinical expression of Alzheimer disease. The Nun Study [see comments]. *J Am Med Assoc* 1997; **277:**813–7.
30. Hachinski VC, Iliff LD, Zilhka E *et al.* Cerebral blood flow in dementia. *Arch Neurol* 1975; **32:**632–7.
31. Moroney JT, Bagiella E, Desmond DW *et al.* Meta-analysis of the Hachinski Ischemic Score in pathologically verified dementias. *Neurology* 1997; **49:**1096–105.
32. American Psychiatric Association. *Diagnostic and Statistical Manual of Mental Disorders*, 3rd edn. Washington, DC; American Psychiatric Association: 1987.
33. American Psychiatric Association. *Diagnostic and Statistical Manual of Mental Disorders*, 4th edn. Washington, DC; American Psychiatric Association: 1994.
34. World Health Organization. *ICD-10 Classification of Mental and Behavioural Disorders: Diagnostic Criteria for Research.* Geneva; WHO: 1993.
35. Chui HC, Victoroff JI, Margolin D, Jagust W, Shankle R, Katzman R. Criteria for the diagnosis of ischemic vascular dementia proposed by the State of California Alzheimer's Disease Diagnostic and Treatment Centers [see comments]. *Neurology* 1992; **42:**473–80.
36. Erkinjuntti T, Ostbye T, Steenhuis R, Hachinski V. The effect of different diagnostic criteria on the prevalence of dementia. *N Engl J Med* 1997; **337:**1667–74.
37. Wetterling T, Kanitz RD, Borgis KJ. Comparison of different diagnostic criteria for vascular dementia (ADDTC, DSM-IV, ICD-10, NINDS-AIREN). *Stroke* 1996; **27:**30–6.
38. Wetterling T, Kanitz RD, Borgis KJ. The ICD-10 criteria for vascular dementia. *Dementia* 1994; **5:**185–8.
39. Erkinjuntti T. Clinical criteria for vascular dementia: The NINDS-AIREN criteria. *Dementia* 1994; **5:**189–92.
40. Rockwood K, Parhad I, Hachinski V *et al.* Diagnosis of vascular dementia: Consortium of Canadian Centres for Clinical Cognitive Research concensus statement. *Can J Neurol Sci* 1994; **21:**358–64.
41. Erkinjuntti T. Vascular dementia: challenge of clinical diagnosis. *Int Psychogeriatr* 1997; **9**(Suppl 1):51–8.
42. Pohjasvaara T, Erkinjuntti T, Vataja R, Kaste M. Dementia three months after stroke. Baseline frequency and effect of different definitions of dementia in the Helsinki Stroke Aging Memory

Study (SAM) cohort. *Stroke* 1997; **28:**785–92.

43. Skoog I, Nilsson L, Palmertz B, Andreasson LA, Svanborg A. A population-based study of dementia in 85-year-olds [see comments]. *N Engl J Med* 1993; **328:**153–8.
44. Erkinjuntti T. Clinical criteria for vascular dementia: the NINDS-AIREN criteria. *Dementia* 1994; **5:**189–92.
45. Lopez OL, Larumbe MR, Becker JT *et al.* Reliability of NINDS-AIREN clinical criteria for the diagnosis of vascular dementia [see comments]. *Neurology* 1994; **44:**1240–5.
46. Verhey FR, Lodder J, Rozendaal N, Jolles J. Comparison of seven sets of criteria used for the diagnosis of vascular dementia. *Neuroepidemiology* 1996; **15:**166–72.
47. Gold G, Giannakopoulos P, Montes-Paixao JC *et al.* Sensitivity and specificity of newly proposed clinical criteria for possible vascular dementia. *Neurology* 1997; **49:**690–4.
48. Gorelick PB. Status of risk factors for dementia associated with stroke. *Stroke* 1997; **28:**459–63.
49. Skoog I. Risk factors for vascular dementia: a review. *Dementia* 1994; **5:**137–44.
50. Skoog I. A review on blood pressure and ischaemic white matter lesions. *Dement Geriatr Cogn Cogn Disord* 1998; **9**(Suppl 1):13–9.
51. Moroney JT, Bagiella E, Desmond DW, Paik MC, Stern Y, Tatemichi TK. Risk factors for incident dementia after stroke. Role of hypoxic and ischemic disorders. *Stroke* 1996; **27:**1283–9.
52. Last JM. *A Dictionary of Epidemiology*, 2nd edn. New York; Oxford University Press: 1988.
53. Skoog I. Possibilities for secondary prevention of Alzheimer's disease. In: *The epidemiology of Alzheimer's disease: from gene to prevention* (Mayeux R, Christein Y, eds), pp 121–134. Berlin; Springer Verlag; 1999.
54. Mortel KF, Meyer JS. Lack of postmenopausal estrogen replacement therapy and the risk of dementia. *J Neuropsychiatr Clin Neurosci* 1995; **7:**334–7.
55. Prince MJ, Bird AS, Blizard RA, Mann AH. Is the cognitive function of older patients affected by antihypertensive treatment? Results from 54 months of the Medical Research Council's trial of hypertension in older adults [see comments]. *Br Med J* 1996; **312:**801–5.
56. Forette F, Seux ML, Staessen JA *et al.* Prevention of dementia in randomised double-blind placebo-controlled Systolic Hypertension in Europe (Syst-Eur) trial. *Lancet* 1998; **352:**1347–51.
57. Wallace RB, Everett GD. Prevention of chronic illness. In: *Maxcy-Rosenau-Last. Public Health and Preventive Medicine* (Wallace RB, Everett GD, Last JM, eds), pp. 805–10. East Norwalk, Connecticut; Appleton & Lange: 1992.
58. Wilson JMG, Jungner G. Principles and practice of screening of disease. *Pub Hlth Pap 34*. Geneva; WHO: 1968.
59. Konno S, Meyer JS, Terayama Y, Margishvili GM, Mortel KF. Classification, diagnosis and treatment of vascular dementia. *Drugs Aging* 1997; **11:**361–73.
60. Meyer JS, Judd BW, Tawaklna T, Rogers RL, Mortel KF. Improved cognition after control of risk factors for multi-infarct dementia. *J Am Med Assoc* 1986; **256:**2203–9.
61. Meyer JS, Rogers RL, McClintic K, Mortel KF, Lotfi J. Randomized clinical trial of daily aspirin therapy in multi-infarct dementia. A pilot study. *J Am Geriatr Soc* 1989; **37:**549–55.
62. Lechner H. Status of treatment of vascular dementia. *Neuroepidemiology* 1998; **17:**10–3.
63. Welch GN, Loscalzo J. Mechanisms of disease: homocysteine and atherothrombosis. *N Engl J Med* 1998; **338:**1042–50.
64. Rother M, Erkinjuntti T, Roessner M, Kittner B, Marcusson J, Karlsson I. Propentofylline in the treatment of Alzheimer's disease and vascular dementia. *Dementia Geriatr Cogn Disord* 1998; **9**(Suppl 1):36–43.
65. Knezevic S, Labs KH, Kittner B *et al.* The treatment of vascular dementia: problems and prospects. In: *Vascular Dementia: Current Concepts* (Erkinjuntti T, Prohovnik I, Wade J *et al.*, eds), pp. 301–12. Chichester; John Wiley & Sons: 1996.
66. Pantoni L, Carosi M, Amigoni S, Mascalchi M, Inzitari D. A preliminary open trial with nimodipine in patients with cognitive impairment and leukoaraiosis. *Clin Neuropharmacol* 1996; **19:**497–506.
67. Görtelmeyer R, Erbler H. Memantine in treatment of mild to moderate dementia syndrome. *Drug Res* 1992; **42:**904–12.
68. Erkinjuntti T. Cerebrovascular dementia: a guide to diagnosis and treatment. *CNS Drugs* 1999; (in press).

19

The role of the neurologist

Cesare Fieschi and Michael G Hennerici

> 'The history of medicine is usually described by a string of dates and names, linked to the discoveries that shaped our present knowledge. The interval between such identifiable advances is measured in centuries when we describe the art of medicine at the beginning of civilisation, but in mere years where our present times are chronicled.'[1]

This is what we have witnessed in less than 30 years (1955–1985) on the prevention of ischemic strokes. The progress comes from many areas of medical research (epidemiology, cardiology, internal medicine, vascular surgery and angiology) but most of all from some of the 'great names' in neurology, whom we wish to praise in this short review.

In 1951 Denny-Brown[2] challenged the old-fashioned theory of 'vasospasm'. C Miller Fisher[3,4] revitalized the pathogenetic relationship between stroke and atheromatous lesions of the carotid bifurcation, and described the occurrence of hemiplegia preceded by attacks of transient monocular blindness in the contralateral eye: 'the wrong eye', later to be identified with the transit of white bodies (platelet–fibrin emboli) passing slowly through the retinal arteries.[5] Millikan and Siekert defined the clinical picture of the 'syndromes of intermittent insufficiency' of vertebrobasilar and carotid artery territories.[6,7]

All this was not really new of course, but what matters is that applications of this knowledge were introduced only in the post-1950s era.

Although classical textbooks clearly reported the concept of embolism secondary to atherosclerosis from the heart,[8] it was only during the 2nd Princeton Conference (1958), that along with other terms such as 'intermittent vascular insufficiency', 'ischemic recurrent attacks', 'recurrent focal cerebral ischemic attacks', and 'transient cerebral ischemia', was the definition of 'transient ischemic attacks' used for the first time.[9]

Transient cerebral ischemic attacks had been known for many years,[10] but the common incidence and clinical relevance of what has been labeled TIAs was introduced in modern times by Kubik and Adams[11] who described in 1946 'warning signs before an occlusion of the basilar artery', and, among others, by Fazio and Loeb[12], Johnson and Walker,[13] Alvarez[14] who coined the definition 'the little strokes', followed later by Alajouanine *et al.*,[15] Hass,[16] Acherson and Hutchinson[17] and of course by others since. However, the role of the Princeton Conferences was instrumental to the codification and validation of this new entity and of its significance. In fact, the concept gained unanimous acceptance at the 4th Princeton Conference in 1965 and the TIA acronym was coined.

The limit of 24 h chosen on that occasion was of course arbitrary and, in fact, in the majority of cases it is much shorter. The same is also true for the absolute harmlessness of the event, since imaging modalities (CT, then MRI and diffusion weighted MRI (DWMRI)) have shown that minute ischemic lesions, or even 'silent strokes', may occur without obvious neurological focal clinical counterpart. Be that as it may, the concept that a major ischemic event can be signaled in advance and hence potentially prevented, is one of the landmarks of this brief history.

The second landmark is the role played by the supra-aortic arterial trunks in the neck, as a frequent source of TIAs on one hand, and of major embolic occlusions and territorial stroke on the other.[18]

The other side of the story is that stroke prevention must take into account—besides correction of the classical and the emergent risk factors—the role of cardioembolic sources and, more recently, the pathogenetic role of aortic plaques.[19] In this, the contribution of neurologists has been based more on technological than conceptual advances.

The contributions reported so far would have had little impact on prevention, were it not for the development of therapies directly derived from the above concepts: anticoagulants, antiplatelet agents, and vascular surgery, to quote the largest ones.

The use of anticoagulants was recognized once again by Miller Fisher and also by Millikan and Siekert. Fisher wrote in 1958: 'in summary, anticoagulants prevent fleeting ischemic attacks, postpone the arrival of an impending stroke, and arrest the progressive downhill course of patients with cerebral thrombosis'.[9] It would be nice if it were as simple as that; however, the above statement prompted the 'national cooperative study' to 'reach a conclusion in a pressing matter of the management of occlusive cerebrovascular disease, sooner than any one centre could hope to accomplish it alone'.[9] In spite of such statements, however, the results of this first randomized, non-blind multicenter study were not as successful as expected.

It was apparent by the early 1970s that the prevention of ischemic strokes by anticoagulants was not the end of the story and they were not universally adopted as 'standard therapy'.

At that time, drugs were available that were known to have an inhibitory effect on platelet functions and had promising preliminary results among patients with cerebrovascular disease.[20,21] This opened the way to controlled trials and mega-trials still being practiced today. Again, there are predecessors[22] but one name stands above all, that of Henry Barnett whose work does not need to be quoted in detail since it is at the basis of this book.[23]

Similar 'waxing and waning' interest has also been raised by carotid surgery. The first successful endarterectomy was performed by DeBakey,[24] and Eastcott *et al.*[25] All of them were vascular surgeons, although clarification on this issue came many years later, with the fundamental collaboration of neurologists.

Combining the concept of TIA in the presence of carotid obstructive lesions as a precondition of stroke, patients were increasingly operated on by vascular surgeons, in particular after the advent of diagnostic facilities for non-invasive demonstration of vascular diseases (ultrasound in particular, but later also MRA and spiral CT), but this type of secondary prevention turned out to be reasonable only 20 years later. Patients with asymptomatic carotid diseases, however, are still unnecessarily exposed to the risks of surgery without the chance of gaining its benefits. Only after the demonstration of the use of extraintracranial bypass surgery for the prevention of stroke in patients with symptomatic, intracranial carotid and middle cerebral artery disease, has this been a subject of a large multicenter trial and finally solved. Again, Henry Barnett and Charles Warlow are to be mentioned for contributing to these large and long-lasting trials.[26,27]

This survey should mention the role of epidemiological studies and of stroke registries.[28–30] Stroke has thus become a preventable condition, and significant steps forward have occurred and are still occurring.

However, this is not enough and we should

discuss what the future role could be for the neurologist in research as well as in practice. The challenging question for the forthcoming century is to identify patients who benefit most and risk least from preventive treatment. This can only be achieved by improved classification of different stroke types and of their pathogenesis, and a refined design of future clinical trials with adequate modeling of experimental conditions prior to clinical studies. Thus, perhaps we will go through a phase of small focused trials, with defined stroke classification to identify effective treatments according to the pathophysiology and heterogeneity of stroke. Examples are trials limited to non-valvular atrial fibrillation as a major stroke risk, which have all resulted in the unanimous evidence of a significant benefit of warfarin vs. aspirin or placebo in primary and secondary prevention of stroke.[23]

On the other hand, if only modest treatment effects are expected, similar to what has been done for aspirin in IST and CAST trials,[31,32] large sample sizes may be appropriate, unless they are too difficult to perform, too costly or too time-consuming.

However, even if such studies had already been performed and results had provided the required evidence, it must be kept in mind that several obvious sources of variability interfere with the translation of the results of pharmacological trials into daily clinical practice. First, differences between patients exist and have to be considered, since some are more seriously ill than others and in chronic-stroke patients several diseases may need different and even contradictory treatment regimens. Second, the course of the disease may be quite variable between patients and need a change of treatment from time to time. Third, some patients may respond differently to a given treatment and individual acceptance of side-effects or compliance may be different.

To conclude, in this era of 'evidence-based' but also of 'cost-effective' medicine it is even more important than in the past that the expert neurologist is able to merge scientific competence and knowledge of the individual patient, in order to guide the appropriate diagnostic steps and to tailor and monitor the best preventive treatment for the particular condition.

REFERENCES

1. Warlow CP, Dennis MS, van Gijn J *et al.* Development of knowledge concerning cerebrovascular disease. In: *Stroke. A Practical Guide to Management*, pp. 4–24. Australia; Blackwell Science: 1996.
2. Denny-Brown D. The treatment of recurrent cerebrovascular symptoms and the question of 'vasospasm'. *Med Clin North Am* 1951;**35:**1457–74.
3. Fisher CM. Occlusion of internal carotid artery. *Arch Neurol Psych* 1951; **65:**346–77.
4. Fisher CM. Transient monocular blindness associated with hemiplegia. *Arch Ophthalmol* 1952; **47:**167–203.
5. Fisher CM. Observations on the fundus oculi in transient monocular blindness. *Neurology* 1959; **9:**333–47.
6. Millikan CH, Siekert RG. Studies in cerebrovascular disease I. The syndrome of intermittent insufficiency of basilar arterial system. *Proc Staff Meet Mayo Clin* 1955; **30:**61.
7. Millikan CH, Siekert RG. Studies in cerebrovascular disease. IV. The syndrome of intermittent insufficiency of the carotid arterial system. *Proc Staff Meet Mayo Clin* 1955; **30:**186.
8. Virchow RLK. Thrombose und Embolie: Gefassentz Ündung und septische Infection. In: *Gesammelte Abbandlungen zur Wissenschaftlichen Medizin* (Virchow RLK, ed.), pp. 219–735. Frankfurt; Meidinger: 1856.
9. Fisher CM. The use of anticoagulants in cerebral thrombosis. *Neurology* 1958; **8:**311.
10. Hunt JR. The role of the carotid arteries, in the causation of vascular lesions of the brain, with remarks on special features of the symptomatology. *Am J Med Sci* 1914; **147:**704–13.
11. Kubik CS, Adams RD. Occlusion of the basilar artery: a clinical and pathological study. *Brain* 1946; **69:**73.
12. Fazio C, Loeb C. Apoplessia transitoria e apoplessia senza focolaio. *Riv Neurol* 1948; **18:**142.
13. Johnson HC, Walker AE. Angiographic diagnosis of spontaneous thrombosis of internal and common carotid arteries. *J Neuro-surg* 1951; **8:**631.
14. Alvarez WC. The little strokes. *J Am Med Assoc* 1955; **157:**199.
15. Alajouanine Th, Lhermitte F, Gautier IC.

Transient cerebral ischemia in atherosclerosis. *Neurology* 1960; **10:**906.

16. Hass WK. A clinical study of cerebral insufficiency: the transient ischemic attack. *Bull NY Acad Med* 1963; **39:**12,774.
17. Acherson J, Hutchinson EC. Observations on the natural history of transient cerebral ischemia. *Lancet* 1964; **ii:**872.
18. Fieschi C, Bozzao L. Transient embolic occlusion of the middle cerebral and internal carotid arteries in cerebral apoplexy. *J Neurol Neurosurg Psychiat* 1969; **32:**236–40.
19. Amarenco P, Duyckaerts C, Tzourio C *et al.* The prevalence of ulcerated plaques in the aortic arch in patients with stroke. *N Engl J Med* 1992; **326:**221–5.
20. Evans G. Effect of drugs that suppress platelet surface interaction on incidence of amaurosis fugax and transient cerebral ischemia. *Surg Forum* 1972; **23:**239–41.
21. Blakely JA, Gent M. Platelets, drugs and longevity in a geriatric population. In: *Platelet, Drugs and Thrombosis* (Hirsh J, Cade JF, Gallus AS *et al.*, eds), pp. 284–91. Basel; S Karger: 1975.
22. Fields WS, Lemak NA, Frankowski RF *et al.* Controlled trial of aspirin in cerebral ischemia. *Stroke* 1977; **8:**301–16.
23. Barnett HJM, Eliasziw M, Meldrum HE. Drugs and surgery in the prevention of ischemic stroke. *N Engl J Med* 1995; **332:**238–48.
24. DeBakey ME. Successful carotid endarterectomy for cerebrovascular insufficiency. *J Am Med Assoc* 1975; **233:**1083.
25. Eastcott HHG, Pickering GW, ROB CG. Reconstruction of internal carotid artery in a patient with intermittent attacks of hemiplegia. *Lancet* 1954; **ii:**994.
26. North American Symptomatic Carotid Endarterectomy Trial Collaborators. Beneficial effect of carotid endarterectomy in symptomatic patients with high-grade carotid stenosis. *N Engl J Med* 1991; **325:**445–53.
27. European Carotid Surgery Trialists. Collaborative Group, MRC European Carotid Surgery Trial: interim results for symptomatic patients with severe (70–99%) or with mild (0–29%) carotid stenosis. *Lancet* 1991; **337:**1235–43.
28. Dawber TR, Kannel WB, McNamara PM, Cohen ME. An epidemiologic study of apoplexy ('strokes'). Observations in 5,209 adults in the Framingham Study on Association of Various Factors in the Development of Apoplexy. *Trans Am Neurol Assoc* 1965; **90:**237–40.
29. Mohr JP, Caplan LR, Melski JW *et al.* The Harvard Cooperative Stroke Registry: a prospective registry. *Neurology* 1978; **28:**754–62.
30. Bogousslavsky J, Van Melle G, Regli F. The Lausanne Stroke Registry: analysis of 1,000 consecutive patients with first stroke. *Stroke* 1988; **19:**1083–92.
31. International Stroke Trial Collaborative Group. The International Stroke Trial (IST): a randomized trial of aspirin, subcutaneous heparin, both, or neither among 19,435 patients with acute ischemic stroke. *Lancet* 1997; **349:**1569–81.
32. Chinese Acute Stroke Trial (CAST) Collaborative Group. CAST: a randomized trial of early aspirin use in 20,000 patients with acute ischemic stroke. *Lancet* 1997; **349:**1641–9.

Index